Colorectal Surgery

Mark Killingback, AM, MS(Hon), FACS(Hon),
FRACS, FRCS, FRCSEd

Colorectal Surgery

Living Pathology in the Operating Room

Springer

Mark Killingback, AM, MS(Hon), FACS(Hon), FRACS, FRCS, FRCSEd
18/1 Lauderdale Avenue
Fairlight 2094
Australia

Library of Congress Control Number: 2006921548

ISBN-10: 0-387-29081-8
ISBN-13: 978-0387-29081-2

Printed on acid-free paper.

Printed in China. (BS/EVB)

9 8 7 6 5 4 3 2 1

springer.com

To Bobbie, my wife of more than 50 years, who has made many sacrifices as the wife of a surgeon and without whom this work would not have been completed.

To Sir Ian Todd, who supported my appointment as a Resident Surgical Officer to St Mark's Hospital in 1960, which determined my career path in surgery.

To my mentors, the late Edward Wilson and the late Sir Edward (Bill) Hughes, who were pioneers in colorectal surgery, master surgeons, prolific authors, innovators, and valued friends.

Foreword

Books addressing the issues of colorectal surgery tend to take a familiar format. Frequently multiauthored, especially for comprehensive presentations on current status of the specialty, there are few single authored texts available. As for this book by Mark Killingback, one is not aware of any comparable treatises devoted to colorectal surgery. So what makes this so unique? And what makes the acquisition and reading of this book so desirable? First, a certain amount of historical perspective. Until this time—and one hopes for sometime yet to come—descriptions of findings at operation, and what was done to correct them, have been considerably augmented—and clarified—by schematic diagrams. (The reference to "sometime to come" is based on the emergence of the e-chart and e-operative note which promises to make such documents entirely paperless).

Dr. Killingback throughout his distinguished and prolific career has practiced the habit of schematically representing his operations—after the intervention—usually with captions. It is a practice he taught many of us. This exemplifies the phrase "a picture is worth a thousand words." However in the course of time, he acquired the skills of an artist and so converted basic line drawings into an art form.

Well, that is nice, you might say. But what does this offer over and above a good photograph of the specimen or of the operative field? This is the distinguishing point. Note how difficult it is to convey the spectrum of the disease or the extent of the difficulty of an operation or show manifestations of a particular syndrome in a photograph—or even a conventional line drawing! How does one adequately convey to the reader, the tapestry, the protean manifestations of Crohn's disease, for example, in a single drawing? In Dr. Killingback's imagery, all the features of thickened, strictured, obstructive, perforative, fistulizing, and ulcerated intestines are shown in one masterful piece of art. Photographic attempts for similar documentation are fortunate to provide two or three such features.

The experienced surgeon will appreciate this book by recognizing the details and exquisitely rendered images that call to mind similar cases encountered. For the surgeon or trainee relatively new to the specialty of colorectal surgery, the graphic presentation of the surgical pathology, with the accompanying succinct and informative text will make the acquisition of this book a valuable one.

Victor W. Fazio, MD
Cleveland, OH
Stanley M. Goldberg, MD
Minneapolis, MN

Preface

This book makes no claims to be a textbook of colorectal surgery, as many aspects of this specialty are not included. It is rather a collection of cases illustrating surgical pathology as encountered by a surgeon performing operations for colorectal disease. The surgeon is the first, in what may be a succession of medical practitioners, to confront the pathology of the disease "face to face." It is a unique opportunity to see the pathology in vivo in its undisturbed state and the interpretation of this morphology is usually vital to the operative technique to follow. In 1907 Moynihan of Leeds General Infirmary (UK) wrote on one of his favorite themes "The Pathology of the Living."[1] He stressed the value of observations of pathology during abdominal surgery and how this influenced diagnosis and treatment. The title of this book is related to this philosophy of surgery proposed by Moynihan. The aim of this work is principally to present illustrations of surgical pathology with artistic merit for surgeons to include in their reference library as a "coffee table book" but the author hopes the art and case history texts will have a significant educational role. Perhaps its main value will be for the younger surgeon who is commencing the journey into unchartered waters of surgical pathology. The author certainly would have valued a forewarning of many of the cases presented in this publication.

Drawing was selected for the illustrations as an art form rather than photography. Illustrative art has the facility to probe into inaccessible areas of the abdomen, to manipulate perspective to include important details, and to emphasise or delete various parts of the subject. Illustration can also combine the internal and external views of a viscus, etc., in the one diagram.

The author has enjoyed a long standing interest in drawing and usually included this aspect in operation report records. The contribution of the medical artist to surgical education was emphasized to the author in 1958–1959 while working as a surgical registrar at the Central Middlesex Hospital London. Ms. Mary Barber was a full-time medical artist employed by the hospital working in a very small cottage in the hospital grounds. With watercolor painting, the artist produced beautiful illustrations of surgical specimens. Most of her work was generated by the senior surgeon, T.G.I. James, who himself had a great interest in recording surgical pathology. The quality of Ms. Barber's work can be seen in her illustration of bowel affected by necrotising colitis[2] (Figure 1). Although this type of artwork has been somewhat overshadowed by color photography, perhaps this book will demonstrate that there is still value in illustrative artwork. The evolution of the illustrations has been presented in three stages. On completion of an operation the author's practice was to open the specimen and pin the bowel to a corkboard for the pathologist. A rough sketch was made to record details. This sketch formed the basis for an improved diagram for the patient's record (Figure 2). Such diagrams have then facilitated third illustrations prepared for this book. The author practiced colorectal surgery as a specialty for 26 of the 39 years of operating experience. Patients described in this book were

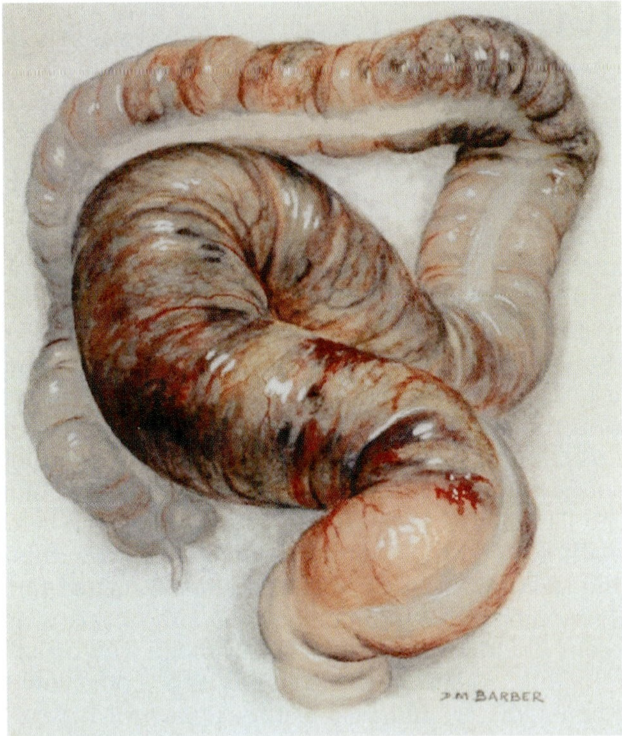

Figure 1: Necrotizing colitis. (Painting by M. Barber, 1959)

managed by the author, who performed the surgery on the pathology depicted in all cases, with the exception of: Case 21, lipomatosis-referred after retirement; Case 49, composite diagram; Case 78, desmoid tumour-no operation and Case 79, pneumatosis-no operation. The observations are therefore personal and prospective. The author has maintained his own detailed records of all patients treated, and this has restricted a minimum need for retrospective searching of patient details in hospital records. Follow-up cases were routine in patients with neoplastic disease, but in many cases not requiring follow-up for management. The patients have been located by the author and follow-up details were established by phone. A number of patients underwent related operations by other surgeons either prior to the author's involvement or subsequently. The stated age of the patient is that at the time of the initial referral.

Many surgeons have an interest in recording operation details by diagrams which can become invaluable in the management of the patient. Victor Fazio attributes his interest in this method of recording operation details, to his mentor the late Rupert B. Turnbull Jr. who was an enthusiastic sketcher of what he observed in the operating room. There are a few publications, however, that feature medical artwork by surgeons. Sir Charles Bell (1774–1842), of London, was a surgeon-anatomist and a talented artist who illustrated many texts with neuroanatomical drawings. His famous paintings of war wounds from the Napoleonic wars are now with the Royal College of Surgeons of Edinburgh.[3] Bateman in his book *Berkeley Moynihan Surgeon* relates that in the early part of the 1900s

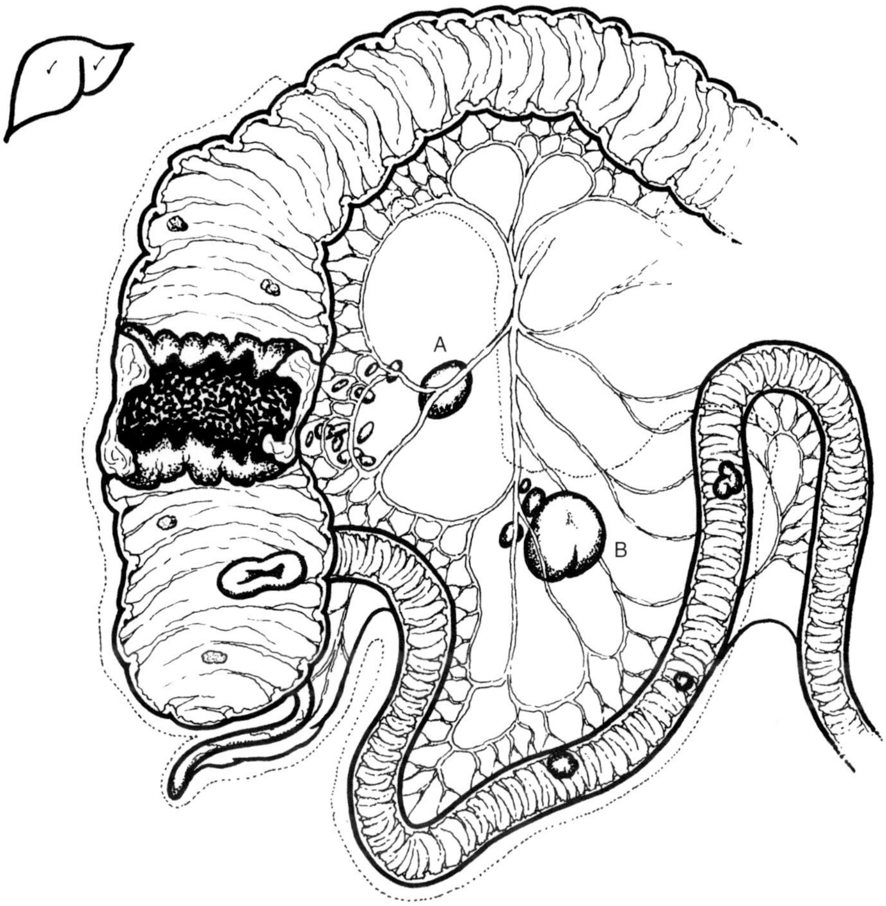

Figure 2: Contemporary diagram (1998) used for patients' records, later used to produce artwork. (Case 23)

this doyen of British surgery was an enthusiastic sketcher of his findings at operation.[4]

At the end of each operation he would draw with coloured crayons upon a thin white sheet of cardboard an exact picture of the abnormalities he had seen while operating. This he would accompany with illustrations and descriptive matter explaining the curative methods he had adopted. He had a swift, light touch that made his drawings very clear in an incisive way they told more than the copious written notes could do. These little sketches were bound in the volumes of his case records.

The location of these records is unfortunately unknown at the present time. During the preparation of this book one other similar publication has appeared describing operative details of 100 personal cases of interest with accompanying diagrams by the surgeon-author M. Trede of Germany.[5] This book contains black/white and color drawings, with accompanying text, that devotes much attention to operative technique. It covers a wide spectrum of surgery including cardiac, pulmonary, vascular and abdominal surgery, the latter concentrating on a unique experience of pancreatic disease. As one reads the book the impact of the personal contribution of the surgeon is obvious.

Colorectal Surgery: Living Pathology in the Operating Room restricts itself to the specialty but should be of interest to those who practice general surgery. There is minimal inclusion of operative technique, which has been well covered by many quality textbooks, but lessons in patient management have been included wherever appropriate in the comment section of each case. The text describes some successes of surgical treatment but errors of judgement and disappointing results are emphasized. All surgeons are aware of the importance of understanding pathology and its relationship to appropriate surgical treatment. There are many prestigious textbooks of pathology to which surgeons may refer, but such publications written by pathologists cannot be expected to link the clinical and operative management to pathology in the one book. This aspect has been a motivation for this publication. The references are not as extensive as might accompany a case report in a journal or a textbook. They have been restricted to suit the needs of the case histories, which are supplementary to the illustrations. An effort has been made to include current references but in relation to some of the uncommon conditions, publications are few and have appeared many years previously.

Philip H. Gordon, a colorectal surgeon from Montreal has written a paper on the problems of producing a medical book.[6] In this he quotes Apley:[7] "... writing is like having a baby: the gestation period is long and the labor painful, but in the end you have something to show for it." I hope what this book has to show will be of interest to my fellow surgeons. The labor of producing the illustrations was not painful but a pleasurable exercise, which has taught me more about the surgical pathology of colorectal disease than I knew previously. I hope the results do the same for the reader.

Mark Killingback, AM, MS(Hon), FACS(Hon), FRACS, FRCS, FRCSEd

References

1. Moynihan BGA. An address on the pathology of the living. *Br. Med. J.* 1907;**2**:1381–5.
2. Killingback M, Lloyd-Williams K. Necrotising colitis. *Br. J. Surg.* 1961;**49**:175–85.
3. Crumplin MKH, Starling P. A surgical artist at war. The paintings and sketches of Sir Charles Bell 1809–1815. Edinburgh, The Royal College of Surgeons of Edinburgh, 2005.
4. Bateman D. *Berkeley Moynihan Surgeon* London, McMillan and Co, 1940.
5. Trede M. The art of surgery: Exceptional cases—unique solutions 100 case studies. Thieme Verlag, Stuttgart, Germany, 1999.
6. Gordon PH. So you want to write a textbook? *J. R. Soc. Med.* 2000;**93**:150–1.
7. Apley AG. So you want to get published. *J. R. Soc. Med.* 1993;**86**:6–8.

Acknowledgments

My surgical colleagues have encouraged me to publish artwork and I thank them for that support. Drs. Victor Fazio and Stanley Goldberg from the United States have been most helpful in supporting the publication of this book and reviewing its contents. My colorectal surgeon colleagues, Drs. P. Chapuis, M. McNamara, and the late W. Hughes assisted at the majority of the operations and their operative skills and counselling while operating was invaluable. I am indebted to pathologists, Drs. Suzanne Danieletto, Stan McCarthy, and Ron Newland for the preparation of the photomicrographs and their advice on many aspects of the pathology. It is important to acknowledge the assistance I had for many years with record keeping and follow-up of patients. Nurse Jenny Searle was responsible for initiating this aspect of my practice, and Prue Barron continued this with meticulous care. Diana Murray has typed the many drafts and final copy of the manuscript. She has done this with considerable expertise and unfailing interest in the project. I am grateful to my art teacher Gwen Kowalski, who has been most encouraging even though some of the sketches unnerved the rest of the art class. I owe a debt of gratitude to Beth Campbell of Springer Science+Business Media, who has been enthusiastic about the book, supported its publication, and assisted greatly in liaising with the publisher. A text cannot be complete without references and I should acknowledge the most helpful assistance I have received over a prolonged period from Ilona Harsanyi, Ann Gilbert, and Eric Gaymer of the Charles Winston Library in Sydney Hospital.

Mark Killingback, AM, MS(Hon),
FACS(Hon), FRACS, FRCS, FRCSEd

Contents

PART VII LYMPHOMA

PART VII ANORECTAL DISEASE

PART IX VARIOUS PATHOLOGY

PART X COMPLICATIONS OF INVESTIGATION AND TREATMENT

PART I

Small Bowel

CASE

1 Lipoma: Terminal Ileum

Male, 81 Years

History

Dark red rectal bleeding and melena occurred over several days, 4 weeks prior to the patient's referral. Chest pain occurred during this period diagnosed as angina. Colonoscopy revealed diverticular disease of the sigmoid colon and a lobulated polyp protruding through the ileocecal valve. The polyp intermittently retracted from view, and examination beyond the ileocecal valve confirmed its attachment to the terminal ileum by a broad pedicle. Biopsy showed nonspecific inflammatory changes. A small bowel series confirmed the polyp in the terminal ileum and suggested this was a solitary lesion.

Operation (12.22.95)

The lesion in the terminal ileum was soft and rubbery on palpation with a broad attachment to the wall of the bowel. There were no enlarged lymph nodes in the mesentery. Eleven cm of terminal ileum was resected and an end-to-end anastomosis performed with a single layer of interrupted polyglactin 910 (vicryl) sutures.

Pathology

The polypoid lesion was pale yellow in color with smooth mucosa covering a lobulated surface. It measured 32 × 28 × 28 mm. There was a vascular ulcer on the distal aspect interpreted as the site of bleeding. The diagnosis of lipoma was confirmed histologically.

Comment

Tumors of the small bowel are uncommon, and Minardi et al. report the incidence of lipomas in the small bowel to be 4.5%.[1] They are usually submucosal but may be subserosal. When symptomatic, the most common presentation is abdominal pain due to intussusception. Bleeding which occurred in this patient is much less common and was probably due to venous congestion and ulceration on the tip of the polyp. Barium enema or CT may demonstrate the lesion.[2] Newer endoscopy techniques and the small intestine camera ("pill cam"),[3] should significantly improve the opportunity for preoperative diagnosis.

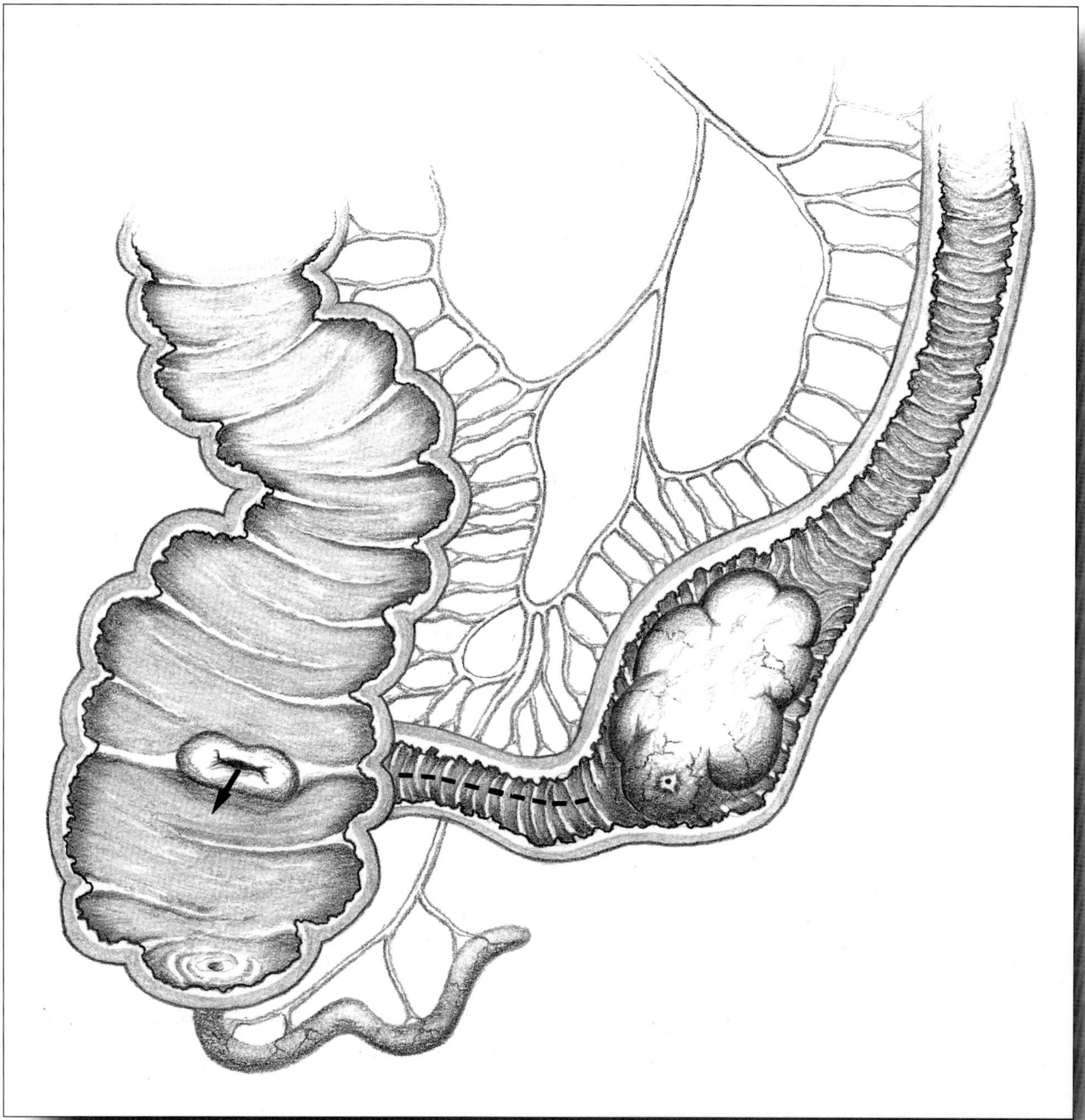

CASE

2 The Intruding Carcinoid

Female, 62 Years

History

The patient was examined by colonoscopy as a routine follow up procedure in view of a past history of three small benign polyps in the ascending colon. There were no gastrointestinal symptoms. Three hyperplastic polyps (3 mm) were removed from the sigmoid (1) ascending colon (2). A polypoid lesion was noted in the partially open ileocecal valve, which was red and smooth. Attempts to biopsy this were unsuccessful. Endoscopy of 10–12 cm of terminal ileum proximal to the polypoid lesion showed no abnormality of the mucosa.

Operation (11.22.93)

A firm mass (30 × 30 mm) was present in the ileocecal angle, attached to the ileum. It appeared to have expanded within the mesentery and was continuous with an intraluminal component within the terminal ileum. The operative diagnosis was leiomyoma. The remainder of the small bowel was normal. A right hemicolectomy was performed which included 90 mm of ileum.

Pathology

The lesion within the lumen of the ileum was a firm "sausage" shaped polypoid tumor, which had extended through the ileocecal valve into the cecum. It was continuous with the extramural mass and on section had a slightly yellowish color. The luminal component was covered with normal mucosa. Histological examination confirmed the diagnosis of carcinoid tumor (Figure 2.1). There were six lymph nodes found in the adjacent small bowel mesentery, the largest of which contained metastatic carcinoid.

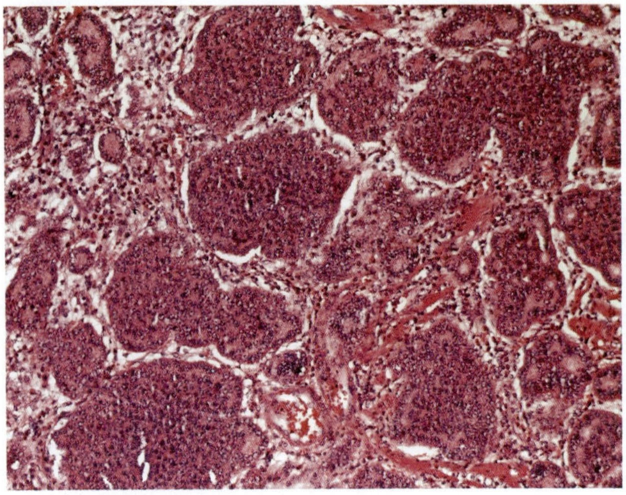

Figure 2.1: Section shows sheets of small bland cells typical of carcinoid.

Follow-Up (2004)

The patient's progress has been monitored with regular clinical examination, abdominal CT, colonoscopy, and urinary assay for 5-hydroxy-indole-acetic-acid excretion. No abnormalities have been detected. The patient remains in good health 11 years since operation.

Comment

This patient's carcinoid tumor was diagnosed by chance during a follow up examination for previous large bowel polyps. Diagnosis by colonoscopy must be very unusual. Incidental diagnosis, usually at laparotomy, has been reported to occur in up to 60% of cases.[1] At laparotomy, the "dumbbell" morphology of the luminal and mesenteric elements suggested the tumor was a leiomyoma. Carcinoids occur mostly in the lower third of the ileum, comprising up to 34% of all small intestinal neoplasms and up to 46% of malignant neoplasms.[2] Most carcinomas of the ileum produce serotonin and substance "P," which is common in the presence of hepatic metastases. It is not unusual for carcinoid tumors to be multiple, and there is a significant association with other types of synchronous primary malignancy, usually in the gastrointestinal tract.[3] The presence of nodal or other metastases is related to the size of the primary tumor. In a literature review Memon et al. found the size:metastasis relationship to be: <1 cm: 20–30%, 1–2 cm: 60–80%, >2 cm: >80%.[3]

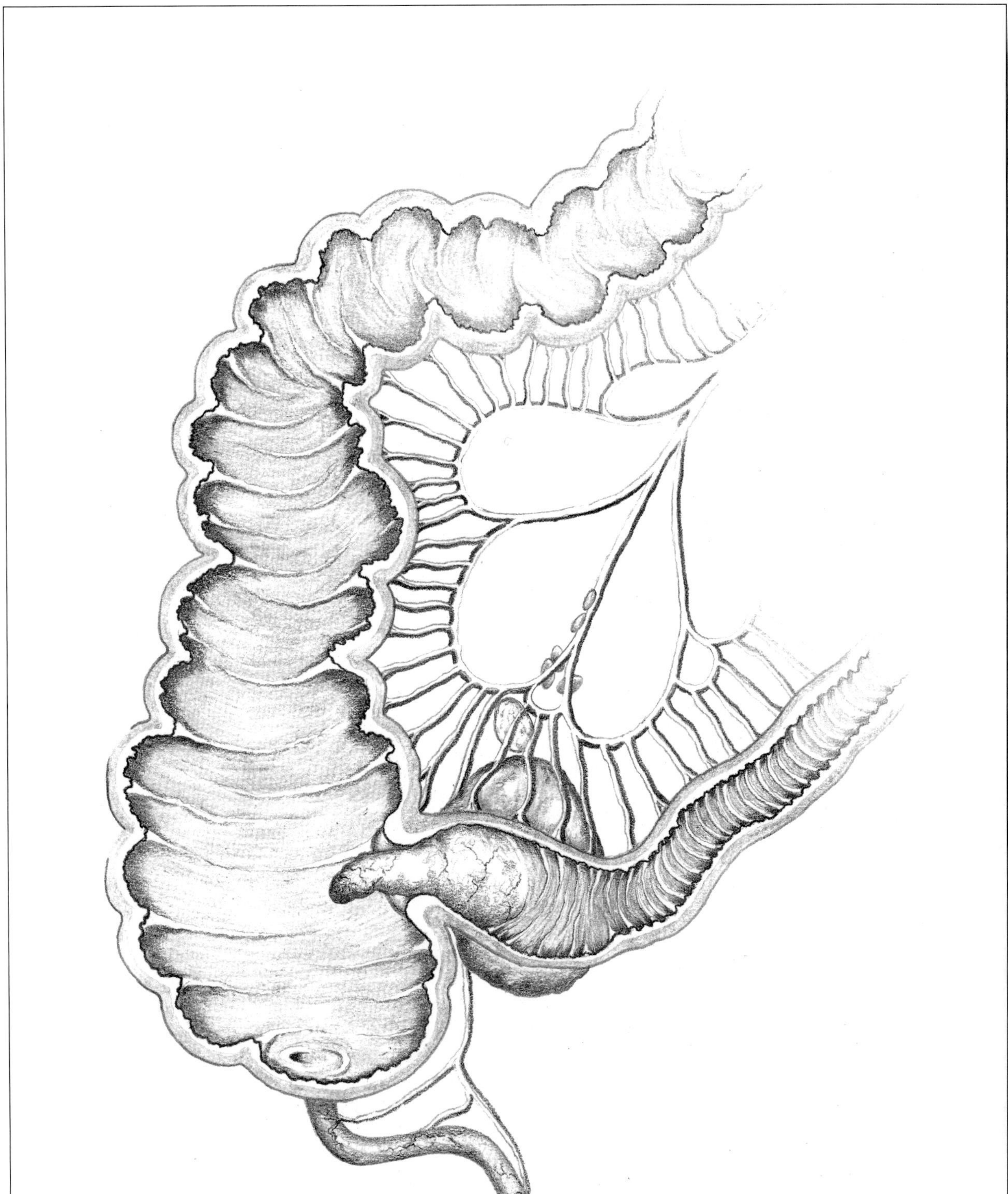

CASE

3 Carcinoidosis of the Ileum

Female, 56 years

History

The patient presented with a family history of colorectal cancer (mother) and recent increase in rectal bleeding. At colonoscopy, seven polyps in the descending and sigmoid colon were removed by diathermy snare. Six polyps were ≤5 mm in size (benign). The largest polyp was situated in the distal sigmoid colon on a short broad pedicle and measured 18 mm. This polyp was a villous adenoma containing infiltrating, moderately differentiated carcinoma. After a detailed discussion with the patient, colon resection was recommended.

Operation (7.24.89)

Laparotomy revealed no obvious pathology in the colon or metastases related to the malignant polyp. On examination of the small bowel, 11 small, firm lesions were palpable over 60 cm of the terminal ileum. The largest "nodule" was associated with puckering on the serosal surface and slightly enlarged hard lymph nodes in the adjacent mesentery. The abnormal area of ileum and mesentery were resected with anastomosis. The site of the malignant polyp was managed by a high anterior resection.

Pathology

The resected colon contained no residual adenocarcinoma. Examination of the mucosal surface of resected ileum revealed an additional 11 nodules previously undetected by palpation during operation. The 22 lesions ranged in size from 2 mm to 12 mm. Histological examination confirmed the diagnosis of multiple carcinoids. Twenty-one of the tumors were confined to the mucosa or submucosa. The largest tumor showed deep extension into the muscularis propria. Three of 5 mesenteric lymph nodes contained metastatic carcinoid tumor.

Operation (3.16.90)

A "second look" laparotomy was performed 8 months after the bowel resections to detect carcinoid tumors that may have been missed at that operation. None were found. There was no evidence of metastatic disease. Appendectomy was performed.

Follow-Up (2004)

Clinical and biochemical assay of urine 5-hydroxy-indole-acetic-acid assessment has shown no evidence of recurrent carcinoid tumor now 14 years, 10 months after resection. Colonoscopy surveillance has continued with the occasional removal of small benign polyps. In October 1997, carcinoma of the left breast was treated by mastectomy and postoperative chemotherapy.

Comment

There have been very few reported cases of this large number of small bowel carcinoids in association synchronously with colorectal cancer (CRCa).[1] The diagnosis of carcinoid tumors of the small bowel is frequently made incidentally during a laparotomy for other abdominal pathology. Early diagnosis is otherwise unusual. There could be some debate about the need for colon resection performed for this patient's adenomatous sigmoid polyp containing a focus of cancer. It certainly facilitated earlier diagnosis of the malignant carcinoid. While multiple carcinoids of the ileum are not unusual, 22 synchronous tumors is a rarity. In Thompson's review from the Mayo Clinic, the largest number of multiple carcinoids in the ileum was 24.[2] The "second look" laparotomy was useful and reassuring, but the use of the intraluminal small bowel camera (capsule video endoscopy) at the present time would be preferred to a "second look" laparotomy.[3]

7.24.89

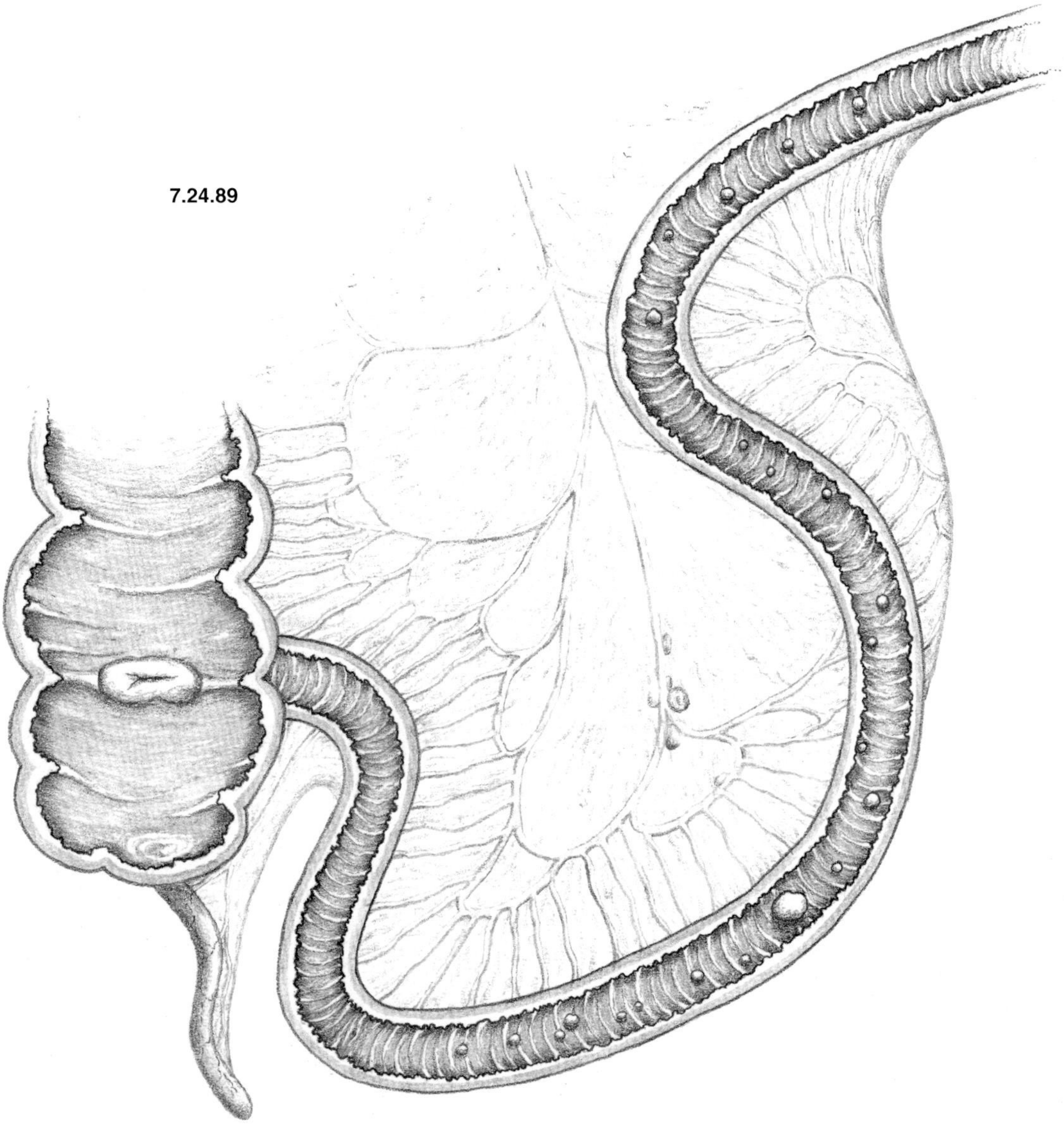

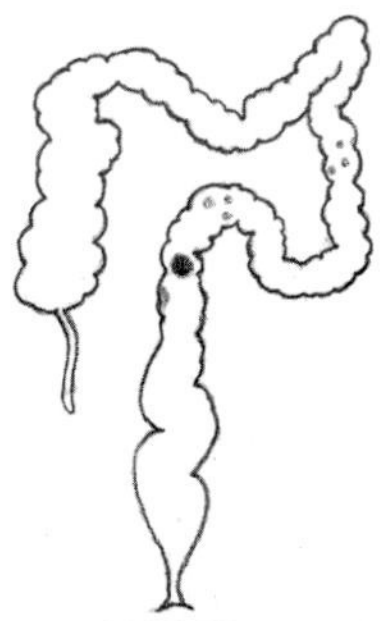

7.11.89

CASE

4 GIST Tumor of Ileum

Female, 67 Years

History

For a few months, the patient had noticed intermittent pain in the right iliac fossa. There were no gastrointestinal symptoms. On referral to a gynecologist, a mobile firm swelling was palpable in the abdomen. The diagnosis of an ovarian tumor was made and operation advised.

Operation (5.22.95)

Laparotomy revealed a soft lobulated tumor attached to the lower ileum over a moderately limited area of the surface of the bowel so that the tumor "flopped" about on manipulation of the ileum. There were no enlarged lymph nodes in the adjacent mesentery or evidence of metastatic disease. Examination of the rest of the small bowel and large bowel revealed no abnormality. The uterus and ovaries appeared normal. At this stage the patient was referred. Resection of 12 cm of ileum and related mesentery was performed. An end-to-end anastomosis was constructed with a single, interrupted layer of polyglactin 910 (vicryl) suture.

Pathology

The tumor measured 60 × 60 × 60 mm. No comment was made on the appearance of the cut surface. Histologically, the lesion appeared to be arising from the muscularis propria of the bowel wall. It was composed of spindle cells with no evidence of atypia (Figure 4.1). The mitotic rate in some areas was 2 mitotic figures per 10 high-power fields. There was no evidence of tumor necrosis, but there were areas of hemorrhage. The report stated the tumor was a "smooth muscle tumor of uncertain malignant potential, but in view of the frequency of mitotic figures, the lesion is best regarded as malignant." Subsequent immunohistochemical staining with CD 117 was positive, therefore classifying the lesion as a gastrointestinal stromal tumor (GIST).

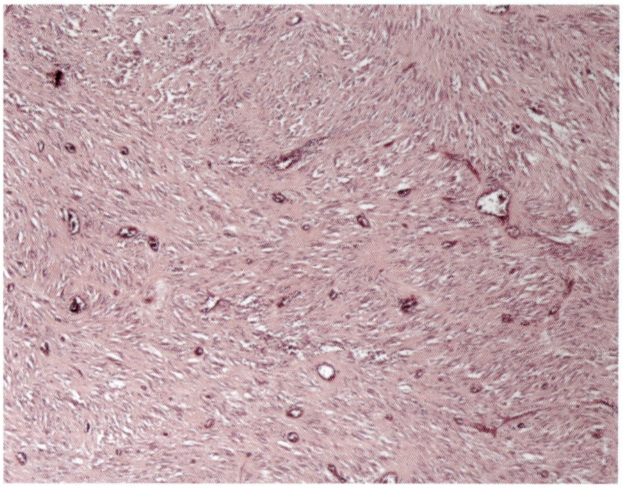

Figure 4.1: Section shows GIST spindle cells within a collagen stroma.

Follow-Up (2004)

The patient has remained well without any gastrointestinal symptoms 9 years and 5 months since operation. The patient is not having follow-up investigations as a routine.

Comment

The GIST is the most common mesenchymal tumor occurring in the small bowel.[1] The diagnosis is made on immunohistochemical investigation with CD 117 proto-oncogenic receptor positive in 100% of cases and CD 34 antigen positive reactivity in 70–80%.[2] The diagnosis can also be made on ultrastructural study.[3] The surgical removal of this patient's lesion proved to be without difficulty as it was not adherent to any other abdominal structure. There were no macroscopic signs of malignancy, but this was inferred on histological examination on the basis of mitoses per high power field. Diagnosis of malignancy in the GIST lesion is difficult and Wolber and Scudamore have suggested that two or more of the following features may confirm malignancy: large size; tumor necrosis; spontaneous coagulation; infiltrative margins; high mitotic count; and nuclear pleomorphism.[4] Clary et al. from the Memorial Sloan-Kettering Cancer Center reviewed 215 patients with stromal tumors of the gastrointestinal tract in which the incidence of malignant behavior was high.[5] They reported a local recurrence rate of 36% and a five year specific survival rate of 28%[5] and emphasize the importance of complete excision of the GIST lesion.

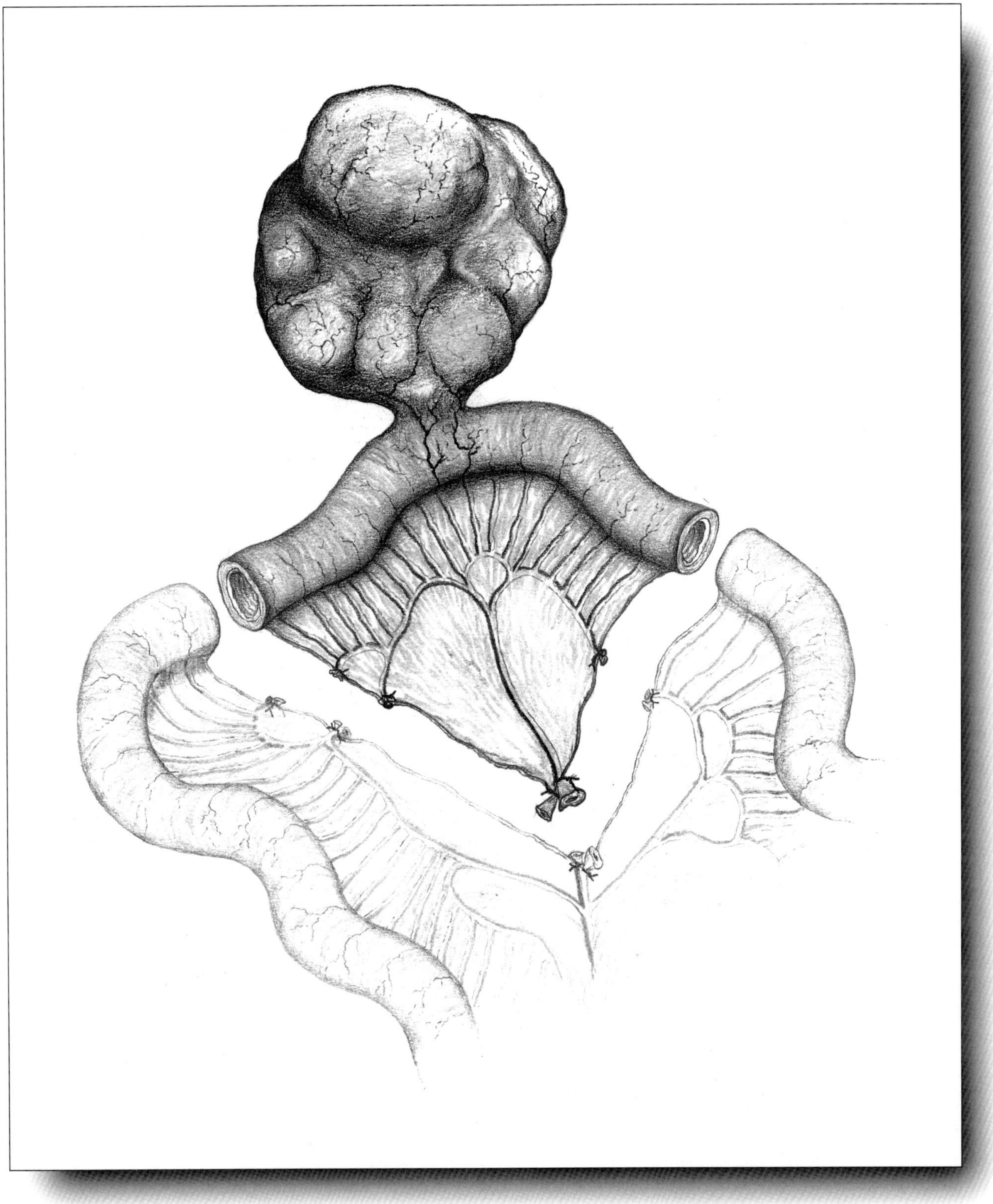

CASE

5 Adenocarcinoma of the Jejunum

Female, 68 Years

History

The patient was referred for investigation of an iron deficiency anemia which bone marrow studies suggested was due to chronic blood loss. Over a period of 6 months the patient had suffered episodic abdominal pain of a colicky type and noticed the onset of fatigue and exertional dyspnea. Panendoscopy and colonoscopy soon after the onset of symptoms revealed no abnormality. These endoscopies were repeated 6 months later and again failed to find a cause for bleeding. A small bowel enema x-ray revealed a stricture of the upper jejunum (Figure 5.1).

Operation (3.22.91)

Laparotomy revealed a neoplastic mass in the upper jejunum with possible involvement of the serosal surface. The associated small bowel mesentery contained several enlarged lymph nodes (the largest measured 20 mm in diameter). There were no other abnormalities on examination of the abdominal viscera or peritoneum. Twenty-five cm of jejunum was resected, with a deep resection of the adjacent mesentery. An end-to-end anastomosis was performed with a single layer of interrupted vicryl sutures and the mesentery closed.

Pathology

Examination of the mucosal surface revealed an annular tumor with proliferative edges and central ulceration. The appearances were similar to that of colon cancer. The cut surface of the tumor was pale with yellowish foci. Histologically, the tumor was a high grade adenocarcinoma (Figure 5.2). The tumor deeply invaded the muscularis propria but did not involve the peritoneal surface. Nine lymph nodes were examined, none of which contained metastases (Dukes A, T_2 N_0 M_0).

Follow-Up (2005)

There has been no evidence of recurrent disease during the 14 years of follow-up.

Comment

The diagnosis of this patient's small bowel malignancy was delayed for 6 months despite the attention of two gastroenterologists. Such delay is not unusual.[1] Although adenocarcinoma of the small bowel accounts for less than 2% of gastrointestinal malignancies, it is the more common cancer affecting the small bowel.[1] Kusumoto et al. report that the small bowel enema x-ray achieved 83% accuracy in diagnosis.[2] Abdominal computerized tomography

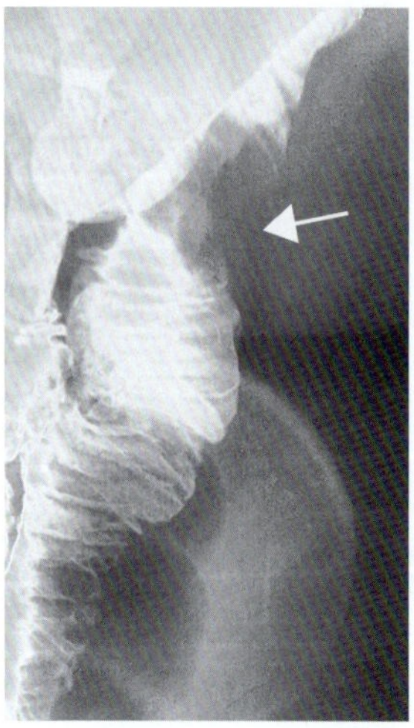

Figure 5.1: Small bowel enema x-ray demonstrates the jejunal carcinoma ("apple core"). See arrow.

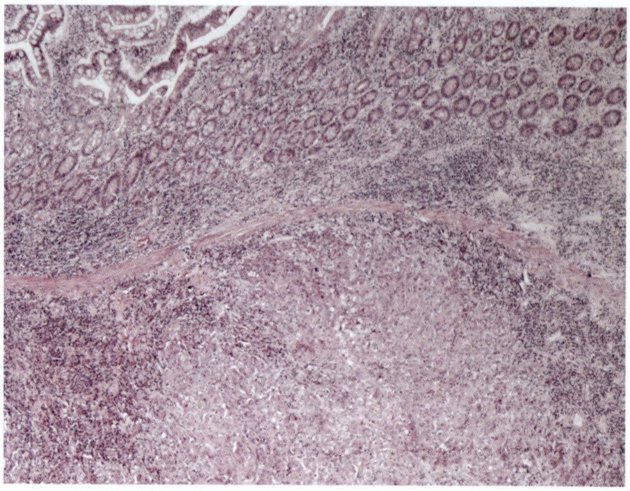

Figure 5.2: This section shows sheets of high grade adenocarcinoma deep to the muscularis mucosae.

(CT) is not proven to be this accurate but may give additional information on the extent of the tumor. Capsule endoscopy may in the future surpass radiological techniques. These lesions, treated by segmental resection, do not usually present a difficult technical challenge. The role of adjuvant chemotherapy is not established at the present time. Howe et al. report from the National Cancer Data Base (USA) the results of 1528 cases of adenocarcinoma of the small intestine from 1985–1995. There were 880 cancers of the jejunum and 648 cancers of the ileum, a ratio of 1.4:1.0. The cancer-specific 5-year survival rate was 37.8%, confirming that the prognosis is less favorable than that of colorectal carcinoma.[3]

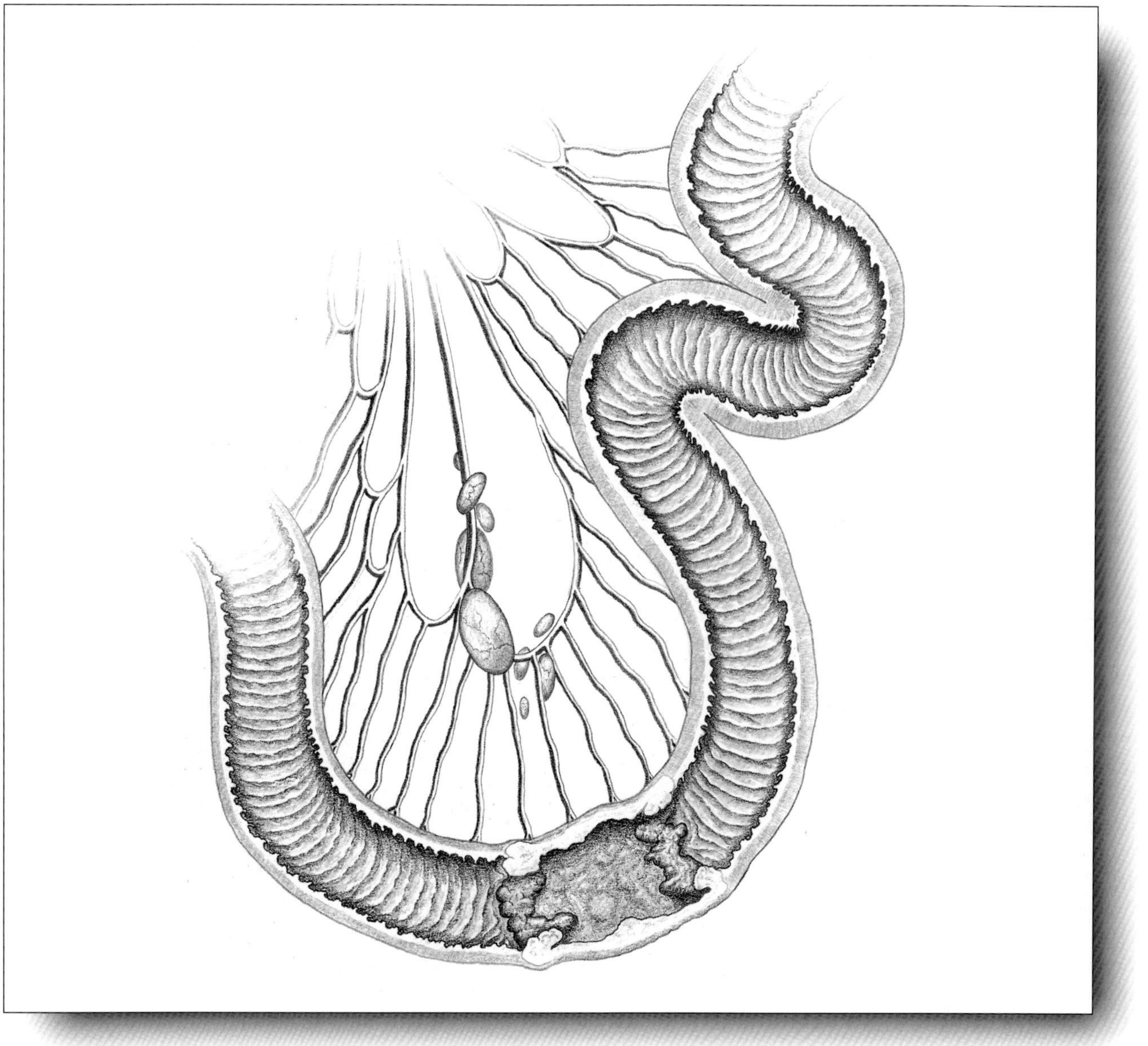

CASE

6 Blind Pouch Syndrome After Bowel Resection

Male, 55 Years

History

At the age of 10 years, appendectomy was performed for intermittent abdominal pain. At 33 years of age, laparotomy was performed for acute bowel obstruction that had been preceded by some years of colicky abdominal pain, and during this period he was found to be anemic. At operation, a fibrous stricture, at the base of a Meckel's diverticulum, was found to be causing the obstruction. This was resected with a side-to-side anastomosis, as the proximal bowel was grossly distended. In 1992, at the age of 55 years, the patient presented with a 9-month history of colicky central abdominal pain and distention. Hematological investigation revealed an iron deficiency anemia. Clinical examination, panendoscopy, and colonoscopy did not reveal significant pathology. A small bowel barium series demonstrated an area of narrowing and dilatation in the lower ileum.

Operation (2.7.92)

Laparotomy identified the side-to-side anastomosis in the terminal ileum. There were long extensions of the closed ends of the afferent and efferent limbs of the anastomosis, with the former showing significant dilatation. The ileum proximal to the anastomosis was dilated with a thickened wall indicating chronic obstruction. The anastomosis, with 18 cm of afferent and 25 cm of efferent ileum, was resected and an end-to-end anastomosis performed with a single layer of interrupted polyglactin 910 (vicryl) sutures.

Pathology

Opening the resected specimen revealed 2 shallow ulcers involving the anastomosis. The mucosa at the edge of each ulcer was hyperemic and the base fibrotic. The mucosa in the remainder of the specimen was normal except for the junction of the distal part of the anastomosis with the efferent limb. The mucosa here was atrophic and fibrotic and associated with a tight fibrous stricture. Histological examination revealed full thickness ulceration of the mucosa. The base of the ulcers was florid inflammatory granulation tissue with chronic inflammation and fibrosis in the submucosa and deeper layers of the bowel wall. The features were nonspecific.

Follow-Up (2005)

No further significant gastrointestinal problems have been reported.

Comment

Blind loop syndrome should be distinguished from the blind pouch (or "pocket") syndrome in that the former is most commonly associated with a bypassed segment of bowel without resection. It may also occur in extensive jejunal diverticulosis and scleroderma. The blind pouch syndrome occurs after resection and side-to-side anastomoses between small bowel or between small and large bowel. An elongated and distended segment of bowel develops which is usually the closed end of the proximal bowel but may also affect the distal closed end if it is jejunum or ileum. Obstructive symptoms are common even in the presence of a widely patent anastomosis,[1] but anastomotic stenosis may occur. Ulceration at the anastomosis or in the pouch[2] may occur and be responsible for microcytic iron deficiency anemia. These symptoms therefore contrast with the blind loop syndrome, which is characterized by diarrhea, steatorrhea, nutritional deficiencies, and a macrocytic anemia, usually in the absence of ulceration. The formation of the distended pouch is thought to be due to altered intraluminal pressure or stagnation of contents in the closed end of the bowel. Walfish and Frankel (1979), at operation, observed preferential flow of small bowel content into the pouch despite a patent anastomosis.[1] It is most likely that the elongated pouch develops from a short closed end of bowel and is not an excessive length of bowel left inadvertently by the surgeon. The incidence of this complication is difficult to estimate. Currently most reports are in the European literature. Frank et al. (1990) report 3 personal cases and review 76 from the literature.[3] Eighty one percent of the patients required operation. The surgery was performed for bleeding (45%), obstruction (40%), and peritonitis (15%). Since the 1980s, with the introduction of the linear stapler, side-to-side anastomosis has been more widely practiced. Is there a legacy to follow? Although the blind pouch may develop and cause symptoms within months,[4] it usually manifests after a long period, as in the patient described in this case report. The necessary treatment is resection with end-to-end anastomosis.

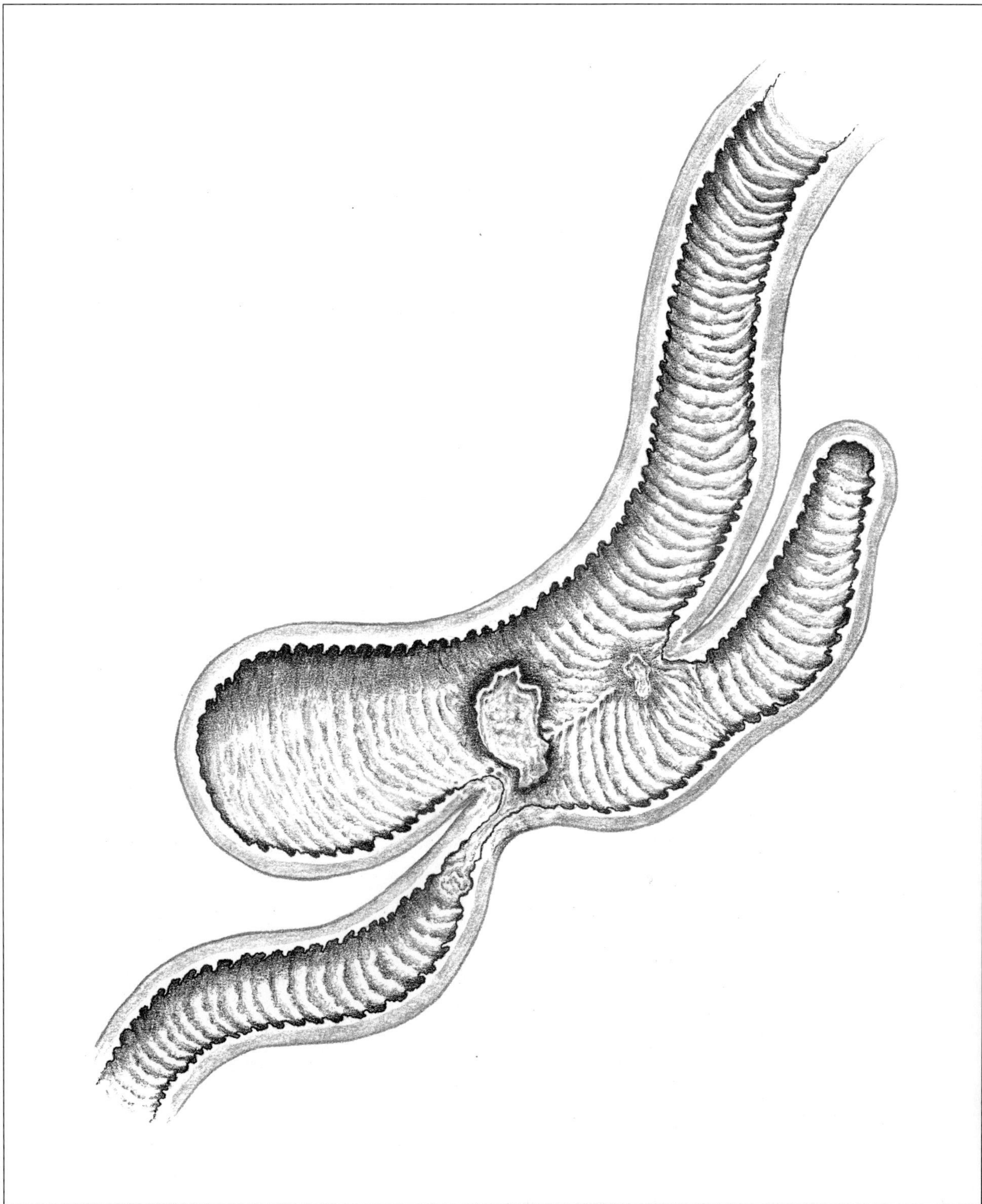

CASE

7 Blind Pouch Syndrome After Ileorectal Anastomosis

Female, 68 Years*

History

Between 1959 and 1974, the patient had suffered 4 episodes of profuse rectal bleeding requiring transfusion. Barium enema examination (1974) revealed diverticulosis throughout the colon. The patient resided some distance from sophisticated surgical services and this influenced the decision to operate.

Operation (11.4.1974)

An elective operation was performed. Many diverticula were present, particularly in the transverse and left colon. There was a focus of induration in the transverse colon in relation to a diverticulum. A colectomy and a high ileorectal anastomosis (IRA) was performed (side ileum-to-end rectum). Microscopic examination of the diverticulum in the transverse colon (Figure 7.1) showed conspicuous dilated vessels.

Follow-Up

Sigmoidoscopy 2 years and 5 months later in 1977 demonstrated a healthy IRA at 13 cm. In 1981, profuse rectal bleeding occurred, and at this time sigmoidoscopy revealed ulceration of the ileum adjacent to the IRA. In 1984, further acute bleeding occurred requiring transfusion. Sigmoidoscopy now revealed a stricture of the IRA in addition to ulceration. A barium enema demonstrated a blind elongated pouch in relation to the IRA (Figure 7.2).

Operation (7.20.1984*)

A large length of ileum (15 cm) was found projecting from the right side of the IRA. It measured 6 cm in width. The IRA and 5 cm of proximal ileum were resected and a further IRA established with an end-to-end anastomosis.

Pathology

There was ulceration and stricture formation of the IRA and adjacent ileum. The mucosa at the apex of the blind loop was intensely hyperemic. Histological examination revealed nonspecific inflammation.

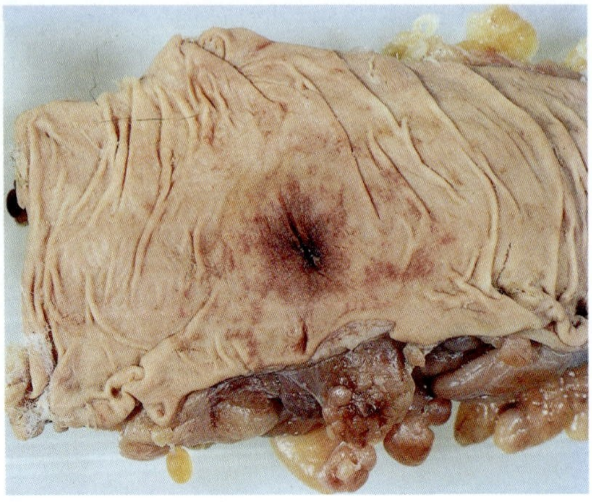

Figure 6.1: Diverticulum in the transverse colon causing bleeding (1974).

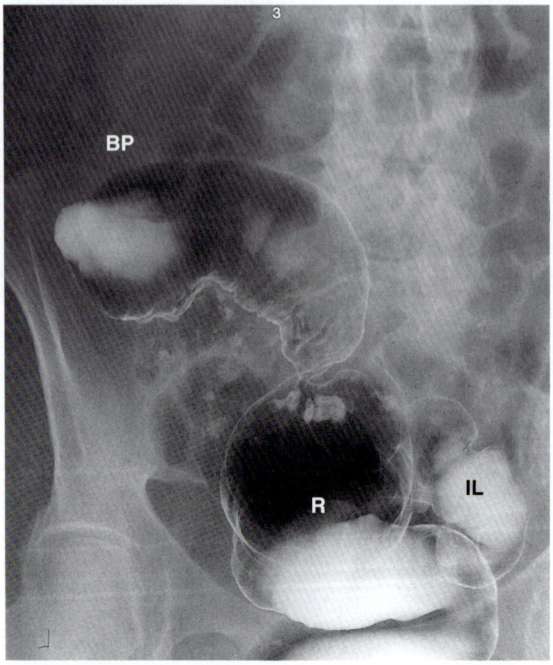

Figure 6.2: A barium enema demonstration of the blind pouch. (1984). BP: blind pouch; IL: ileum; R: rectum.

Postoperative Course

The patient's gastrointestinal recovery from the operation was slow but satisfactory. She was, however, suffering from persistent angina. Investigation revealed severe, inoperable coronary artery disease and poor left ventricular function. The patient suffered a fatal myocardial infarct 29 days after the operation.

Comment

This patient is another example of the blind pouch syndrome which, in contrast to Case 6, was a complication of a side-to-end anastomosis between ileum and large bowel. It has more frequently been reported as a complication of ileo-colic anastomosis after right hemicolectomy.[1,2,3] Although there was anastomotic stenosis, the symptoms were due solely to bleeding from the ulceration, which commenced 7 years after the ileorectal anastomosis. At this first operation (IRA), the closure of the terminal end of the anastomosis was adjacent to the anastomosis, proving the large blind pouch developed subsequently. The ulceration in such a case can be resolved only by surgery. It is unfortunate that operation was not performed 3 years earlier (1981), which may have avoided the fatal consequences of her cardiovascular disease.

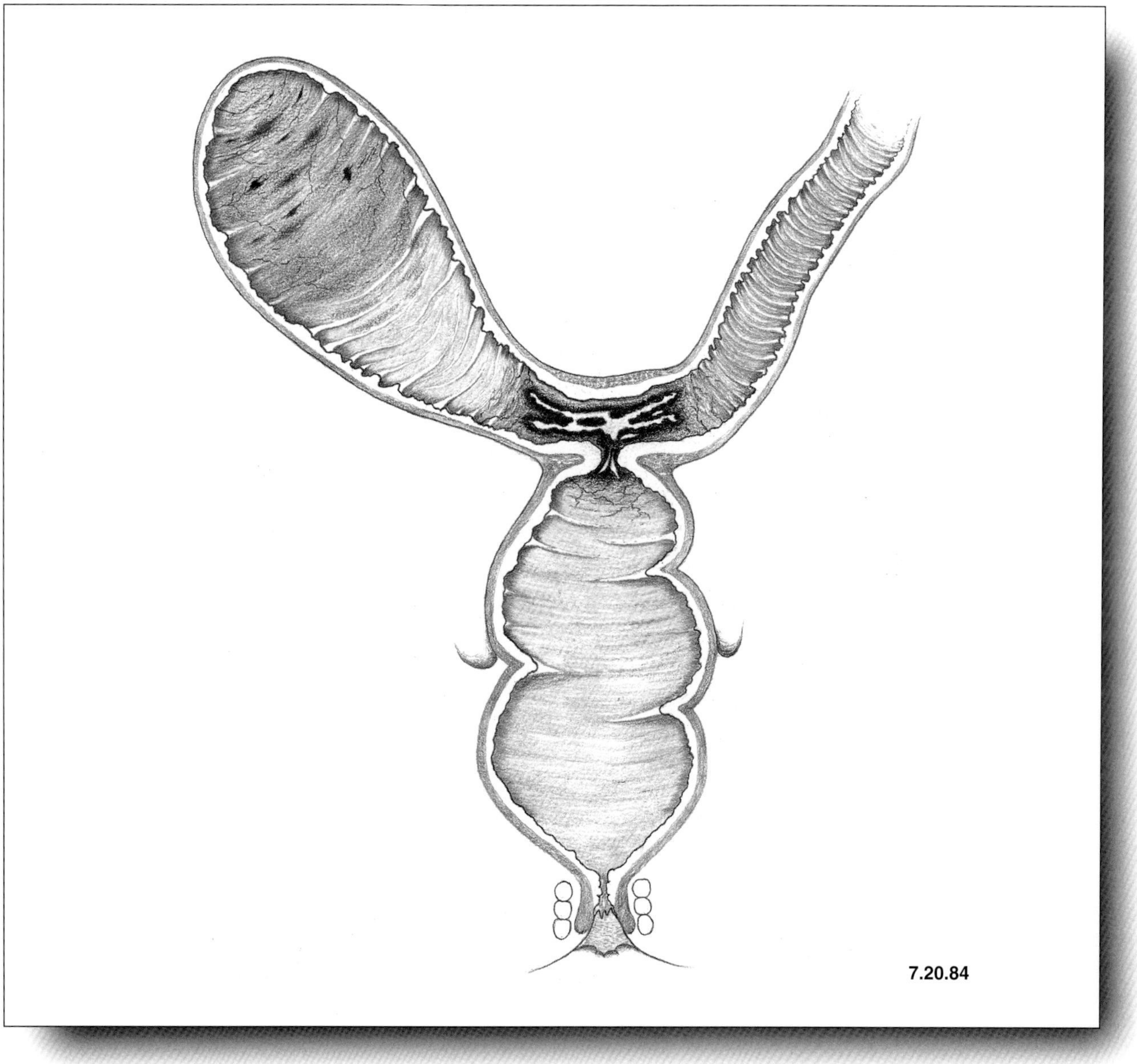

PART II Appendix

CASE

8 Acute Appendicitis: Diagnosis at Colonoscopy

Male, 59 Years

History

The patient suffered recent acute pain in the right iliac fossa. Admission to hospital was necessary, and a plain x-ray of the abdomen revealed loops of dilated small bowel. A gastrograffin enema indicated deformity of the ileocecal region. The patient's condition settled and he was discharged from hospital and transferred for further investigations.

Colonoscopy

Colonoscopy revealed a "beehive" shaped polypoid lesion at the base of the appendix (Figure 8.1). It appeared to be inflammatory rather than neoplastic, and appendicitis was suspected.

Operation (8.7.98)

At operation, recent acute appendicitis was confirmed with retrograde intussusception induced by a tense and distended appendix. The distal cecum with the appendix was resected.

Comment

This is a rare mode of acute appendicitis diagnosis. The smooth surface, the inflammatory changes, and the site of the lesion suggested the diagnosis.

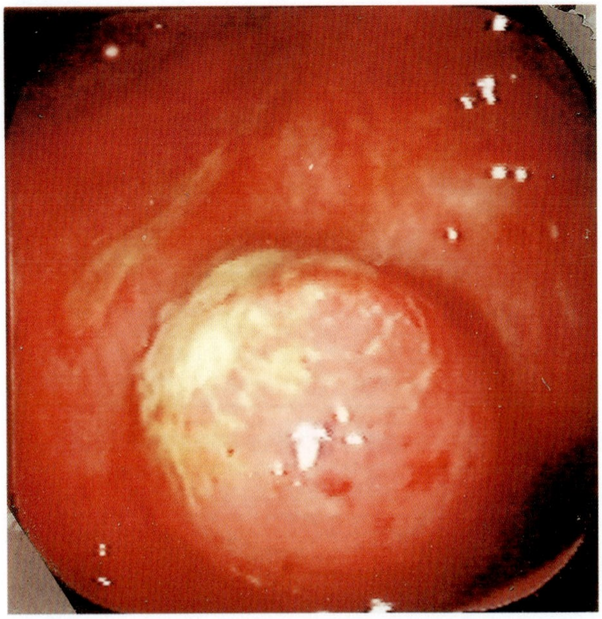

Figure 8.1: The inverted inflamed appendix seen at colonoscopy.

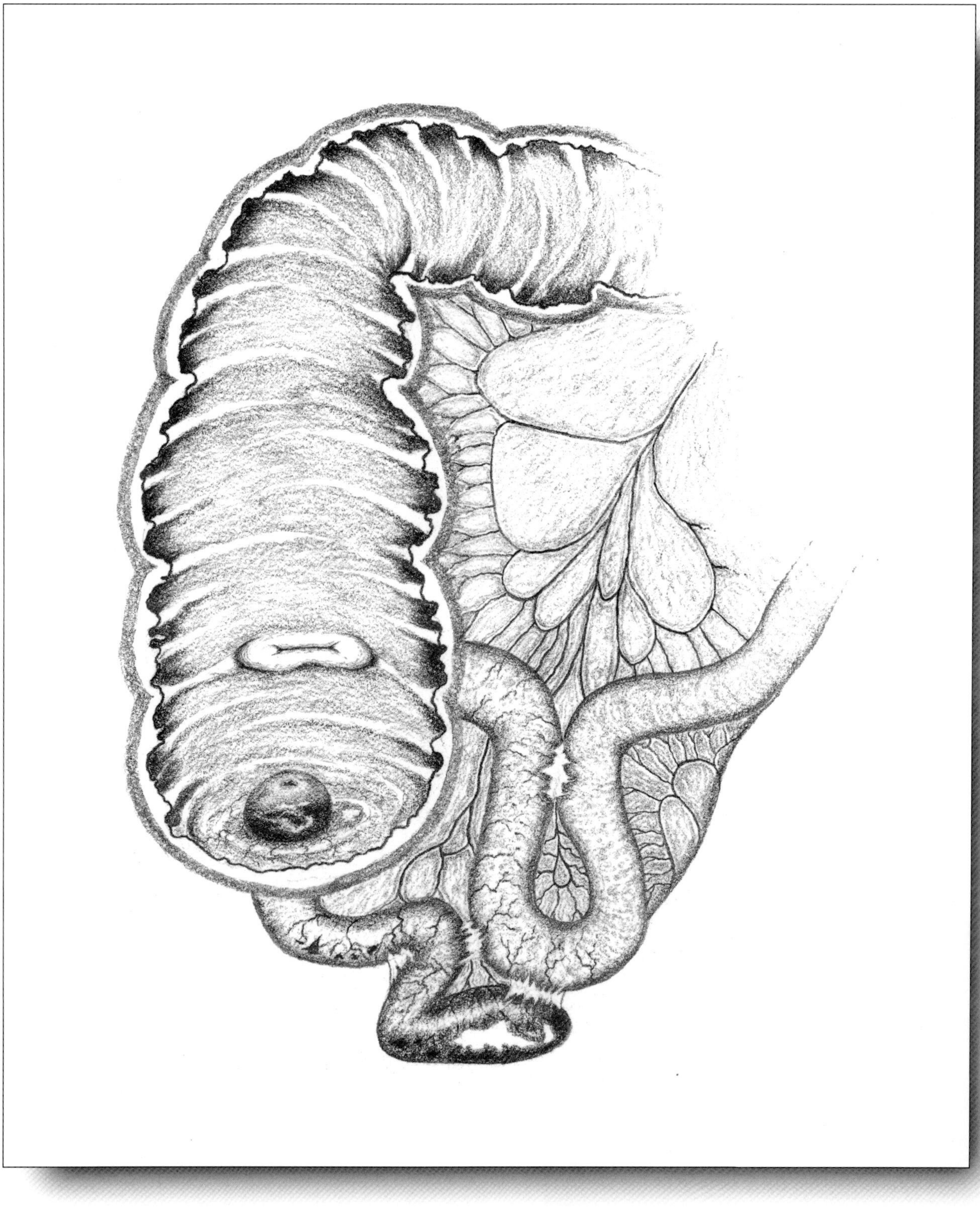

CASE

9 Mucocele of the Appendix

Female, 51 Years

History

The patient was examined by colonoscopy in view of a family history of colorectal cancer (mother). There were no previous or current gastrointestinal symptoms. In the base of the cecum there was a smooth hemispherical swelling covered by normal mucosa (Figure 9.1). This was diagnosed as a mucocele of the appendix by the colonoscopist. A computerized tomography (CT) examination demonstrated that the lesion was continuous with the appendix, which was dilated (Figure 9.2).

Operation (7.28.97)

The findings at operation confirmed the diagnosis. The proximal appendix was significantly dilated and continuous with a palpable intracecal swelling. The distal half of the appendix was pale, reduced in caliber, and firm in consistency, suggesting fibrosis. There was no evidence of malignancy or other intra-abdominal abnormality. A limited right hemicolectomy was performed in preference to a local excision, since an occult cystadenocarcinoma could not be excluded.

Pathology

The appendix was 60 mm in length. Distally its caliber was 6 mm, whereas proximally it was dilated to 20 mm. The appendix ostium was obstructed. The lumen contained clear mucoid material. Histologically there were areas of both mucosal hyperplasia and atrophy. There was extravasation of mucin into the wall of the appendix (Figure 9.3). This extravasation was devoid of cells.

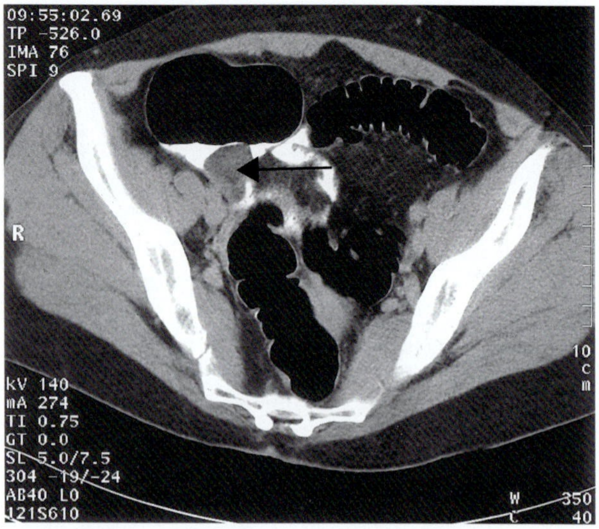

Figure 9.2: The CT with contrast clearly shows the lesion in the cecum.

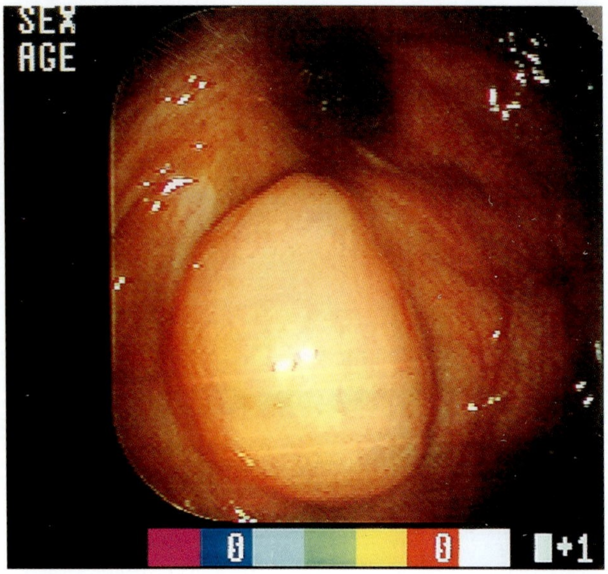

Figure 9.1: The endoscopic view of the mucocele.

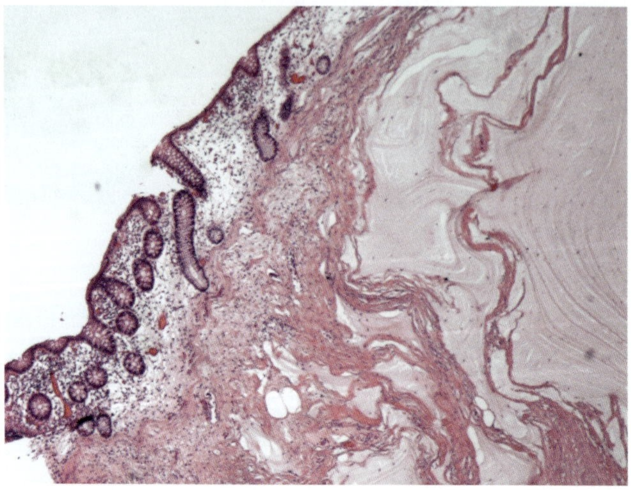

Figure 9.3: Pools of mucus are present within the wall of the appendix.

Comment

Rokitansky is credited with first description of this entity in 1842.[1] Woodruff and McDonald reported 146 mucoceles in over 43 000 appendectomy specimens examined at the Mayo Clinic.[2] The pathology is frequently not diagnosed until laparotomy. The first report of a colonoscopic diagnosis was by Ponsky in 1976.[3] Surgical treatment is necessary to confirm the diagnosis and to prevent the complication of pseudomyxoma peritonei which may follow perforation of a mucocele if the primary pathology is a cystadenoma or cystadenocarcinoma.

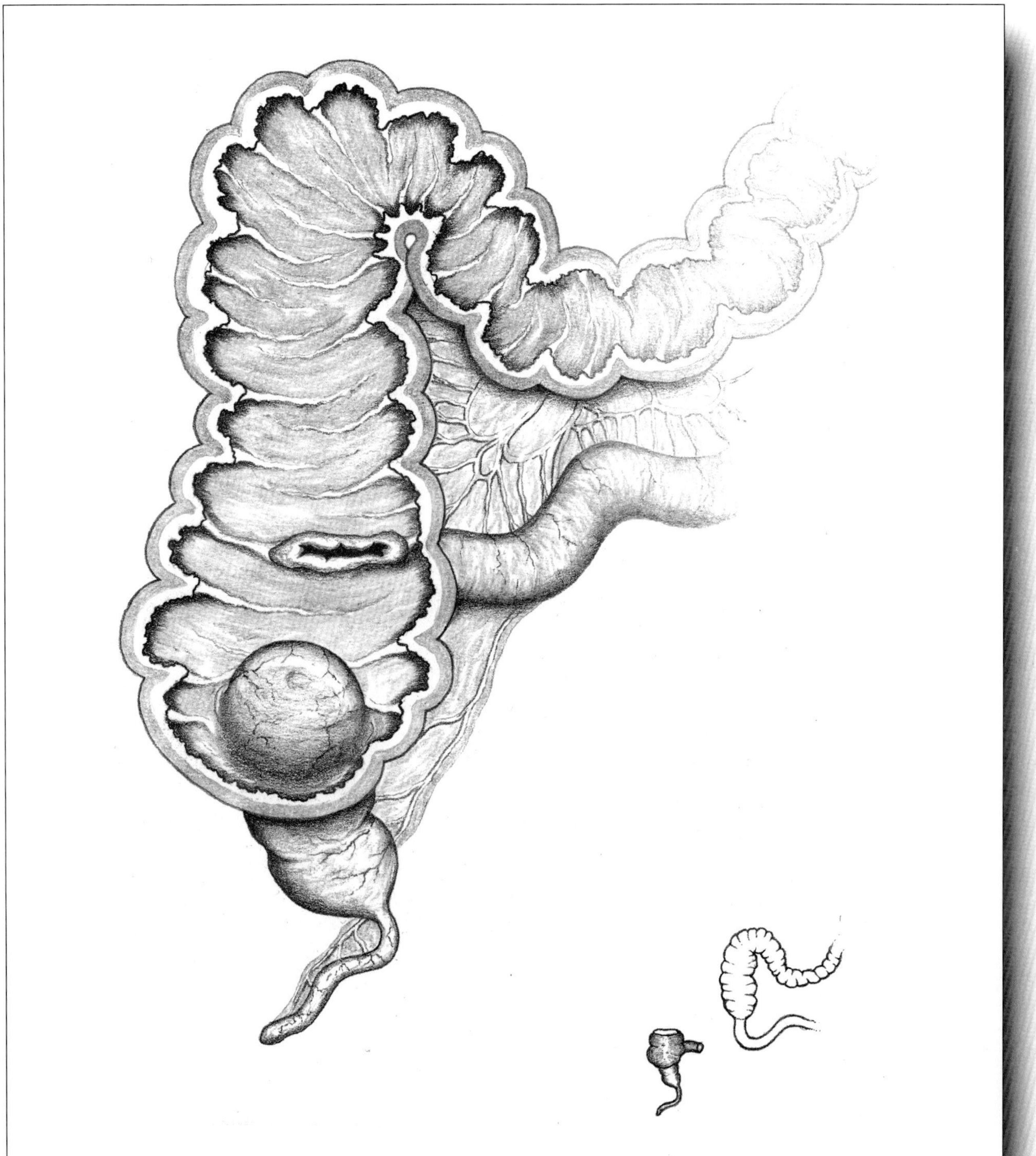

CASE

10 Cystadenoma: Appendix

Male, 70 Years

History

Following an "influenza type illness," the patient complained of pain in the right sacral region. A white cell count of 19,000 returned to normal after antibiotics. A computerized tomography (CT) examination of the pelvis revealed a 4.0 × 6.5 cm cystic mass, thick walled and partly calcified. The mass was intimately related to the right side of the sigmoid colon and contained multiple septations (Figure 10.1). A calculus was demonstrated in the right ureter. Examination under anesthetic revealed a mobile soft mass in the pelvis. Three small hyperplastic polyps at 20 cm were the only abnormalities seen on colonoscopy. The indirect hemagglutination test (IHA) for hydatid disease was negative.

Operation (11.4.96)

A ruptured mucocele of the appendix was diagnosed, revealing a collection of green mucoid material in the pelvis. Appendectomy was performed. The ureteric calculus was removed from the lower part of the right ureter by a urological colleague.

Pathology

There was focal calcification in the wall of the cystic mass. Foci of atypical mucinous epithelium (Figure 10.2) and occasional papillary configuration were present. The appearance was consistent with a mucinous cystadenoma.

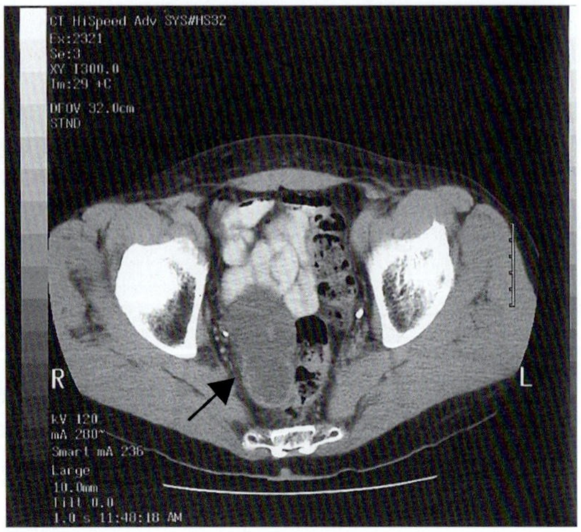

Figure 10.1: The CT examination demonstrates the pelvic mass.

Comment

Mucus producing pathology of the appendix is rare, and the diagnosis is not usually made prior to operation.[1] In this patient a second radiological opinion prior to operation suggested the diagnosis was a mucocele of the appendix, in view of the calcification in the wall of the cystic mass.[2] Unfortunately the lesion had already ruptured at the time of laparotomy, thereby increasing the risk of peritoneal dissemination. Clinical and CT examination have been normal 8 years since operation. Mucocele of the appendix is divided into 4 distinct pathological entities: (i) nonneoplastic mucocele due to luminal obstruction; (ii) mucosal hyperplasia; (iii) mucinous cystadenoma with villous adenomatous change; and (iv) malignant mucinous cystadenoma.[3] Histologically there can be difficulty in distinguishing between categories (iii) and (iv). These lesions can produce a refractory mucinous ascites, which has been referred to as pseudomyxoma peritonei. Ronnet et al., in a review of 109 cases, have suggested subdividing this entity into **disseminated peritoneal adenomucinosis (DPAM)** for benign disease and **peritoneal mucinous carcinomatosis (PMCA)** for malignant mucinous ascites.[4]

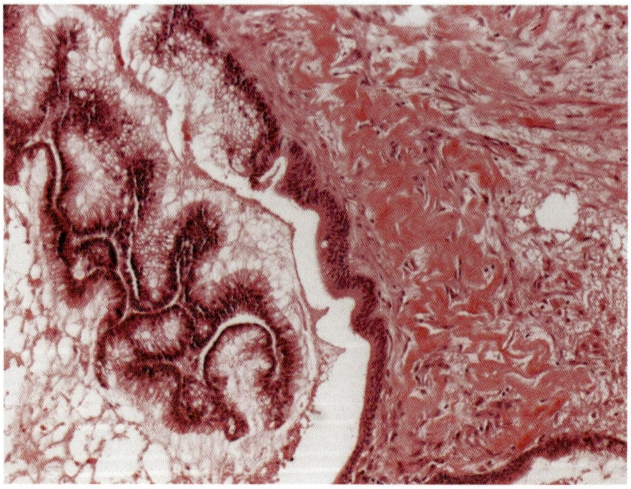

Figure 10.2: Atypical stratified columnar epithelium consistent with the diagnosis of a cystadenoma. Mucus present in lumen of the appendix (left).

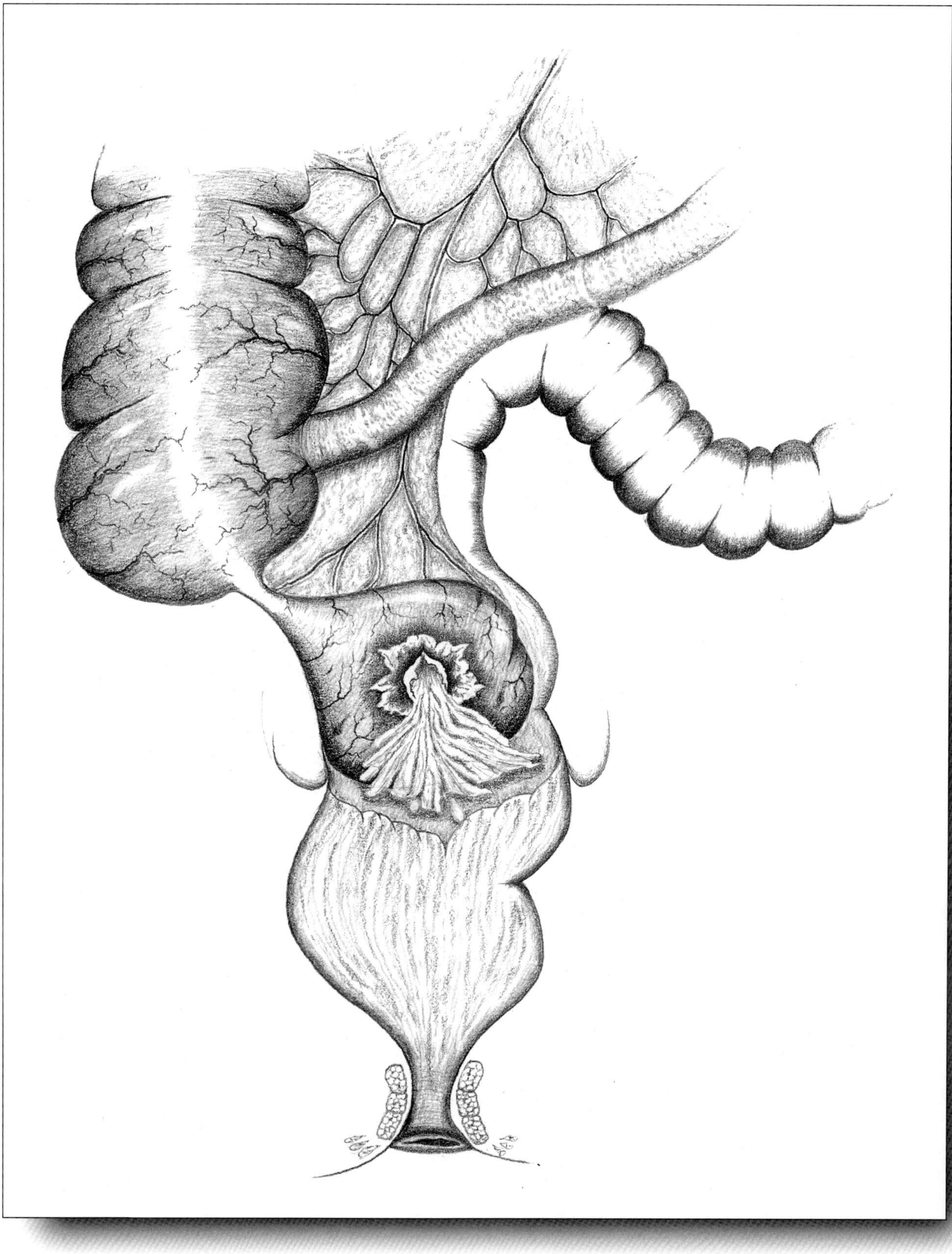

CASE 11 Carcinoma of the Appendix

Female, 53 Years

History

For 6 months the patient had noted an increase in the frequency of bowel function. For this reason the patient took part in a community bowel screening program (Hemoccult II) for bowel cancer. The stools were positive for occult blood. Colonoscopy revealed a "convoluted bowel". In "the mid ascending colon" there was a 1.5 cm ulcerated lesion, which on biopsy revealed moderately differentiated adenocarcinoma. A computerized tomography (CT) scan showed a mass related to the right colon, extending posteriorly into the psoas muscle (Figure 11.1). No metastatic disease was detected in the liver. The patient was referred for surgical treatment.

Operation (10.9.95)

Through the anterior wall of the cecum a mass was palpable, fixed to the retroperitoneal tissues. The appendix formed part of the mass, but only its proximal 2–3 cm was recognizable. There were no enlarged mesenteric lymph nodes or any metastases identified. The tumor mass was "dumbbell" shaped, as illustrated on the CT (Figure 11.1), with the posterior extension deeply penetrating the psoas muscle. Adequate access to this area was not possible until the colon distally and the ileum proximally had been transected. Despite this improved access, the thin "isthmus" of the "dumbbell" fractured during dissection so that the deeper part of the tumor was excised separately from the main specimen. The tumor bed in the psoas muscle was extensively treated with diathermy. An ileo-transverse colon anastomosis was completed with a circular stapler.

Pathology

Below the ileocecal valve there was a malignant ulcer surrounded by a thin rim of friable tumor which merged with the appendix to form the tumor mass. Histologically the lesion was a moderately differentiated mucinous adenocarcinoma. The tumor was seen lining the appendiceal lumen and extending through the wall. "The lumen of the appendix has been completely blocked: the sections confirm that it is the primary site" (Figure 11.2). The margin of tumor clearance of the deep part of the tumor (within the psoas muscle) was satisfactory. There were no metastases in 11 mesenteric lymph nodes examined (Dukes B, T_3 N_0 M_0).

Follow-Up (2004)

In view of the risk of local recurrence, the patient was treated with adjuvant chemotherapy (5 Flourouracil and Folinic acid) for 6 months. The

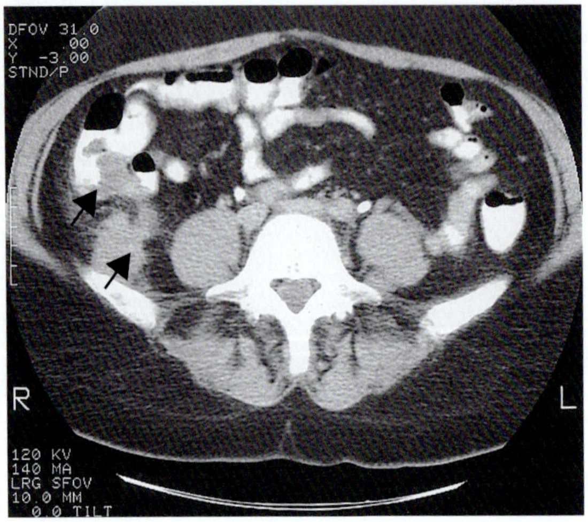

Figure 11.1: The CT demonstrates the cecal mass with posterior extramural extension.

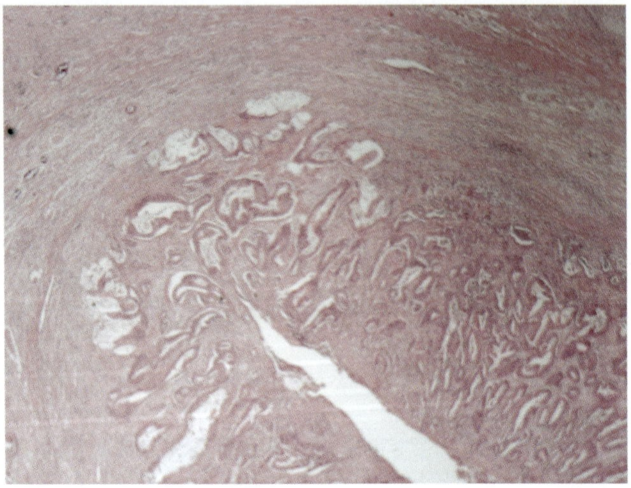

Figure 11.2: Adenocarcinoma is shown filling the lumen of the appendix.

patient remains free of recurrent or metachronous disease 9 years after operation.

Comment

Although the pathology was thought to be a carcinoma of the cecum at operation, the pathology evidence favors a malignancy developing in a retrocecal appendix and subsequently ulcerating into the cecum. Appendiceal carcinoma is rare and it is not unusual for the diagnosis to be made first by the pathologist. Nitecki et al studied 94 patients treated at the Mayo Clinic and found that a correct intraoperative diagnosis was made in only 32% of patients.[1] The mucinous variety of appendiceal carcinoma occurs in approximately half the appendiceal malignancies (if carcinoids are excluded). Its spread is to the peritoneum (pseudomyxoma peritonei) rather than to lymph nodes or liver. Increasing depth of local invasion has an adverse effect on prognosis.[1,2] Dukes B, T_3 N_0 M_0 tumors have been reported to have a 67%, 5-year survival.[1] Right hemicolectomy is the recommended treatment.[1,2]

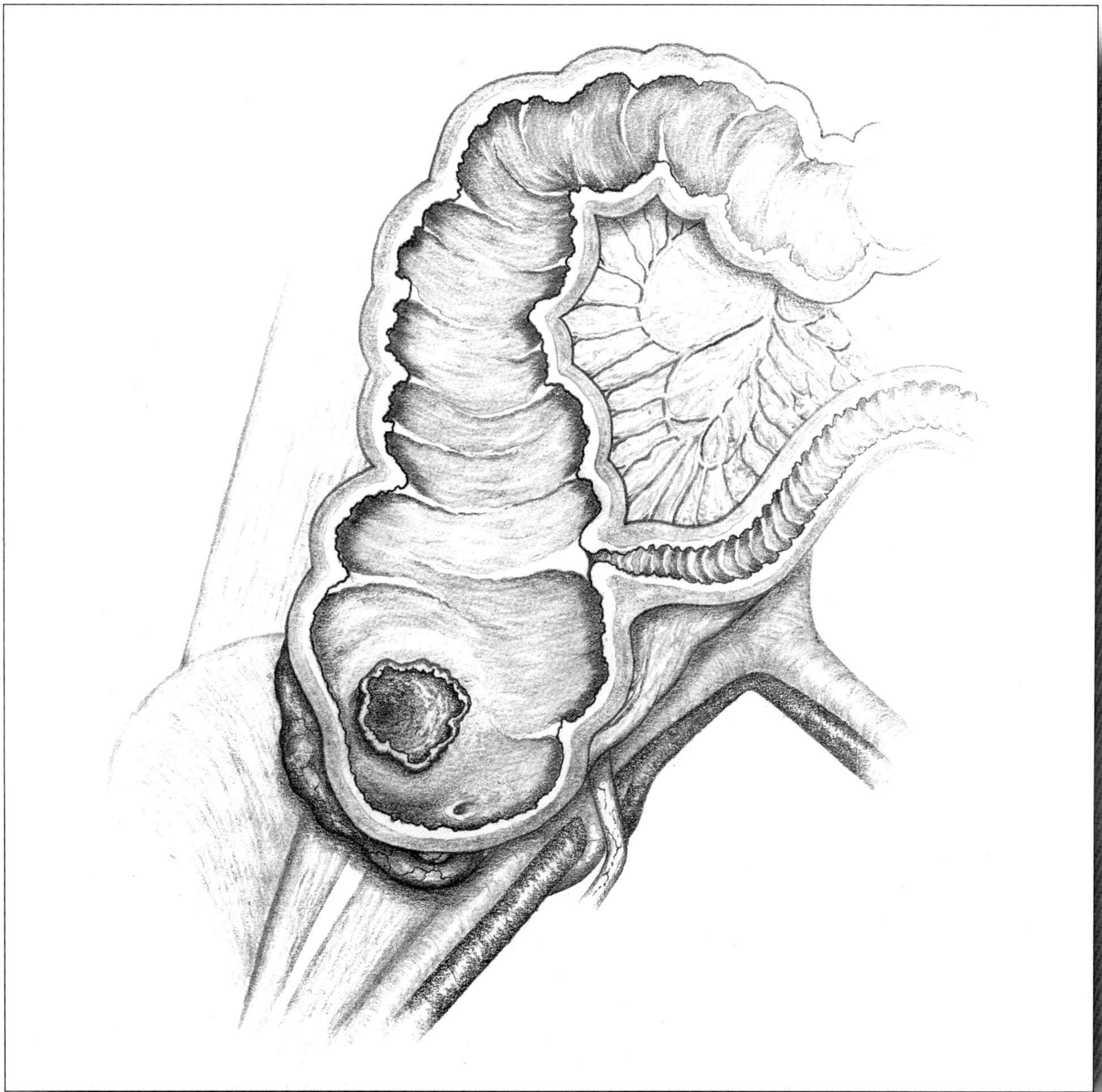

PART

III Polyps-Polyposis

CASE

12 A Mega Polyp Associated with a Micro Cancer

Male, 61 Years

History

A barium enema was performed in this patient to investigate the recent onset of constipation, abdominal distention, and weight loss. The x-ray demonstrated a large irregularity of the sigmoid colon and no other colonic pathology (Figure 12.1). On referral, examination of the abdomen revealed a large asymptomatic distention of the urinary bladder wall above the umbilicus. Flexible sigmoidoscopy revealed a large soft polypoid tumor at 22 cm. Urological investigations indicated the need for prostatectomy, which was performed prior to the colorectal surgery.

Operation (3.2.98)

At laparotomy the only abnormality was the large soft polyp in the mid sigmoid colon. There was no obvious enlargement of mesenteric lymph nodes in relation to the sigmoid colon. The appendix was markedly kinked by congenital adhesions. The lower two thirds of the sigmoid colon was resected with a sutured end-to-end anastomosis. Appendectomy was performed.

Pathology

The polyp extended over 80 mm of the sigmoid colon and "carpeted" the entire circumference of the lumen, forming a "tube" of polyp tissue. Most of the lesion was flat, the proximal edge of which merged with normal colon mucosa. There were raised polypoid areas within the polyp, but, on careful palpation, no firmness in consistency was detected. The histological examination of the polyp showed a tubulovillous adenoma with areas of severe dysplasia but no evidence of invasive malignancy. Five lymph nodes were examined, 1 of which contained a deposit of metastatic adenocarcinoma, (Figure 12.2) Dukes C, pTNM stage 3[1] (assuming the nodal metastasis is related to the sigmoid tumor).

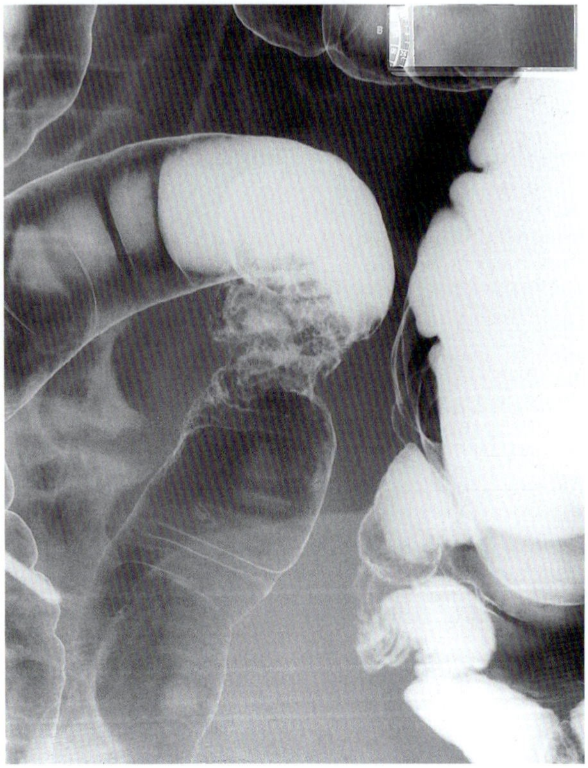

Figure 12.1: The barium enema shows the more proliferative bulk of the sigmoid polyp.

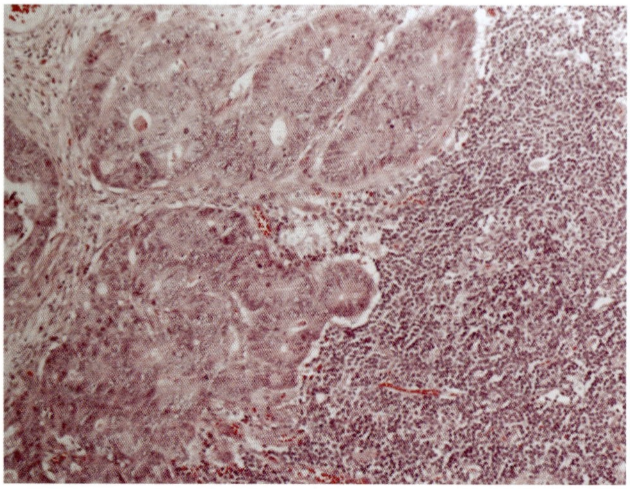

Figure 12.2: Deposit of adenocarcinoma in one mesenteric lymph node.

Follow-Up (2004)

In the past 6 years 2 small benign polyps have been removed by colonoscopy. There is no evidence of recurrence of the colon cancer, but the patient developed non-Hodgkin's lymphoma in 2003, which appears to have responded to chemotherapy.

Comment

This tumor is an example of "large polyp occult carcinoma" that showed no evidence of the primary focus of malignancy on operative, macroscopic, or microscopic examination. The malignancy was not identified in the polyp despite the reexamination of a further 27 blocks of tissue. The incidence of invasive carcinoma in a polyp is known to be directly related to size,[2] and, therefore, giant polyps such as this case can be associated with a high incidence of carcinoma. Sakamoto et al reported recurrent malignancy after excision of a "benign" villous adenoma.[3] Where possible, these lesions are best treated by bowel resection as this and Cases 13 and 14 demonstrate.

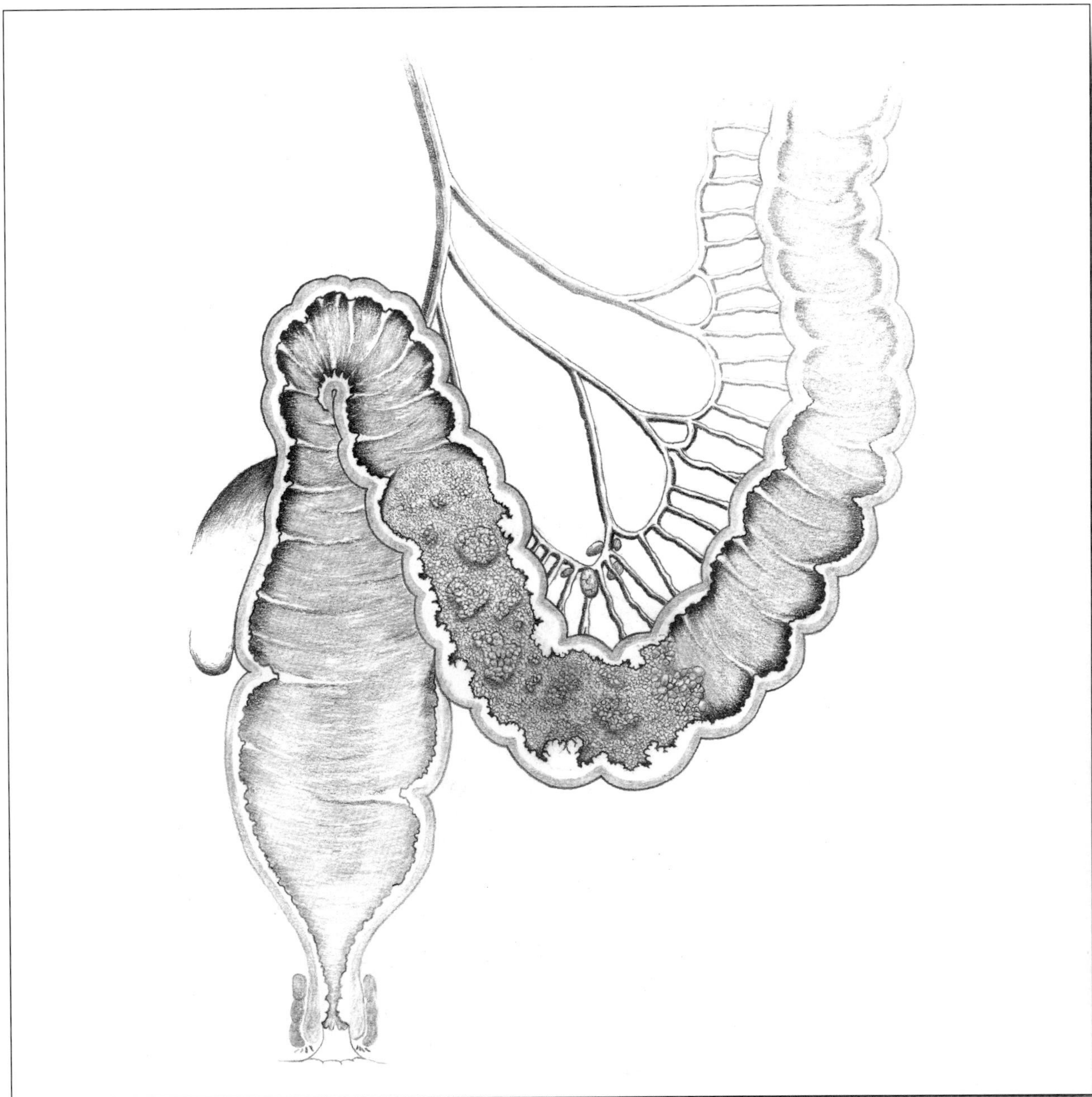

CASE

13 Extensive "Benign" Polyp of the Rectum and Sigmoid Colon

Male, 69 Years

History

The patient complained of diarrhea for 10 years. Sigmoidoscopy revealed an extensive flat polyp with polypoid areas which extended from the anal canal to the lower sigmoid colon, reaching a level of 20cm. There were no obvious features of malignancy. A barium enema showed diverticulosis proximal to the lesion.

Operation (2.4.77)

Laparotomy and loop transverse colostomy.

Operation (2.18.77)

Via a posterior transsphincteric approach, submucosal dissection removed the tumor from the rectal muscle. The rectum and sphincter were repaired.

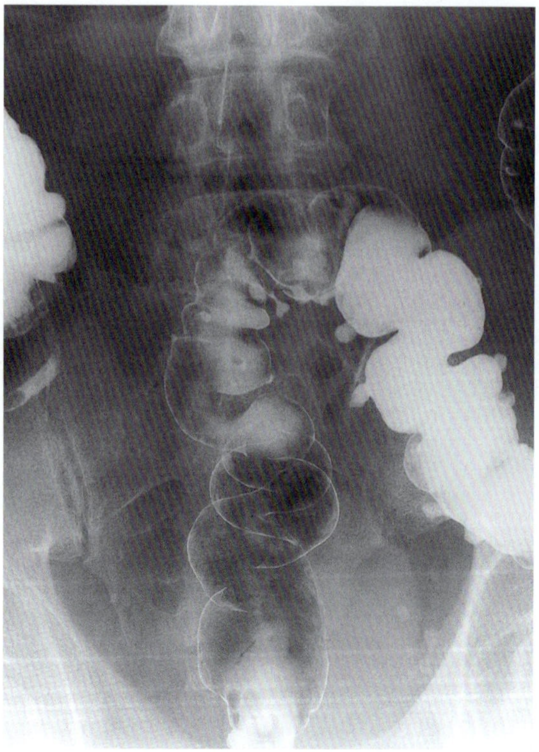

Figure 13.1: Complete resolution of postoperative stricture.

Pathology

Examination of the specimen (23.0 × 18.0cm) revealed a villous adenoma with no evidence of malignancy.

Follow-Up

The colostomy was closed 3 months after the excision of the polyp. A rectal stricture resolved spontaneously (Figure 13.1). Bowel function was satisfactory. No abnormality was detected on regular follow up until March 1986. A presacral cystic swelling, 11.0 × 7.0cm, was apparent on computerized tomography (CT) examination of the pelvis. Transrectal exploration of the cyst produced a copious discharge of mucus, which on histological examination contained clusters of mucoid adenocarcinoma cells. Palliative chemotherapy or radiotherapy was decided against. The patient's health steadily deteriorated until he died (1.8.87), 10 years after removal of the "benign" polyp.

Comment

The extensive lesion would be best classified as a giant polyp. The surgical options for such a polyp should be considered differently to those for smaller

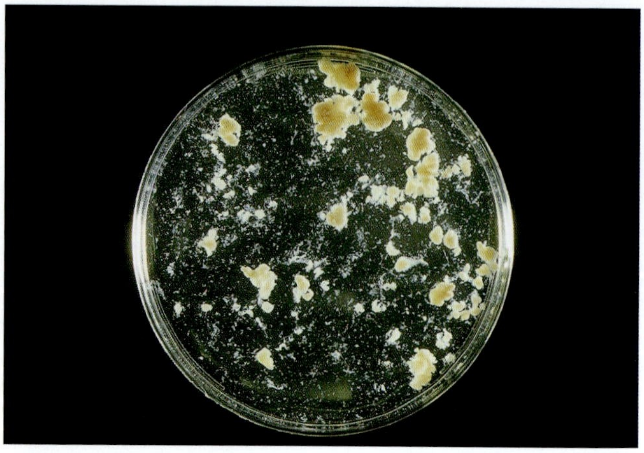

Figure 13.2: Free polyp fragments in washings from the operative field of another patient, also treated with posterior transsphincteric surgery.

flat polyps occurring in the rectum. The treatment should be based on the probability of invasive carcinoma rather than the technical feasibility of local excision. The focus of invasive carcinoma in such polyps may remain undetected despite multiple sections. Galandiuk et al, in reviewing 1049 patients with villous and tubulo-villous polyps, clearly demonstrated an increasing incidence of invasive carcinoma with larger lesions.[1] Polyps larger than 4 cm had a 32% incidence of invasive carcinoma.[1] One can only speculate the risk of carcinoma in polyps 10–20 cm in size. A number of technically clever transanal operations are available for local excision.[2,3] The posterior transsphincteric operation, first performed by Harrison Cripps in 1880,[4] was revived by York Mason in the 1970s, but a review of this operation has highlighted the unacceptable complication rate.[5] The mode of the local recurrence may have been cell implantation, since the presacral space was exposed throughout the operation. Figure 13.2 shows the tissue debris in the wound irrigation fluid from another patient undergoing the same operation for a giant "benign" polyp. This patient also succumbed to recurrent cancer in the presacral space. Both patients were fit enough for resection with coloanal anastomosis.

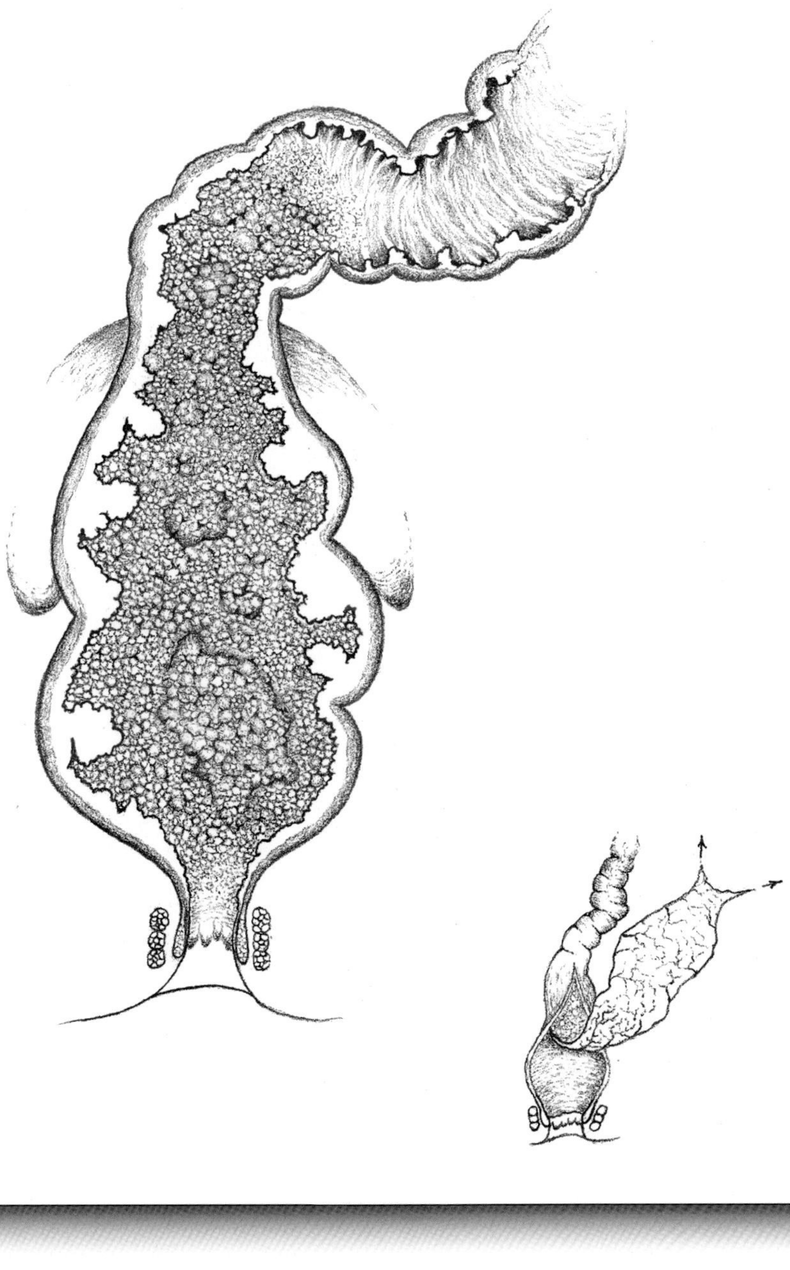

2.18.77

CASE

14 A Bad Result from a Successful Operation for a Polyp in the Sigmoid Colon

Male, 54 Years

History

The patient presented with a 3-year history of rectal bleeding and "explosive" diarrhea. Flexible sigmoidoscopy revealed a large polyp at 22 cm and 4 small polyps at lower levels. Colonoscopy identified 4 small polyps between the large lesion and the splenic flexure.

Operation (3.19.90)

With an operating sigmoidoscope and snare, the polyp was removed "piecemeal" until a "clean" mucosal defect was obtained with no visible residual polyp.

Pathology

The polyp fragments were soft, and placed together they measured 70 × 70 mm. Histological examination showed a villous adenoma with no evidence of malignancy.

Follow Up

The smaller polyps were removed at subsequent colonoscopy (12.12.91) when the diathermy scar of the large polyp site was identified. The patient delayed his next colonoscopy for almost 3 years. At this time he was asymptomatic. Colonoscopy revealed an ulcer adjacent to the scar at 22 cm which, on biopsy, showed adenocarcinoma.

Operation (9.16.94)

At laparotomy a large mass of lymph nodes of the sigmoid mesentery was identified adjacent to the lower third of the sigmoid colon. There was a 15 mm node at the origin of the inferior mesenteric artery. Four small metastases (confirmed on biopsy) were present in the liver. A high anterior resection with anastomosis was performed.

Pathology

Examination of the lumen of the colon revealed a malignant ulcer 23 mm in diameter at the level of the lymph node mass and continuous with it. It was adjacent to but not continuous with the diathermy scar. The extracolic mass had formed a "dome shaped" deformity beneath the malignant ulcer. Histological examination confirmed the diagnosis of adenocarcinoma (moderately differentiated) with extensive lymph node involvement.

Follow-Up

The patient was treated with 5 flourouracil and folinic acid but failed to show any response. He died of metastatic disease 18 months after the palliative resection.

Comment

The morphology of the resected lesion was consistent with the lymph node mass having "erupted" into the lumen of the colon to produce a malignant ulcer. If so, the apparently benign polyp must have contained an undiagnosed focus of carcinoma. A metachronous primary carcinoma at the same site seems less likely but cannot be excluded. Although the challenging diathermy snare of a large polyp at 22 cm was a technical success, in hindsight this patient would have been better managed by resection.

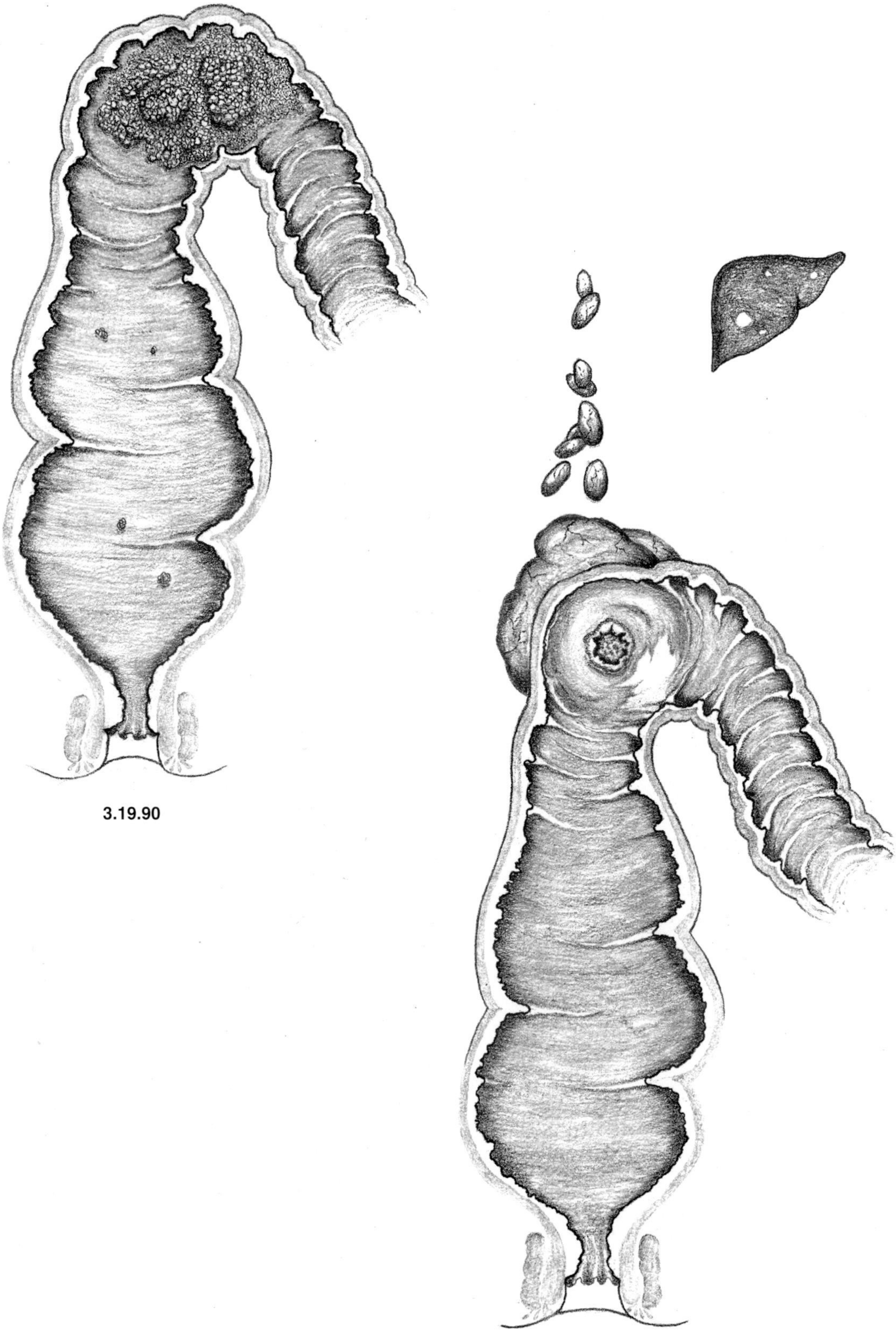

3.19.90

9.16.94

CASE

15 One Operation for Double Pathology

Female, 78 Years

History

The patient complained of diarrhea and mucous discharge for 13 years. There had been intermittent rectal bleeding. Prolapse of the rectum had been noted for a period of 12 months. There had been recent weight loss and general weakness. On digital rectal examination, a soft polyp encircling the rectum was easily palpable at the 7 cm level. Complete rectal prolapse was present on straining. There was laxity of the anal sphincter. Sigmoidoscopy revealed an extensive rectal polyp with a combination of flat and polypoid contours. The upper limit of the polyp was 20 cm from the anal verge. There were no macroscopic features to suggest malignancy. There were abnormalities of biochemistry on blood examination: Na, 125 mmol/L (N-134–143); K, 3.8 mmol/L (N-3.5–5.0); Urea, 28.9 mmol/L (N-2.0–7.0); and creatinine, 0.21 mmol/L (N-0.05–0.11).

Operation (1.16.87)

A Delorme operation was performed in view of the patient's poor general health. The excised mucosa measured 15 × 13 cm.

Pathology

The histological examination showed both villous and tubulovillous adenoma with several submucosal "lakes" of mucin which were interpreted as early proctitis cystica profunda.

Follow-Up

The postoperative assessment was satisfactory 2 months after operation. The patient did not return for further examination.

Comment

In this frail patient the surgical approach was satisfactory treatment for the coexisting giant rectal polyp and the rectal prolapse. The submucosal dissection of the polyp by the Delorme technique allowed very precise separation of the polyp from the muscular layer of the rectum. This was greatly facilitated by infiltrating the submucosal plane with the vasoconstrictor (ornipressin). The alternative operation in this patient was a low anterior resection, decided against, as the patient was a poor risk for abdominal surgery. In this group of patients the Delorme operation for rectal prolapse is well tolerated, but the results are inferior to abdominal surgical repair. Oliver et al found a recurrence rate of 22% in 41 operations in 40 poor risk patients and attributed the failures to weak or absent sphincter tone.[1] Tobin et al regarded the operation as most suitable for the medically unfit patient.[2] In 43 of 49 poor risk patients who were reviewed, the recurrence rate was 26%. There was an improvement in anal continence in 50% of the 40 patients documented with preoperative sphincter disability.[2]

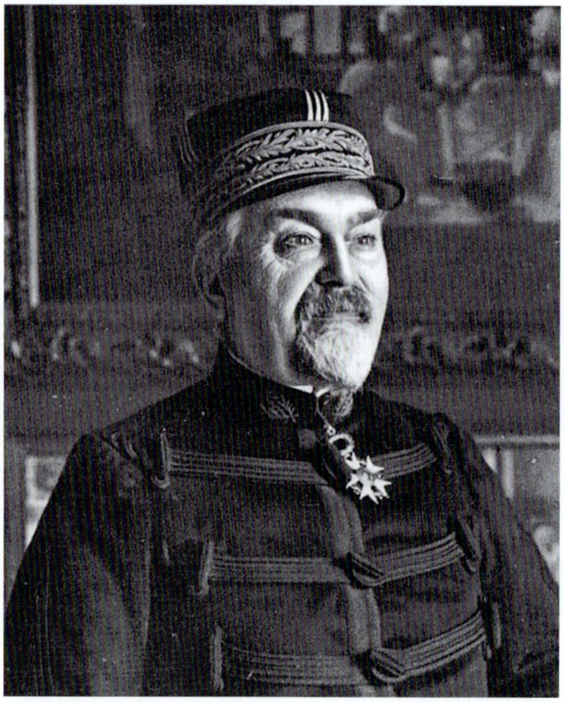

Figure 15.1: Edmond Delorme (1847–1929). (Courtesy of Prof. M. Corman.)

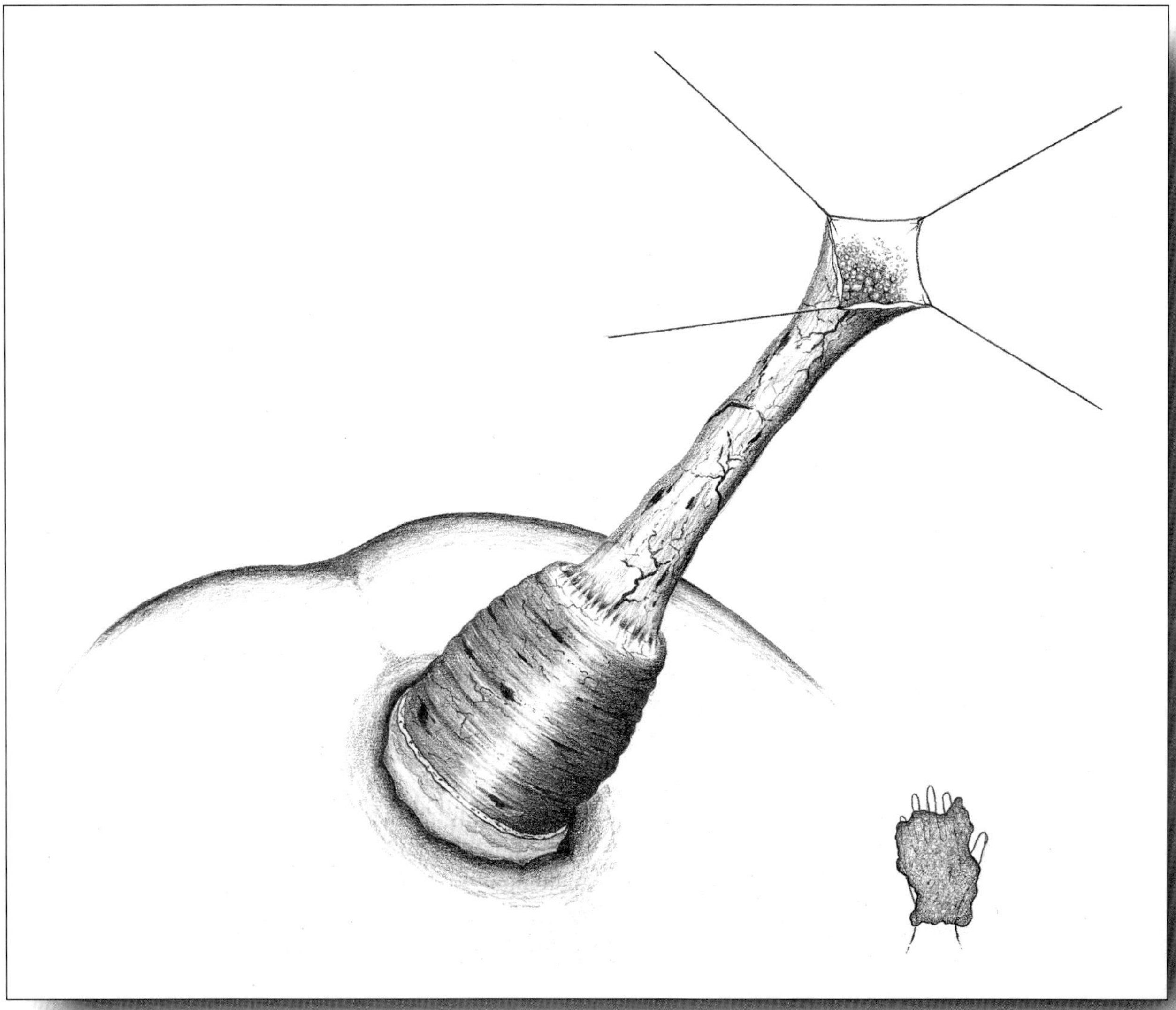

CASE

16 Juvenile Polyposis and Rectal Prolapse

Male, 13 Years

History

The male patient aged 13 years had noticed rectal bleeding for 15 months. A prolapsed rectal polyp had been observed. A barium enema showed no evidence of other polyps.

Operation (initial procedure) (3.24.78)

Examination of the rectum under anasthesia revealed multiple polyps in the lower rectum. Sigmoidoscopy noted the upper level of involvement was 9 cm. The polyps were deeply congested, smooth with a glistening surface. They were fragile and fractured readily. The pedicles were vascular and varied in size. There were approximately 20 polyps of moderate size (5–10 mm) removed by diathermy snare. There were many small polyps (1–8 mm), which were fulgurated.

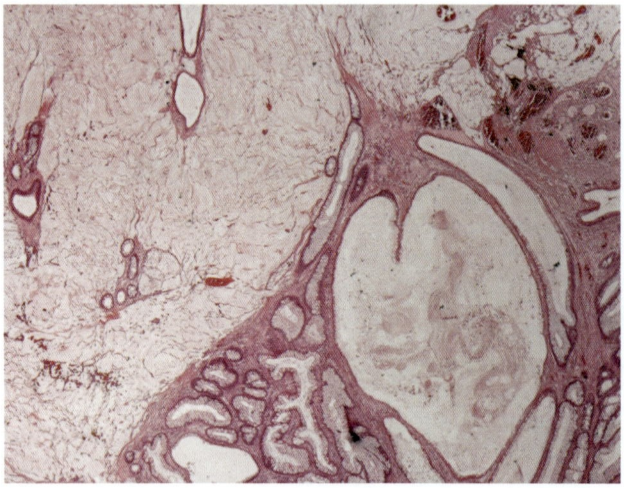

Figure 16.1: Within the vascular stroma there are dilated glands lined by normal epithelium and containing mucus.

Pathology

Histological examination showed typical appearance of juvenile polyp (Figure 16.1).

Follow-Up

Twenty months after the initial removal of rectal polyps, 40 polyps (5–20 mm) were removed by diathermy snare and fulguration. Twelve months later a further 83 polyps were removed, and at this time rectal prolapse was diagnosed while the patient was anesthetized. Over the next 20 years further removal of polyps was undertaken on an additional 14 occasions. The polyps remained typical in appearance and consistency and, subsequent to 1993, were never larger than 6 mm. Colonoscopy examination revealed no polyps proximal to those described. A rectopexy (Ripstein) was performed for the rectal prolapse in 1995 at the age of 30 years. In excess of 400 polyps had been removed by July 2001.

Comment

The patient's juvenile polyposis (JP) was confined to the lower rectum over a period of 33 years. The histology of the polyps remained typical of juvenile polyps. The incidental occurrence of rectal prolapse with juvenile polyposis is unusual. McColl et al from St Mark's Hospital, London reported that 11 of 131 patients (8.4%) with polyposis of the colon had JP, the rectum being the commonest site of the polyps in the large bowel.[1] Smilow et al were the first to report the familial nature of the disease,[2] which can also be sporadic. The potential for upper or lower gastrointestinal malignancy has been reported since 1975 and may be a cumulative risk as high as 50% in familial JP.[3] Because of the potential distribution of the polyps, screening of patients should include the gastrointestinal tract (GIT) from stomach to rectum. Family members can now be screened for mutations in the SMAD4 gene.[3]

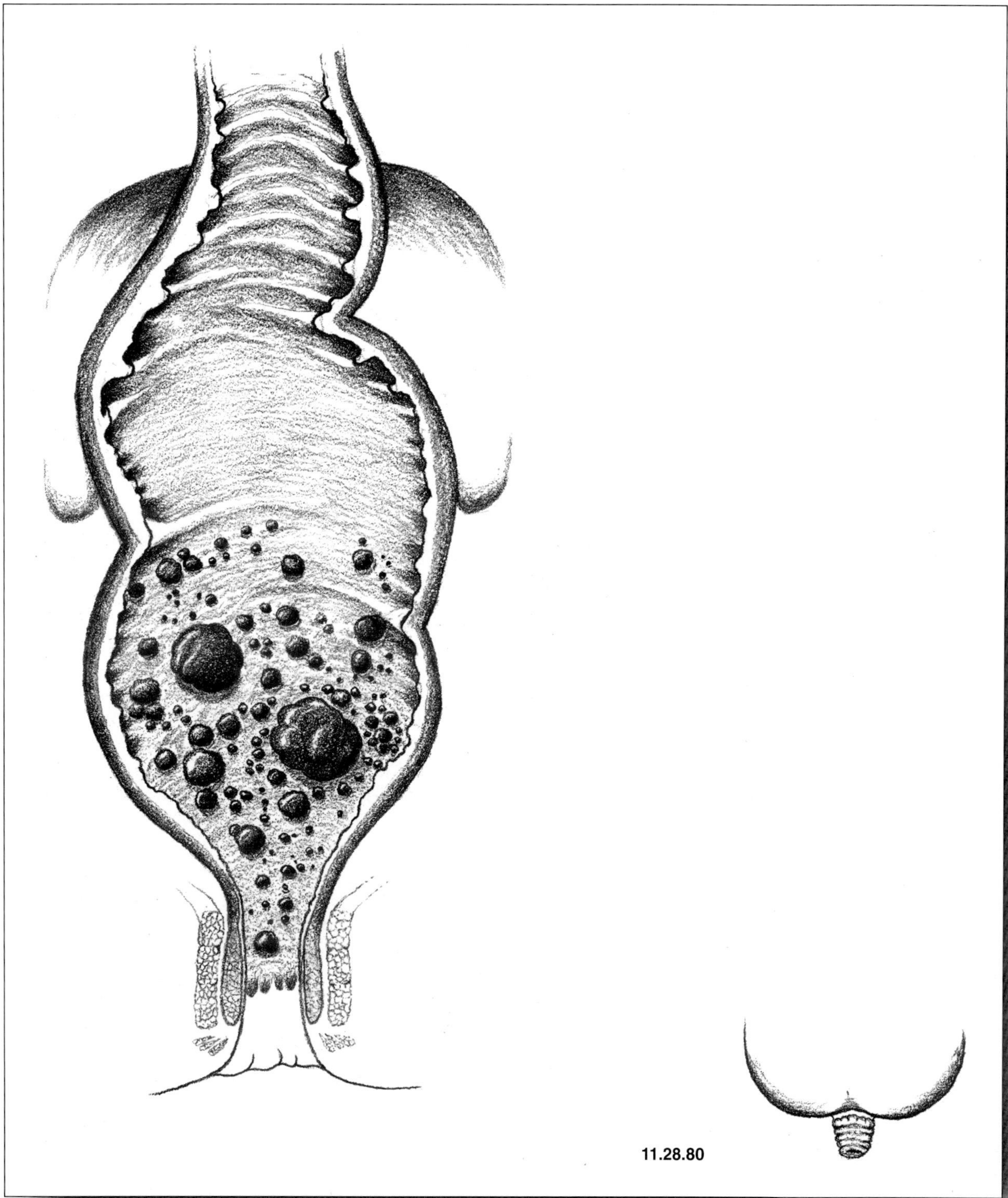
11.28.80

CASE

17 Juvenile Polyposis in an Adult

Female, 31 Years

History

In 1981, approximately 40 polyps were identified in the colon and rectum by colonoscopy. At least 30 of the polyps were situated in the right colon. Initially 6 excised polyps were thought to be the Peutz Jegher variety, but subsequently the diagnosis of juvenile polyposis (JP) was established.

Operation (3.8.81)

At laparotomy soft polyps were palpable in the right and transverse colon, the largest of which was situated in the cecum. A right hemicolectomy was performed with the distal level of resection in the mid transverse colon. An end-to-end anastomosis was completed with a single layer of interrupted sutures.

Pathology

The resected colon contained 30 polyps that were characterized by long pedicles of up to 30 mm in length and frequently branched, giving a "tree-like" appearance. The polyps were soft, the largest being a lobulated mass 48 mm in diameter: histological sections of all polyps showed the typical features of JP. There was no evidence of malignancy.

Follow-Up

Since operation a further 29 polyps have been removed during surveillance colonoscopies; most of these have been JP and a few have been adenomas. A family history emerged in 1986 when the patient's daughter, aged 9 years, was found to have JP of the colon treated by colonoscopic excision and right hemicolectomy.

Comment

The multiple polyps in juvenile polyposis were first described by Verse,[1] but it was not until the 1980s that the increased risk of colorectal carcinoma in these patients was well established.[2] Jass et al[3] have reported 18 patients with colorectal carcinomas occurring in 87 patients with JP, and they suggested the cumulative risk could be as high as 50%. The colon polyposis may be associated with polyps in the stomach and small bowel as well as extracolonic abnormalities.[3] The polyps may be typical (81%) with dilated cystic glands and inflammatory infiltrate in the lamina propria, atypical (16%) or adenomatous (2%).[4] The disease may be sporadic or familial, and the latter is inherited as an autosomal dominant. An abnormality predisposing one to JP has been identified on chromosome 18q21.1.[5] Treatment is varied according to the number and distribution of the polyps and therefore may be endoscopic, resection, or a combination of these methods. When polyps are too numerous or difficult to control endoscopically, colectomy and ileorectal anastomosis (IRA) or restorative proctocolectomy are the operations of choice.[6] Long term follow up by endoscopy is necessary in these patients subsequent to initial treatment. It is also recommended that first degree family members undergo screening for colorectal carcinoma in addition to screening for polyps.

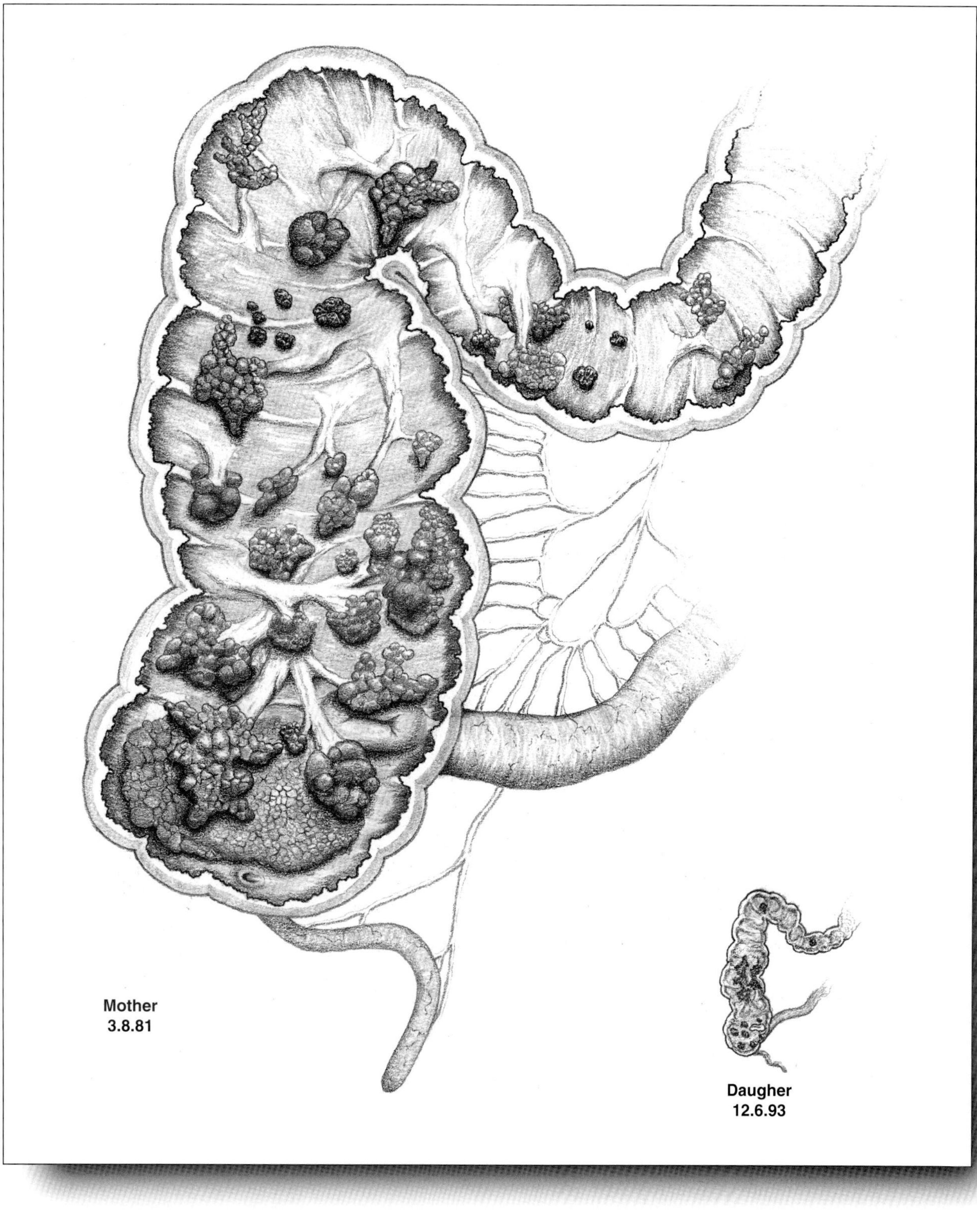
Mother
3.8.81
Daugher
12.6.93

CASE
18 Chronic Intussusception of the Colon Due to Peutz-Jeghers Syndrome

Male, 24 Years

History
The patient presented in May 1965 with an established family history (mother and sister) of the Peutz–Jeghers syndrome (PJS). He had suffered epigastric lower abdominal colic for 2 years, then daily for 2 months. The pain was accompanied by loud borborygmi, and black stools appeared after the more severe attacks. The only abnormality on physical examination was the presence of pigmented spots, typical of PJS, on the eyelids, lips, buccal surfaces, and fingers (Figure 18.3). A barium meal follow-through demonstrated a round filling defect in the first part of duodenum, the "size of a marble;" the small bowel appeared normal.

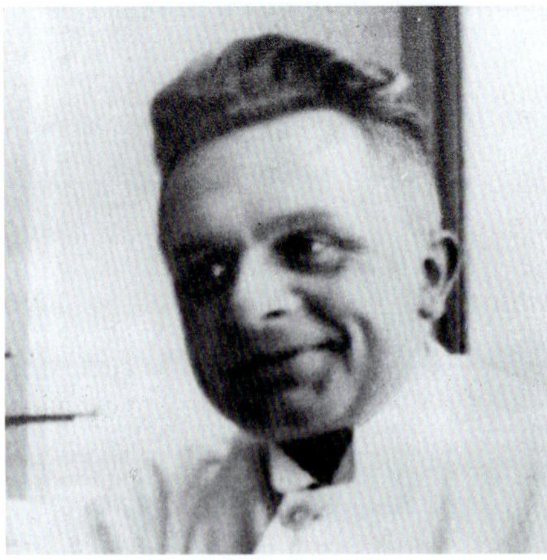

Figure 18.1: J.L.A. Peutz (1886–1957).

Operation (7.8.65)
At laparotomy chronic colocolic intussusception of the transverse colon was found, fixed by adhesions. The intussusception had reached the lower descending colon but was easily reduced after division of adhesions. A large mass of confluent polyps in the mid transverse colon was exposed by colotomy and removed by ligature transection of a broad pedicle. The colon between this site and the rectum was examined with a rigid sigmoidoscope to exclude the presence of other polyps. Feces in the proximal colon precluded intraoperative enteroscopy, but a polyp detected in the cecum by palpation was removed via a colotomy. A small, branched polyp in the terminal ileum and a spherical polyp in the duodenum, adjacent to the pylorus, were removed via enterotomies. A normal appendix was removed.

Pathology
The polyps were soft in consistency with prominent lobulation. Both the polyp mass in the transverse colon (45 mm) and the ileal polyp (14 mm) exhibited a characteristic branched morphology. Histologically the polyps were typical of PJS (Figure 18.4).

Follow-Up
During the subsequent 23 years the patient required laparotomy on 3 occasions: small bowel obstruction requiring division of adhesions (1966), resection of 20 cm of ileum containing a benign 34 mm polyp (1978), and resection of 50 cm of ileum for a gangrenous intussusception caused by a benign 30 mm polyp (1988). In 1990 he was diagnosed with lung cancer and died later that year aged 49 years. (It is not known if the lung cancer was primary or metastatic.)

Comment
This rare autosomal dominant disease has been estimated to occur in 1:120000 births.[1] Hamartoma-

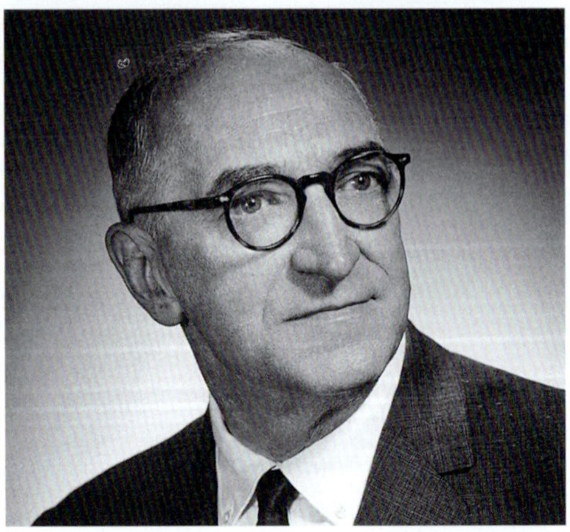

Figure 18.2: H.J. Jeghers (1904–1990).

tous and adenomatous polyps may occur from stomach to rectum. The predisposition to malignancy in the gastrointestinal tract (GIT) and extra-GIT sites was debated for some years, but evidence for this now exists.[2] Treatment should avoid bowel resection where possible, as surgery for further polyps is often necessary. Asymptomatic polyps are best removed before the complications of bleeding and intussusception occur. Spigelman et al recommend the removal of such polyps over 1.5 cm in size by endoscopy or operation.[2] St Mark's Hospital and the Cleveland Clinic recommend that during a laparotomy for PJS, all polyps, irrespective of size, should be removed (endoscopically or by enterotomy) to effect a "clean sweep"[3] and thus reduce the need for subsequent surgery.[2,3] Follow-up for life is important for these patients in order to detect metachronous polyps and cancers. It is likely that small bowel surveillance will be best achieved by the use of video capsule endoscopy (VCE) as it becomes more widely available. Two recent studies have shown VCE to be superior to radiographic investigation with impact on clinical management.[4,5] The 2 family members of the patient who were affected by PJS died of the disease. His sister, aged 8 years, died of small bowel intussusception, and the mother, aged 54, years succumbed to pancreatic cancer. Primary lung cancer complicating PJS is rare, and to 2005 only 7 cases have been published.[6]

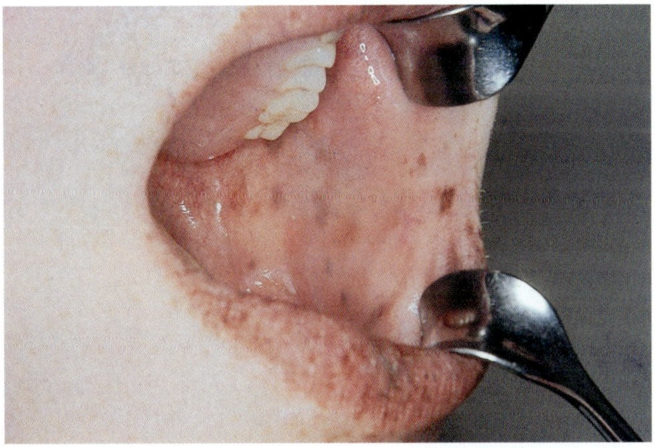

Figure 18.3: Buccal pigmentation.

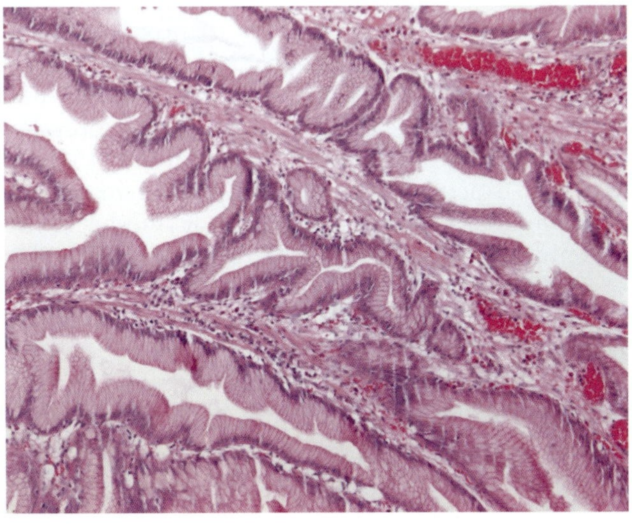

Figure 18.4: Polyp showing muscle strands between glands, characteristic of PJS.

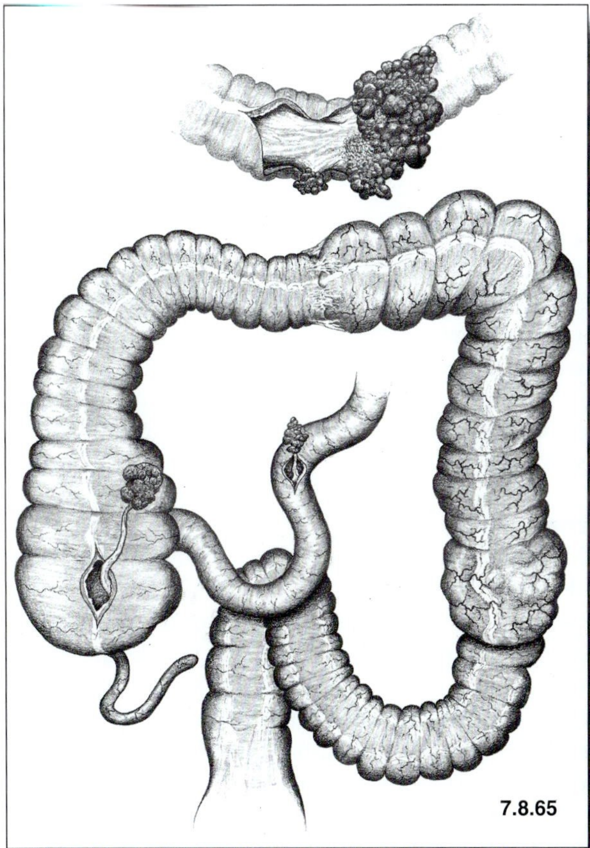

For a full-page image of this figure see the appendix.

CASE

19 Carcinoma of the Rectum: FAP and Rectovaginal Fistula

Female, 46 Years

History

The patient, who suffered from morbid obesity, and denying any bowel symptoms presented with a 7-week history of a fecal vaginal discharge. There was no family history of bowel cancer. Examination revealed a large fixed carcinoma of the rectum with a lower edge at 5 cm. There was a small malignant ulcer on the posterior wall of the vagina, discharging flatus and fecal liquid. The narrow lumen of the tumor prevented endoscopic examination beyond the lower edge. A barium enema was contraindicated due to the possibility of initiating bowel obstruction. Biopsy showed a well differentiated adenocarcinoma. Computerized tomography (CT) examination showed perirectal extension of the tumor with adherence to the uterus and vagina. There was no pelvic lymphadenopathy or evidence of extra pelvic metastases. The patient was treated with a 5-week course of radiotherapy (40 Gy), and after 4 weeks CT examination showed "an overall reduction in size" of the tumor.

Operation (12.9.85)

Laparotomy revealed the surprise finding of multiple, palpable polyps throughout the colon. The rectal tumor was adherent to the uterus with extension to the deep aspects of the pelvis on the right side. Proctocolectomy with en bloc radical hysterectomy and excision of the posterior wall of the vagina was performed.

Pathology

The mucosa of the colon and rectum contained hundreds of sessile and pedunculated polyps, the largest measuring 40 mm in diameter. Polyps examined histologically were tubulovillous. The rectal carcinoma was annular, deeply excavated, 48 mm in axial dimension, and showing malignant infiltration of the uterus as well as vagina. Histological examination of the right aspect of the tumor confirmed that despite the concern at operation, the margin of excision was satisfactory. The tumor was a mucinous adenocarcinoma. There were "nodules" in the perirectal fat containing mucus and epithelial cells, regarded as metastatic nodes, attenuated by radiotherapy (Dukes C, T_3 N_2 M_0).

Follow-Up

In 1992, panendoscopy revealed a 20 mm adenomatous polyp in the second part of the duodenum. In 1994 cholecystectomy and transduodenal polypectomy was performed by open abdominal surgery. No abdominal metastases were identified. In 1998 a cerebral tumor was diagnosed but considered to be inoperable. Biopsy was not performed. There was no response to chemotherapy or radiotherapy. The patient died in August 2000.

Comment

The patient and 1 of 2 children were confirmed as suffering from familial adenomatous polyposis (FAP) with positive gene testing. They appear to be the first FAP patients in the family line. Rectovaginal fistula is uncommon in patients with rectal cancer. It is difficult to believe this extensive tumor was not accompanied by bowel symptoms. Restorative proctocolectomy was not regarded as a safe option in this patient. The recommended operation for a low rectal carcinoma and rectovaginal fistula is the one performed on this patient as illustrated by Keighley and Williams.[1] The patient's survival for nearly 15 years was not expected. The cerebral tumor may have been coincidental, a metastasis, or another extra colonic manifestation of FAP syndrome. Kropilak et al have reported 13 patients with brain tumors and a family history of FAP. Six of the patients had documented FAP. Although the brain tumors appeared at an early age (mean 15 years) the age range was $1\frac{1}{2}$ to 59 years.[2]

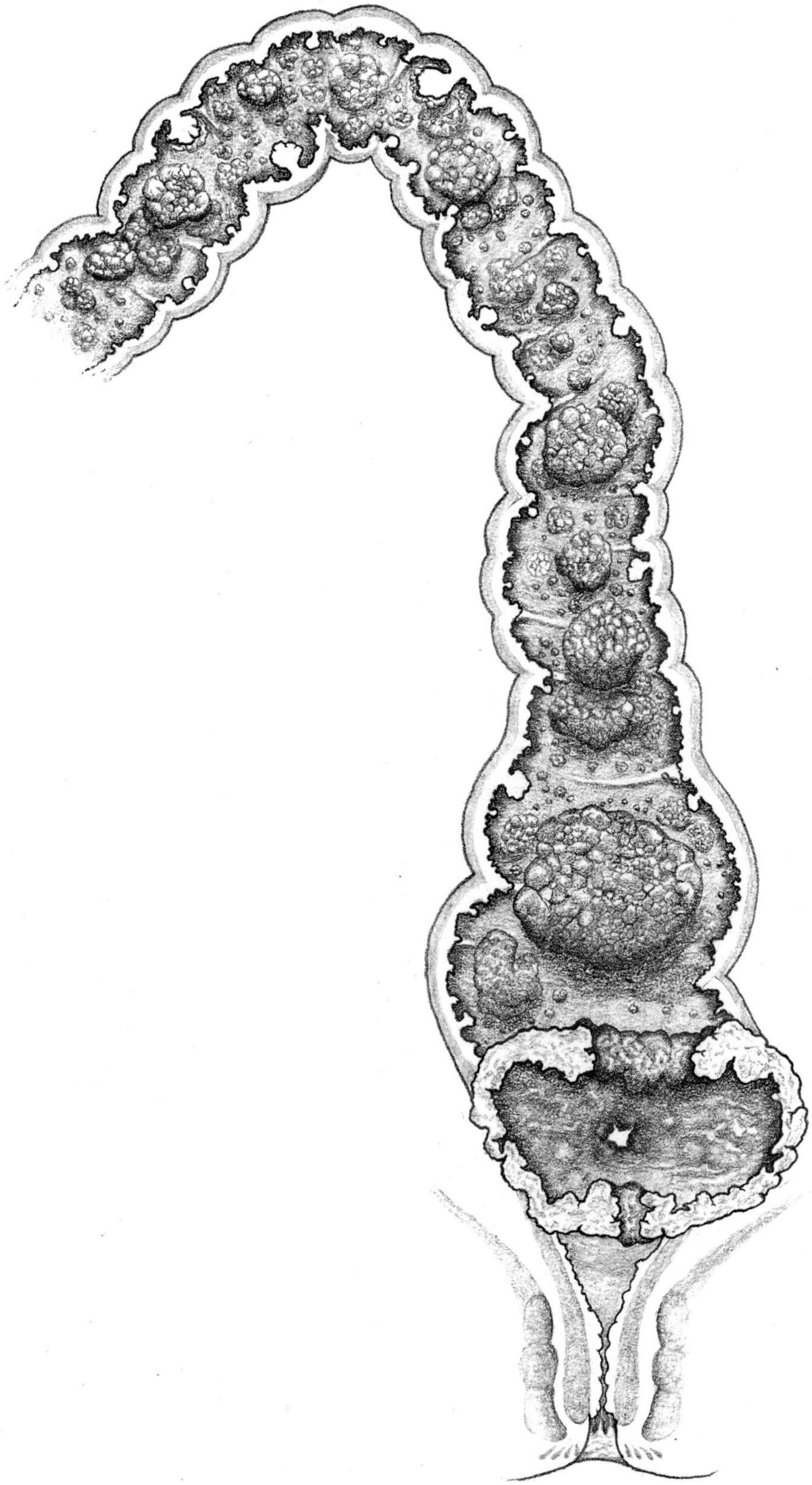

Posterior aspect

CASE

20 Ileorectal Anastomosis for FAP: Rectal Cancer

Female 35, Years

History
In July 1970 the patient underwent colectomy and ileorectal anastomosis for the treatment of familial adenomatous polyposis (FAP). At follow up, villous adenomata had been removed by diathermy snare on 10 occasions. The surgeon supervising the follow up referred her in 1994 for a restorative proctocolectomy, since he was concerned about future malignant change in the rectum. Flexible sigmoidoscopy identified the ileorectal anastomosis (IRA) at 20 cm and multiple flat polyps in the rectum. No obvious carcinoma was identified on endoscopy or digital examination. Operation was advised to anticipate the onset of carcinoma.

Operation (3.27.95)
Laparotomy revealed adhesions involving the small bowel, particularly in the region of the side ileum:end rectum anastomosis. Projecting to the left of the anastomosis was a blind pouch 10 cm in length. There was no evidence of metastatic disease within the abdomen. The ileum was disconnected from the anastomosis and the rectum excised to the level of the pelvic floor. The operation was performed with coagulating diathermy dissection, laterally to the endopelvic pelvic fascia, anteriorly posterior to the Waldeyer's fascia and posteriorly via a thin fascial presacral anatomical plane. A J-pouch and a proximal loop ileostomy was constructed.

Pathology
Examination of the rectum revealed multiple sessile polyps and an extensive soft sessile polyp up to 12 cm in length. This polyp was predominantly flat with polypoid areas. Its shape was patchy with islands of normal mucosa within it, suggesting that coalescing of multiple polyps had occurred. Situated in its center was an ulcerated tumor 25 × 25 mm. In the upper part of the rectum there was a smaller ulcerated lesion (8 × 8 mm). Histological examination of the polyps showed a tubulovillous pattern. The larger ulcer was a moderately differentiated adenocarcinoma associated with villous adenoma. This tumor extended through the bowel wall to perirectal fat (T_3). The smaller ulcer was also a moderately differentiated adenocarcinoma with invasion limited to the submucosa (T_1). Seventeen perirectal lymph nodes were examined, 2 of which contained metastatic carcinoma. The tumors were probably Dukes C, T_3 N_1 M_0 and Dukes A, T_1 N_0 M_0.

Operation (5.22.95)
Closure of loop ileostomy.

Follow-Up (2004)
Postoperative radiotherapy was not administered, to avoid the risk of post irradiation pouch dysfunction. The patient was treated with adjuvant chemotherapy (flourouracil and folinic acid) for 12 months. She remained well until May 1998 when computerized (CT) examination demonstrated a large solitary mass in the right lobe of the liver. A right hemihepatectomy was performed. Progress was satisfactory until May 2004 when pulmonary metastases were detected. At last follow-up the patient's well being did not appear to be affected by this latest spread of the disease. There has been no evidence of local pelvic recurrence.

Comment
In FAP patients the risk of rectal cancer is known to increase with length of follow up after IRA. This patient's carcinomas were diagnosed 25 years after the IRA was performed. In patients treated entirely or predominantly before the ileal pouch surgery commenced, the risk of rectal cancer has been reported as: 3.6% (St Mark's Hospital),[1] 12.9% (Cleveland Clinic),[2] 13.1% (Leeds Castle Polyposis Group),[3] and 32% (Mayo Clinic),[4] Church et al have highlighted a change in indication for IRA since the advent of pouch surgery and suggest that IRA is a satisfactory operation if the rectum is not severely affected by polyposis.[2] Church et al report that since 1983, 135 patients treated at the Cleveland Clinic with IRA with a median follow up of 135 months have remained free of rectal cancer.[2] The patient reported here had a longer rectal segment remaining than the recommended 12 cm level of anastomosis. A lower IRA would not have prevented the development of the cancer in the mid rectum. It is of interest that this carcinoma was not diagnosed prior to operation.

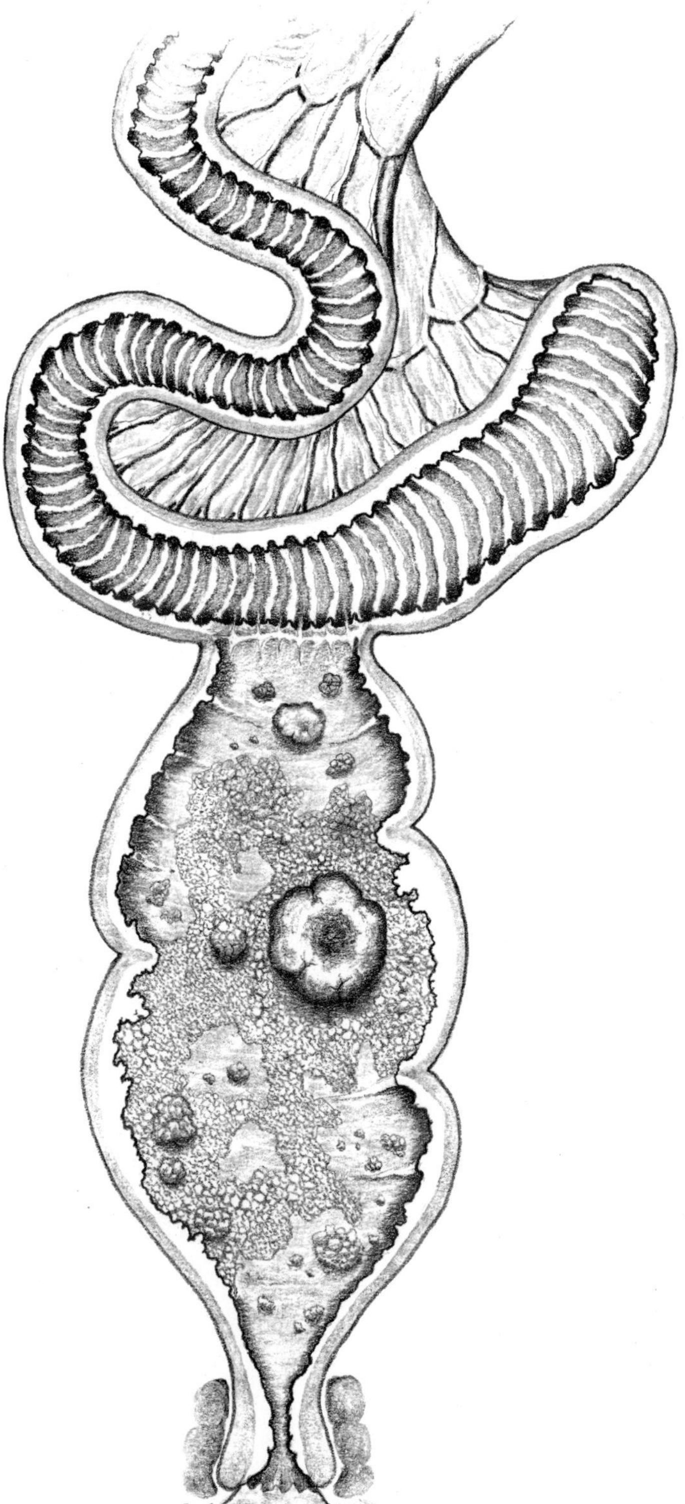

CASE 21 Large Bowel Lipomatosis

Female, 53 Years

History

In 1990 colonoscopy revealed multiple lipomas in the left colon and rectum. There was also a central lower abdominal mass reaching the level of the umbilicus. Laparotomy revealed a deep abdominal wall tumor (12 × 9 cm) attached to the sigmoid colon, bladder, and a tube-ovarian mass containing a cystadenoma (14 × 14 cm). These lesions were removed. An ulcerated polypoid lipoma (6 × 2.5 cm) was removed from the splenic flexure by colotomy. The histology of the abdominal wall tumor revealed a fibroblastic pattern (no mitoses) and chronic inflammatory cells. Diagnosis: inflammatory pseudotumor

Follow-Up Investigations (10.8.98)

In 1998 colonoscopy and barium enema revealed lipomatous polyps in the rectum and colon as far as the mid descending colon (Figures 21.1 and 21.2). They varied in size from 3 mm to 65 mm.

Operation (1.18.99)

The colon was obscured by extensive "fat wrapping" and large appendices epiploicae. Resection-anastomosis was performed. The small lesions were lipomas, tubular adenomas, and hyperplastic polyps. The larger polyps were lipomas.

Follow-Up (2005)

Colonoscopy has subsequently revealed small lipomas in the transverse and ascending colon. Some of the small rectal polyps removed are "stromal polyps" showing increased smooth muscle fibers in the submucosa.

Comment

The true nature of the "inflammatory pseudotumor" removed in 1990 remains unclear and may be similar to the case reported by Kunakemakon et al.[1] Its relationship to the lipomatosis of the colon is not established. While lipomas are the second commonest benign "tumor" of the colon, lipomatosis is rare. The age range at presentation in the few reports available is 2–58 years. The condition may be asymptomatic or be the cause of abdominal pain, diarrhea, or rectal bleeding. Surgical treatment is not obligatory and will depend on the extent of the colon disease and the clinical significance. It does not appear to be a familial disease. The lipomas are usually submucosal but may be subserosal as well, forming "dumb-bell" lesions.[2] Marked fatty infiltration of the appendices epiploicae may be associated with the condition.[3,4,5]

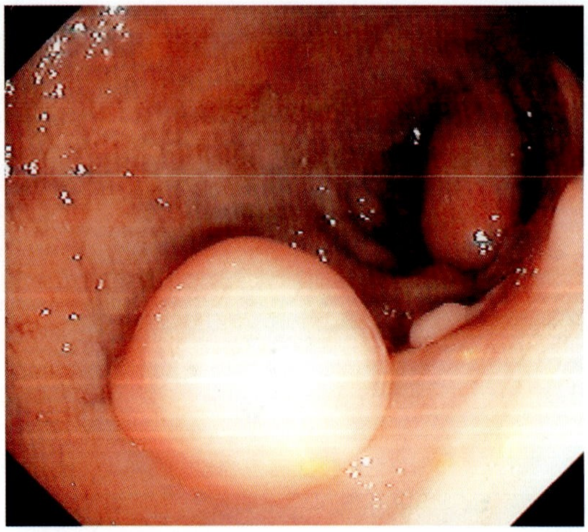

Figure 21.1: Lipomas seen on colonoscopy.

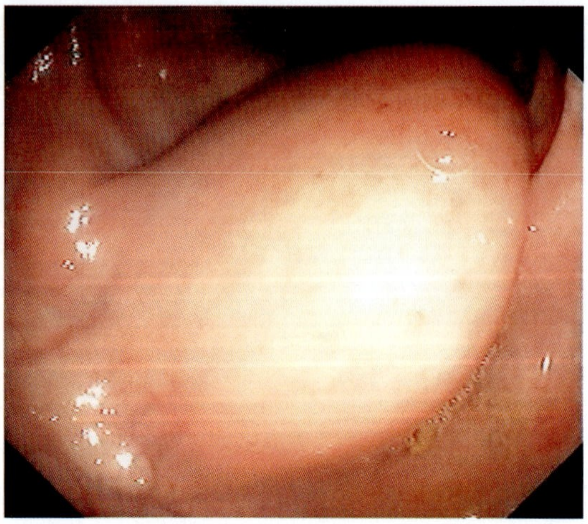

Figure 21.2: Lipoma in sigmoid colon.

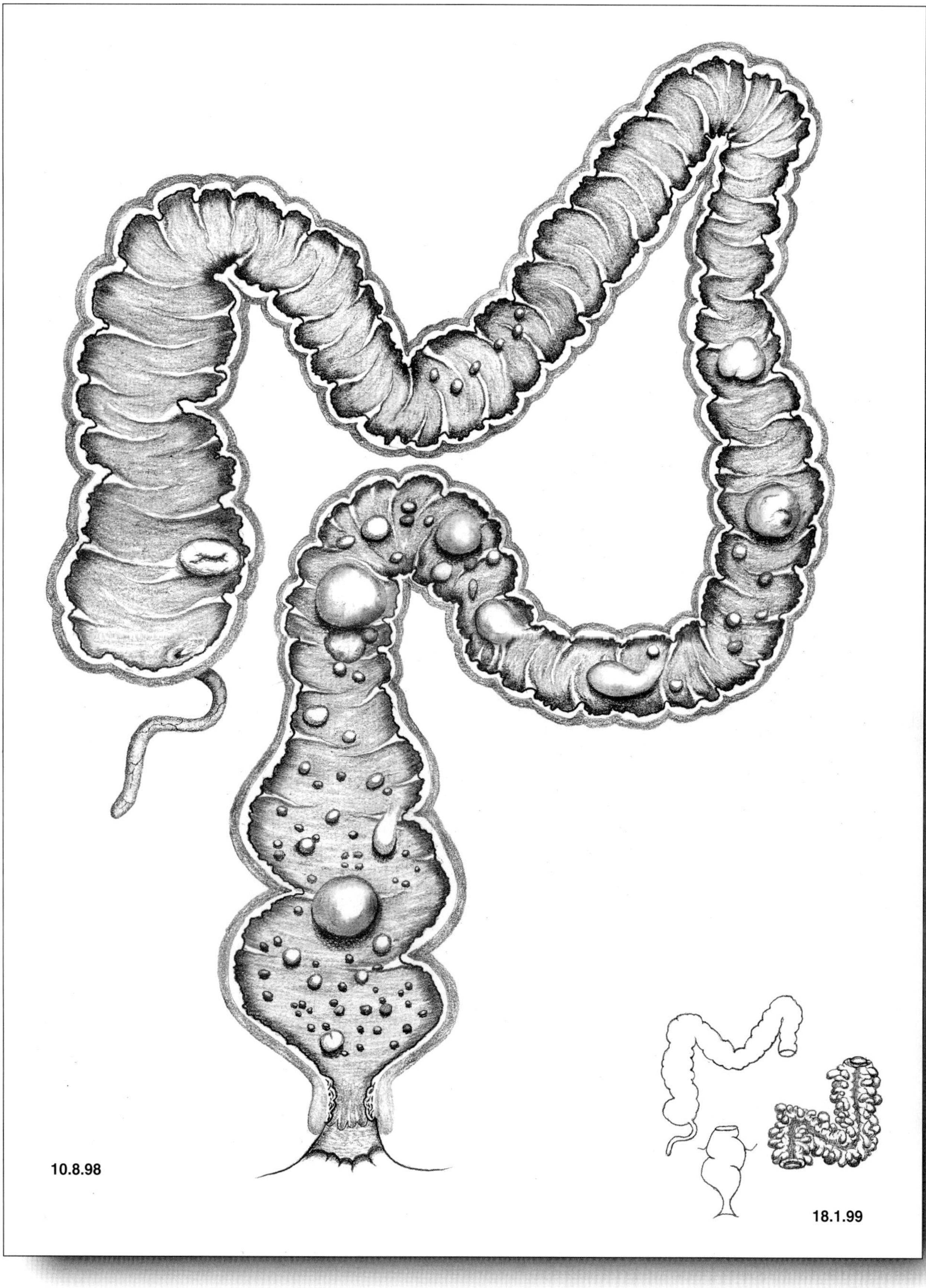
10.8.98
18.1.99

CASE

22 A Polypoid Lesion in the Sigmoid Colon

Male, 46 Years

History

The patient had a family history of colorectal cancer (father). He presented with a 10-day history of central abdominal pain, anorexia, and fever. A rapid loss of weight had occurred during this period. He was admitted to a hospital where colonoscopy revealed a polypoid mass at 30 cm. This was diagnosed as a carcinoma and the patient was referred for operation. A further colonoscopy to the cecum was performed. The lesion was of an intense red color, lobulated, and with a smooth surface (Figure 22.1). Immediately proximal to it there was a less prominent but similar change in the mucosa. Diverticula were present in the sigmoid and descending colon. There was no other mucosal abnormality. Biopsy revealed mucosal inflammation. On rectal examination, there was a fixed left-sided pelvic mass. A preoperative diagnosis of diverticulitis was made.

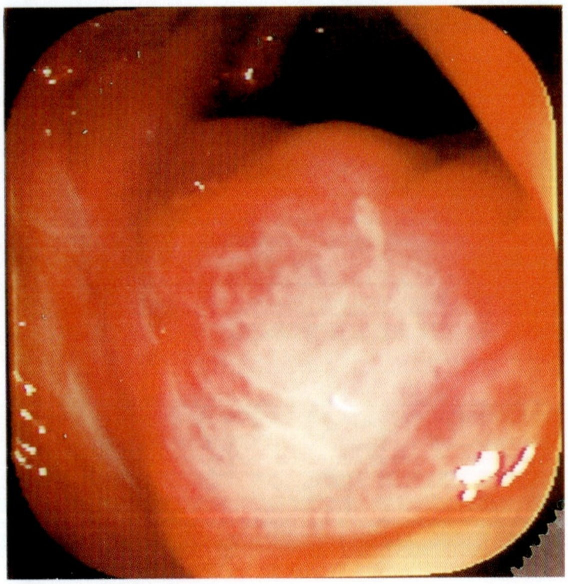

Figure 22.1: Colonoscopy reveals a lobulated polypoid lesion at 30 cm, the surface of which is intensely red, smooth, and shiny.

Operation (7.7.97)

Laparotomy revealed a pelvic abscess contained by an inflamed segment of sigmoid colon, the left side of the upper rectum, and the side wall of the pelvis. There was marked diverticulosis proximal to the inflammatory mass, which affected most of the descending colon. The upper rectum, sigmoid, and descending colon were resected. An extraperitoneal anastomosis was performed with a circular stapler (later measured at 9 cm). Irrigation suction drains were placed in the "bed" of the previous abscess. Postoperative recovery was satisfactory.

Pathology

The diagnosis of diverticulitis was confirmed and there was no evidence of malignancy. The colon was grossly thickened by inflammation. The polypoid mucosal lesions were due to marked edema. An intramural abscess was anticipated to be the cause of the unusual mucosal mass but no such pathology was found.

Comment

While the differential diagnosis of sigmoid diverticulitis and carcinoma can be very difficult on the basis of clinical and radiological findings, if colonoscopy can negotiate the lesion, the diagnostic problem is usually resolved. The prominent polypoidal mass was an unusual manifestation of diverticulitis (the author has seen only one previous similar case). The smooth shiny surface of the lesion was the principal endoscopic finding that distinguished it from carcinoma. Schnyder et al report a similar but much larger polypoidal mass caused by mucosal edema associated with divcerticulitis.[1] The distal level of resection was extraperitoneal to obtain a healthy rectal wall for anastomosis. The proximal level of resection was determined by the extent of the diverticulosis in a relatively young patient.

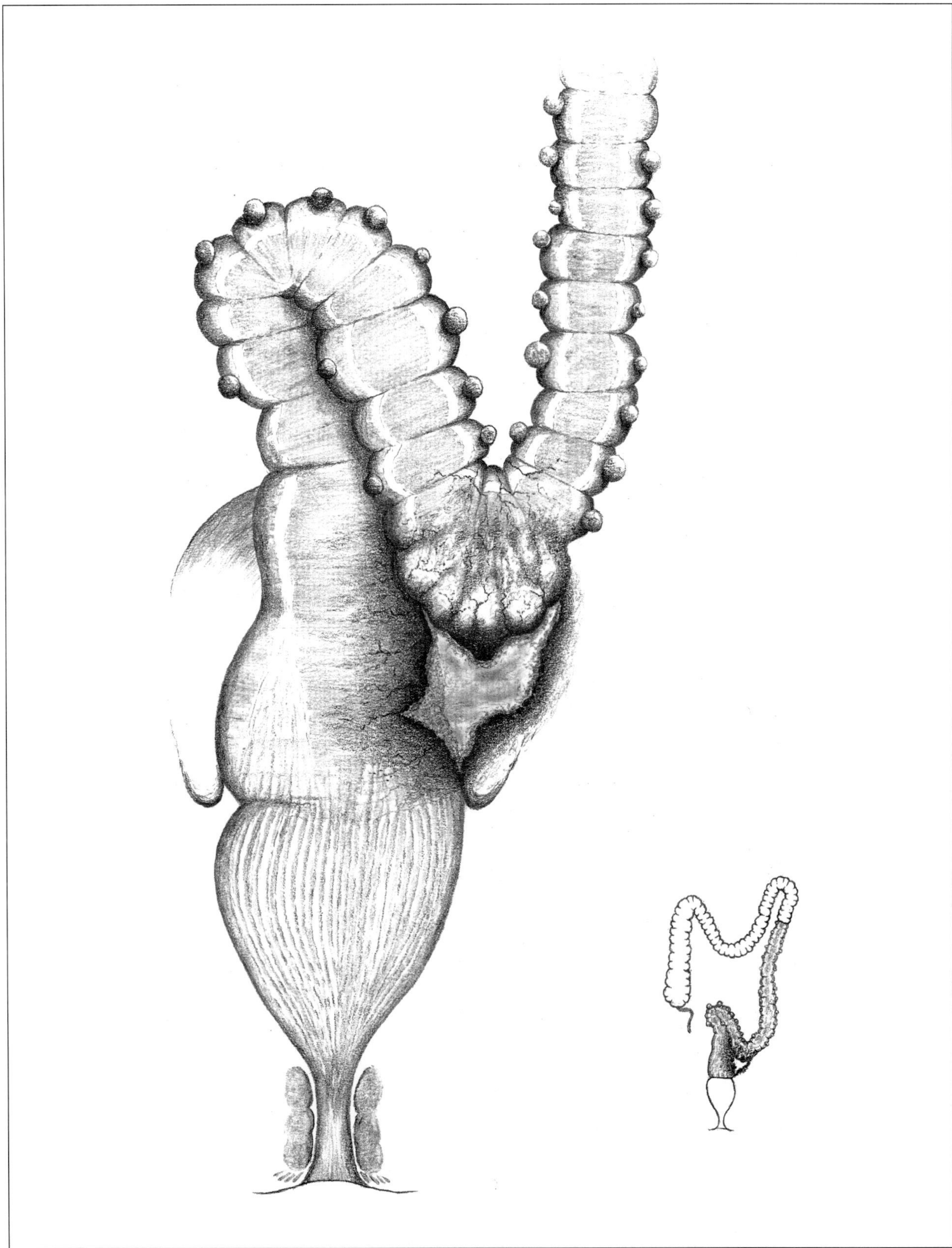

PART IV Cancer of the Colon and Rectum

CASE

23 Synchronous Colon Carcinoma and Malignant Carcinoid

Female, 80 Years

History

The patient was found to be anemic (hemoglobin 8.0 g/L) when investigated for an episode of syncope. Fecal occult blood test was positive. Colonoscopy identified an annular carcinoma in the ascending colon and a large pedunculated polyp at the 15 cm level in the rectum.

Operation (8.7.98)

The carcinoma in the mid ascending colon was confirmed with enlargement of adjacent lymph nodes. There was also a large hard lymph node related to the superior mesenteric vessels, which was thought to be related to the colon pathology although its anatomical position seemed unusual. There was no evidence of metastases beyond the suspicious lymph nodes in the mesentery. The right colon with 70 cm of terminal ileum was resected. An end-to-end anastomosis was performed with a circular stapler.

Pathology

The colon cancer was deeply ulcerating and involved the pericolic tissues. Histological examination revealed a poorly differentiated signet ring carcinoma (Figure 23.1). The largest adjacent "lymph node" was a metastatic nodule composed of signet ring carcinoma with no identifiable lymph node tissue (Dukes C, T_3 N_1 M_0). On the luminal aspect of the ileum, there were 3 yellow submucosal nodules. Histologically they were carcinoids. The largest of these measured 11 mm in diameter and extended through the muscularis propria. The large "ectopic" node and 2 smaller nodes related to the superior mesenteric vessels were yellow on the cut surface and contained metastatic carcinoid tumor.

Operation (10.8.98)

The snare removal of the rectal polyp (20 mm) and 2 smaller polyps nearby was performed subsequent to the resection to minimize the risk of implantation from the proximal carcinoma. Histological examination of the largest polyp showed severe dysplasia in a tubular adenoma.

Follow-Up (2004)

No adjuvant chemotherapy was administered in view of the patient's age. In 2003 a left hemicolectomy was performed for a metachronous colon carcinoma in the sigmoid colon (Dukes A, T_2 N_0 M_0). The patient has no evidence of recurrent malig-

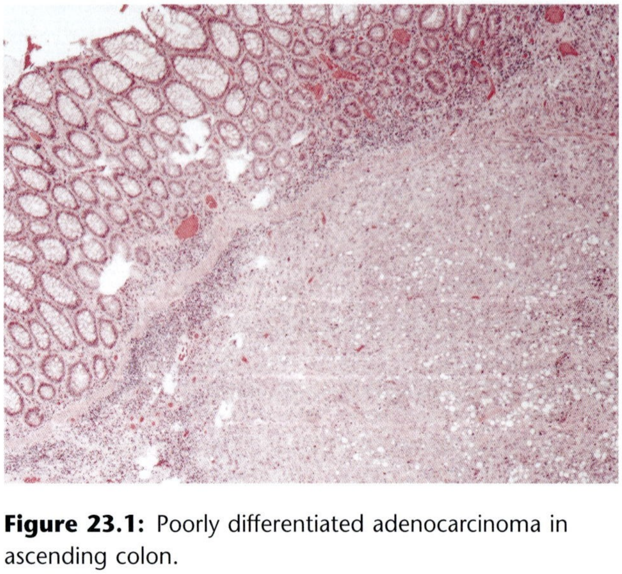

Figure 23.1: Poorly differentiated adenocarcinoma in ascending colon.

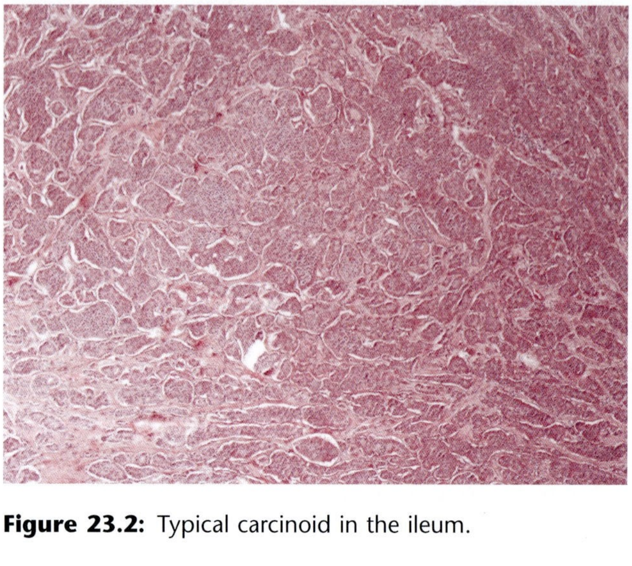

Figure 23.2: Typical carcinoid in the ileum.

nancy 5 years and 8 months since the first bowel resection.

Comment

It is not uncommon for carcinoids of the ileum to be multiple.[1] Carcinoid tumor may be associated with other malignancies of the gastrointestinal tract (29%–53%).[2] The combination of colorectal carcinoma and *multiple* carcinoids of the small bowel is rare.[3] The largest lymph node in the small bowel mesentery in this patient was misinterpreted as a colorectal cancer (CRC) metastasis and, to include it in the resection, 70 cm of ileum was removed. The carcinoid tumors were thus resected fortuitously. The small bowel was not assessed adequately at operation since the carcinoids should have been detected by palpation. Three mesenteric lymph nodes contained carcinoid metastases and are presumed to relate to the largest primary in the ileum, 11 mm in diameter. Thompson et al report an 18% incidence of lymph node metastasis in carcinoids of the ileum less than 10 mm in size.[1] This patient's long term survival from a poorly differentiated signet ring carcinoma was not expected. There was some reluctance to subject her to routine colonoscopic surveillance in view of her age. Nevertheless the patient's metachronous cancer was diagnosed at the Dukes A, T_2 N_0 M_0 stage.

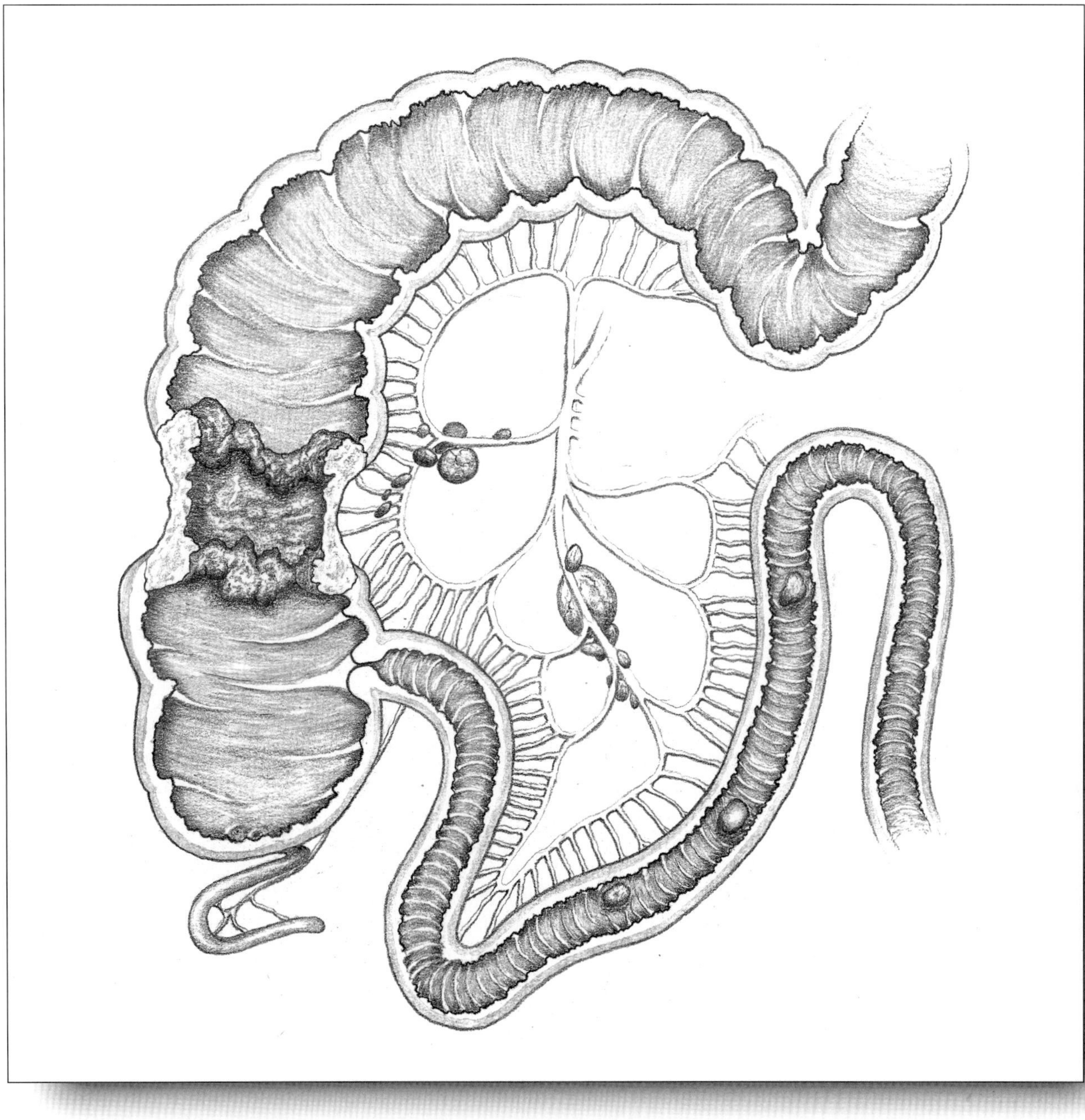

CASE 24 Coexistent Cancer and Diverticulitis

Female, 78 Years

History

The patient's complaint was an aggravation of prolapsed "hemorrhoids" for 2 months. She had noted occasional constipation but no other gastrointestinal symptoms. Physical examination revealed circumferential mucosal prolapse and a large mass, readily palpable in the pelvis. Sigmoidoscopy identified the proliferative edge of a rectal carcinoma at 16 cm, confirmed by biopsy. Further examination of the bowel proximal to the tumor was not possible. Computerized tomography (CT) examination identified an abnormality at the rectosigmoid area with extensive thickening of the bowel wall and diverticular disease. There was dilatation of the right ureter. The liver showed no evidence of metastases.

Operation (10.22.93)

At laparotomy there was a large fixed mass in the pelvis formed by the upper third of the rectum and distal sigmoid colon, the latter showing evidence of chronic inflammation. The mass was hard, appeared to infiltrate the posterior surface of the uterus, and involve the right ureter which was dilated. There was no evidence of extra pelvic metastases. Proximal to the mass, there was obvious diverticulosis that reached the lower descending colon. It was thought the cancer was solely responsible for the pelvic mass, and therefore the resection included a radical hysterectomy en bloc. It was thought prudent not to resect the ureter in this 78-year-old frail patient, and the ureter was "peeled" away from the mass. A low anterior resection was performed with a proximal loop ileostomy.

Pathology

The annular carcinoma was ulcerating with a proliferative edge, causing significant constriction of the lumen and invasion of the perirectal tissues. The uterus was adherent to the mid sigmoid colon by benign adhesions that were related to a diverticular abscess confined to the pericolic fat. There were other foci of inflammation in diverticula in this part of the sigmoid colon. There was narrowing of the lumen with redundant mucosa typical of chronic diverticular disease. The excision margin of the resected cancer was negative for malignancy and examined lymph nodes did not contain any metastases (Dukes B, T_3 N_0 M_0).

Postoperative Course

Initially the patient's recovery was satisfactory until the second week, when an unexplained episode of tachycardia and peripheral cyanosis occurred. Contrast radiological assessment of the anastomosis showed no evidence of impaired healing. CT examination of the abdomen demonstrated thrombosis of the splenic vein and a major infarct of the spleen, which was managed conservatively. Routine prophylactic heparin therapy had been administered during the postoperative period. A follow up CT examination 1 week later revealed infarcts of the liver and kidney, and within a few days the patient suffered a stroke with a right hemiparesis. CT of the brain confirmed an infarct in the postero-inferior part of the left occipital lobe. Despite increasing return of motor function, the patient remained aphasic, depressed, and refused all attempts at oral feeding. At the request of the family, total parentral nutrition (TPN) was eventually discontinued. The patient died 11 weeks after operation.

Comment

The patient suffered from synchronous major pathologies of the large bowel and yet was virtually without related symptoms. "Silent cancer" is well recognized as a clinical entity, but not so with diverticulitis of this severity. The diverticulitis was not diagnosed until the resected specimen was examined. At operation, difficult decisions were required in relation to the attachment of the pelvic mass to the right ureter and uterus. If the benign nature of the attachment to the uterus had been appreciated, then hysterectomy would have been avoided. This is the only case of postoperative multiple visceral infarcts encountered by the author. Its etiology remained obscure. In a series of 208 elective resections for diverticular disease, the incidence of coexistent carcinoma of the sigmoid colon or upper rectum was 2 (1.0%).[1]

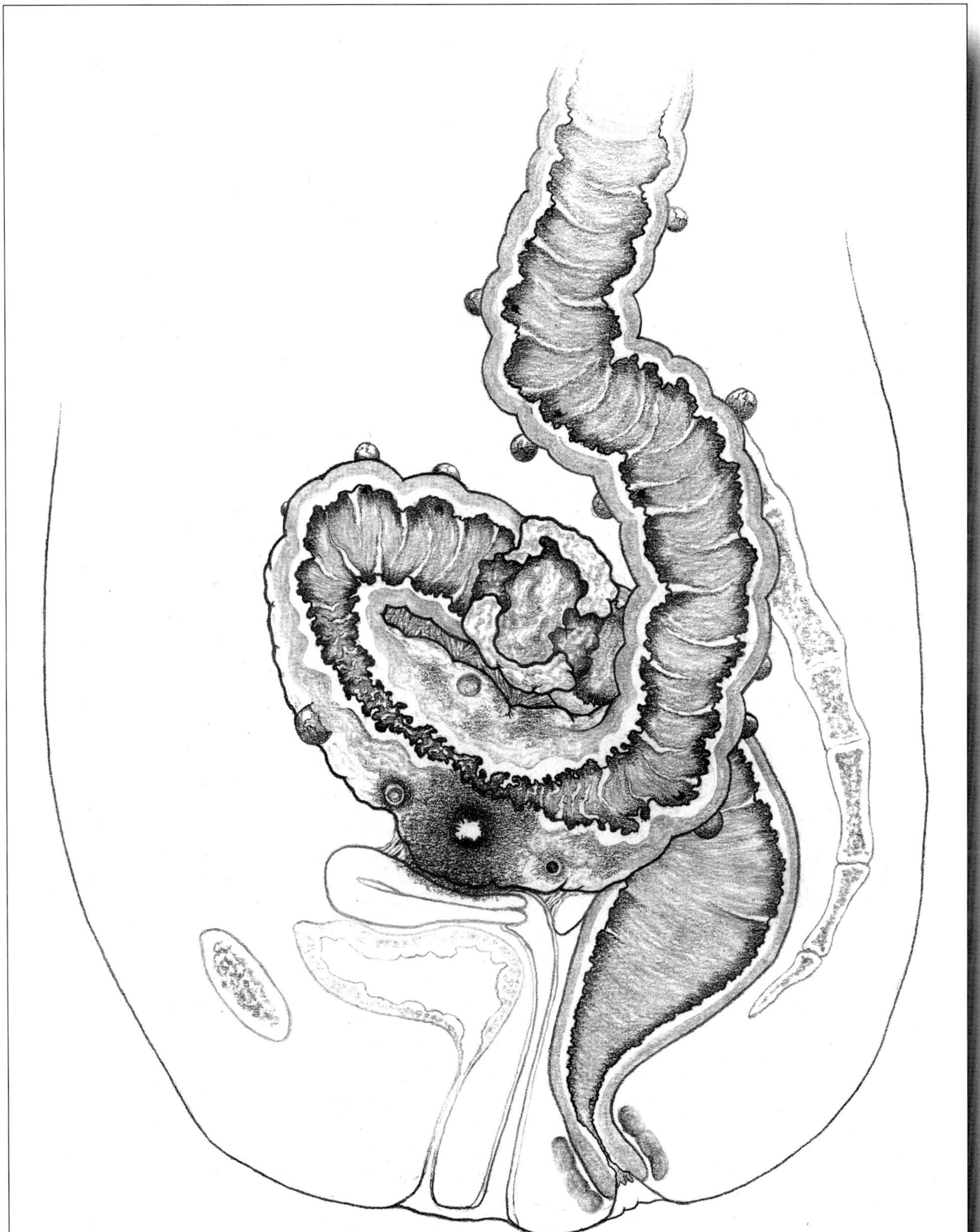

CASE

25 Sigmoid Carcinoma and Serosal Cysts

Female, 54 Years

History

During a 2-month period, the patient had noticed a loss of weight, abdominal "wind" pain, and diarrhea. Rectal examination revealed a mobile mass in the pelvis, and sigmoidoscopy was normal to 19 cm. A barium enema showed complete retrograde obstruction in the lower sigmoid colon consistent with a neoplasm. Flexible endoscopy was not performed.

Operation (5.30.79)

A large sigmoid carcinoma, 6 cm in diameter was resected, with an anastomosis in the intraperitoneal rectum. There were no obvious metastases.

Pathology

Over the peritoneal surface of the bulky tumor, there were 3 thin-walled sacs, 2–3 cm in size, containing a clear straw colored fluid. They were related to pale areas overlying transmural infiltration by the cancer. The tumor was a fungating ulcer 6.5 cm in length. The depth of invasion was limited to the muscle layer. Twenty-six lymph nodes were examined and no metastases were found (Dukes A, T_2 N_0 M_0). There was an inflammatory reaction in the muscle of the bowel wall, which was more acute in the outer layers with small abscesses. There were no histological features to suggest the tumor was anaplastic. The 3 cystic structures appeared to arise from the serosal tissue and were lined by squamous epithelium.

Follow-Up

The patient remained well for a year. The onset of dysphagia was investigated with a barium swallow that showed a mediastinal mass deforming the middle third of the esophagus. Esophagoscopy revealed an area of inflammation but no ulceration. Thoracotomy revealed a large tumor mass arising in the muscle layer of the esophagus. It was not resectable. A biopsy confirmed the diagnosis of metastatic undifferentiated carcinoma consistent with a primary colon tumor. The patient did not return for further visits and subsequently succumbed to metastatic disease.

Comment

The serous cysts attached to the tumor were most unusual. No reference to such lesions has been found in the literature. The intramural metastasis of the esophagus is also a very uncommon hematogenous spread from an extrathoracic site. Primary malignancies that have metastasized to the esophagus in this way are breast, stomach, pancreas, kidney, testes, prostate, and uterus.[1,2]

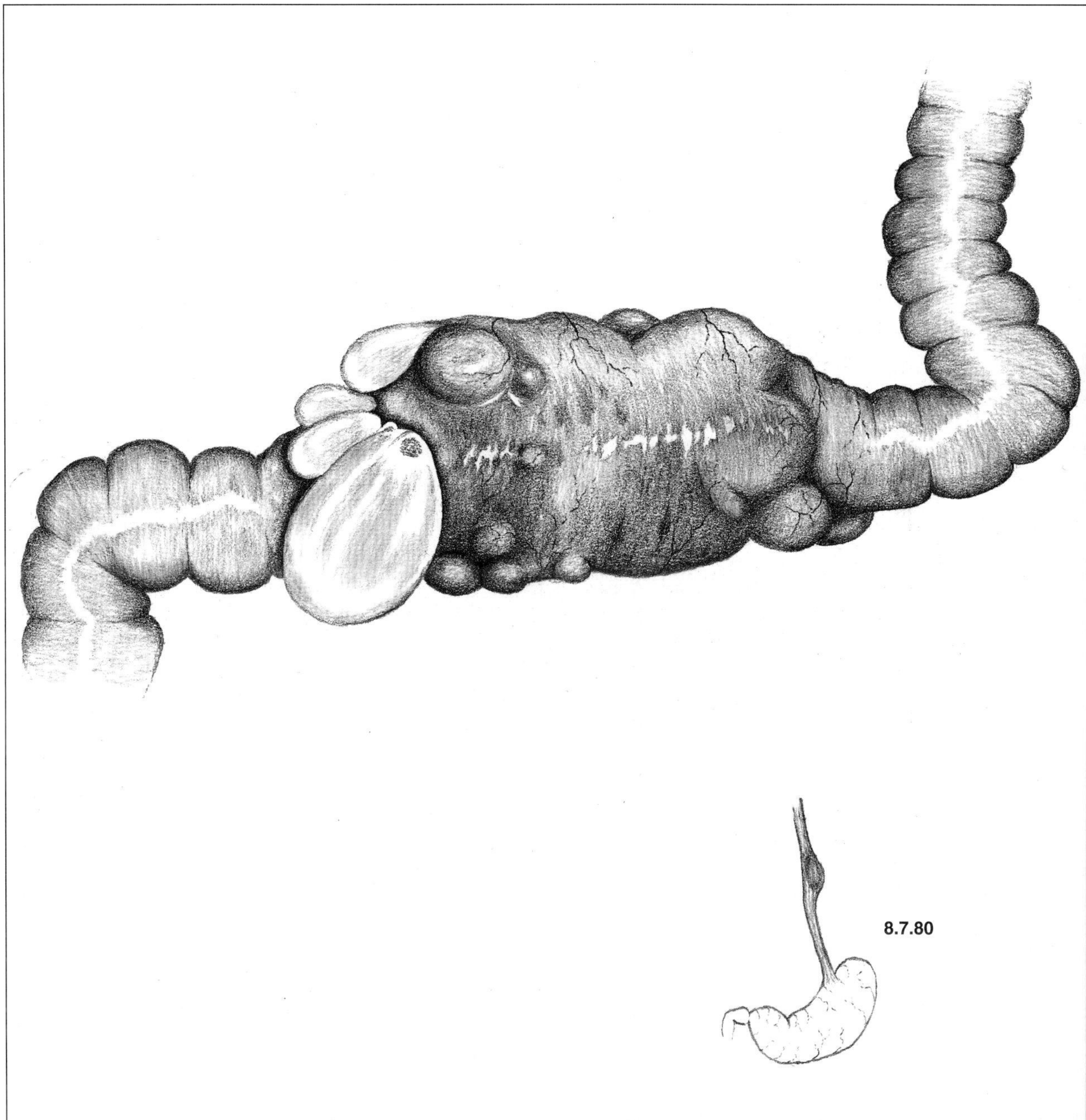
8.7.80

CASE

26 Cavitating Cancer of the Transverse Colon

Male, 67 Years

History

This patient presented with symptoms due to iron deficiency anemia (Hb: 59g/L) made worse by his chronic bronchitis and emphysema, which required oxygen administration at home. A barium enema showed a large carcinoma of the transverse colon. Short colonoscopy to the distal extent of the tumor revealed 3 small polyps in the left colon and sigmoid colon diverticulosis.

Operation (5.18.95)

At laparotomy there was a large spherical mass (13 × 13 cm) involving the mid transverse colon. The serosal surface was lobulated and gray in color. Enlarged lymph nodes were apparent along the course of the middle colic vessels. There was no evidence of metastatic disease beyond the intended perimeter of surgical excision. An extended right hemicolectomy was performed. An end-to-end anastomosis was made with a circular stapler via a colotomy.

Pathology

On sectioning the specimen, the tumor was seen to occupy the entire circumference of the lumen with malignant stenosis at its proximal and distal limits. The tumor had formed a huge malignant cavity contained within a "shell" of tumor. Several polypoid elevations projected from the surface. Histological examination revealed a moderately to poorly differentiated mucinous adenocarcinoma, which extended beyond the muscularis propria to involve the serosa. There were no metastases identified in the lymph nodes (Dukes B, T_3 N_0 M_0). Seven small polyps in the resected colon (3–10 mm) were benign tubular adenomata.

Postoperative Follow-Up

With intensive care support of the patient's respiratory problems, his postoperative course was uncomplicated. The patient survived the malignancy beyond 5 years and died of respiratory failure.

Comment

The morphology of this type of tumor, which forms a large cavity within an outer "shell" of neoplasm, is a definite entity, although not often encountered by the surgeon. It is possible that these are rapidly growing neoplasms which are accompanied by significant tumor necrosis, thus producing a large hollow mass. No description of this morphological variety of colorectal cancer (CRC) has been found in the literature. While the morphology appeared ominous in this patient, the cancer survival was better than expected.

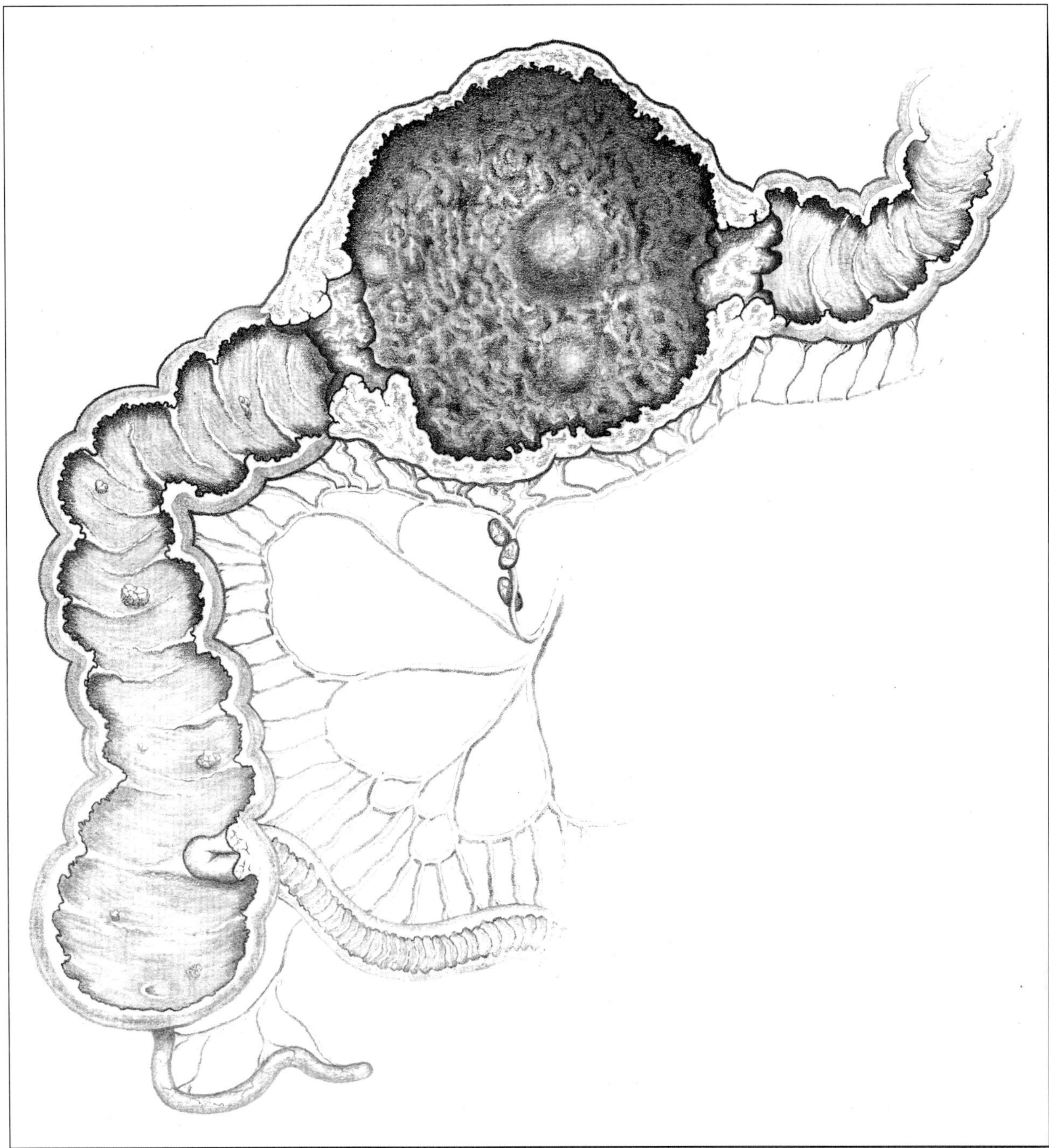

CASE 27 The Wagging Tongue of a Sigmoid Cancer

Female, 56 Years

History

The patient's prior medical history included hypertension, a myocardial infarct, and diabetes. For 1 year, frequent episodes of diarrhea had been present. For 3 months, she complained of lower abdominal pain, worse after meals, abdominal distention, audible bowel sounds, anorexia, and loss of weight. A barium enema examination demonstrated a large lesion of the distal sigmoid colon. On examination, there was abdominal distention and an irregular, immobile pelvic mass. Sigmoidoscopy revealed a polypoid tumor of the rectum at 10 cm. Biopsy confirmed the lesion to be a moderately well differentiated adenocarcinoma.

Operation (4.13.89)

There was a large mass involving the distal sigmoid colon and mesentery. A loop of terminal ileum was adherent to the mass. The liver appeared normal. No intraabdominal metastases beyond surgical excision were identified. A low anterior resection was performed including 30 cm of ileum in continuity. The wide excision compromised the blood supply of the ovaries, which were therefore removed.

Pathology

The primary lesion was an ulcer measuring 6 cm in length. There was extensive spread locally to form a large mass in the mesentery that had also spread distally to then breach the wall of the upper third of the rectum and "re-enter" the lumen. This mass of neoplasm measured 11 cm in length, its distal part protruding like a "tongue," freely movable within the lumen of the rectum. The mesentery of the resected ileum was invaded by carcinoma. None of the 12 lymph nodes showed metastases. The tumor was moderately well differentiated adenocarcinoma (Dukes B, T_3 M_0 N_0).

Follow-Up

The patient lived for 7 years, 5 months without evidence of recurrent disease. Death was the result of cardiac disease.

Comment

It is of interest that adenocarcinoma of the large bowel can develop locally to form an extensive primary mass without metastasizing to lymph nodes. It is unusual to find extraluminal spread "bursting" back into the bowel. This may have been related to the large extra rectal component being impacted in the pelvis. The "eruption" of the lesion to reenter the rectum suggested incorrectly that two primary cancers were present.

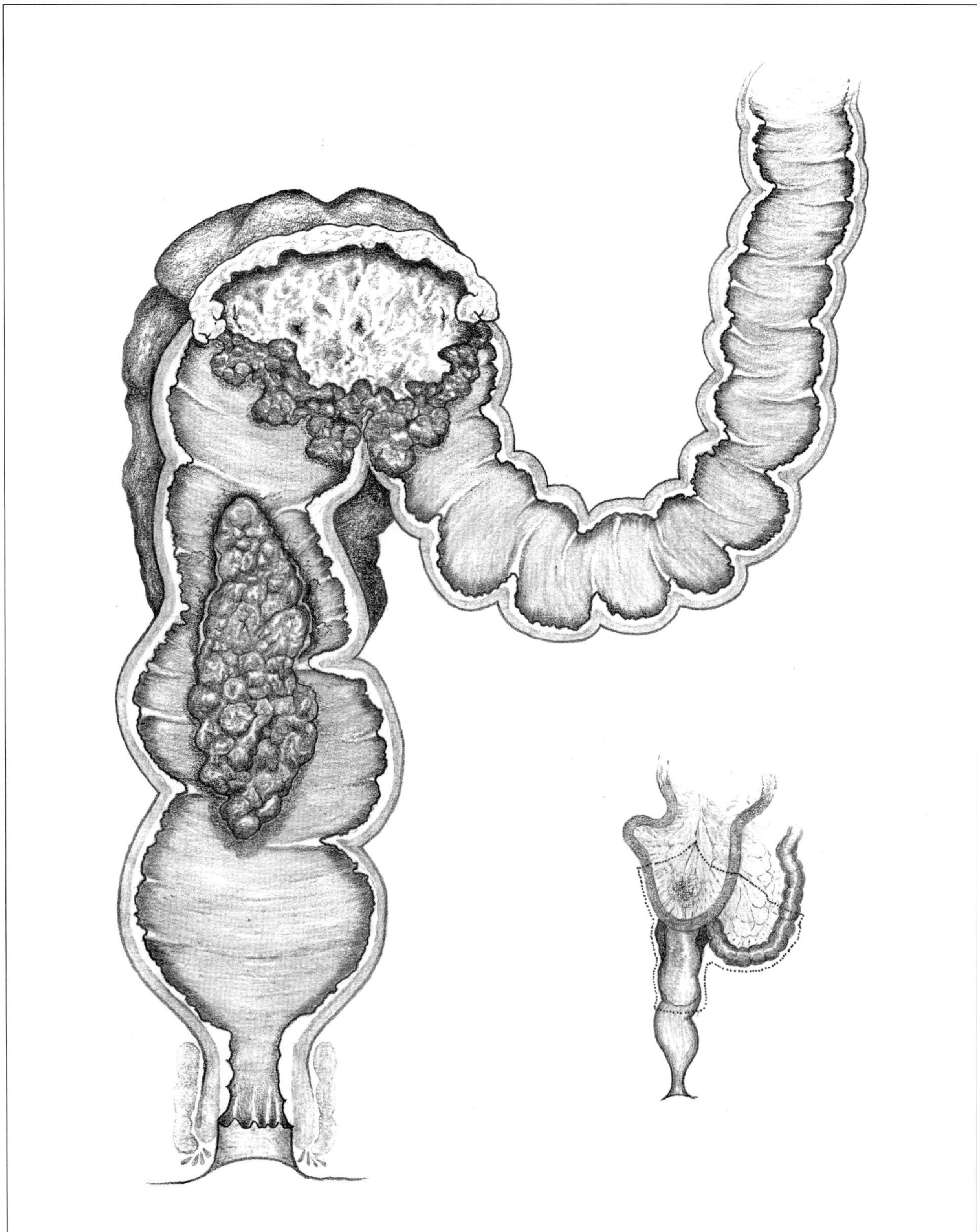

CASE

28 Protracted Recurrence of Mucoid Cancer

Male, 51 Years

History

In 1981 the patient (aged 37 years) underwent colectomy and ileorectal anastomosis for chronic ulcerative colitis complicated by mucoid carcinomas (2) of the ascending colon that had penetrated beyond the muscularis propria (Dukes B, T_3 N_0 M_0). He remained well until 1995, when he presented with a 3-month history of abdominal pain and localized distention on the left side of the abdomen. Examination revealed a firm mass in the left iliac fossa accompanied by distended loops of small bowel. The findings were confirmed by computerized tomography (CT) examination.

Operation (7.17.95)

Laparotomy revealed a mass in the posterior aspect of the left abdomen that was intimately involved with the mesentery of the small bowel. Mucoid material was erupting from the surface of the mass, and similar deposits were in the left "paracolic" gutter and pelvis. The liver appeared normal. Extensive adhesions to the small bowel were not completely dissected. The mass was dissected free of the left ureter and removed in continuity with 20 cm of the small bowel. All visible mucoid deposits were removed.

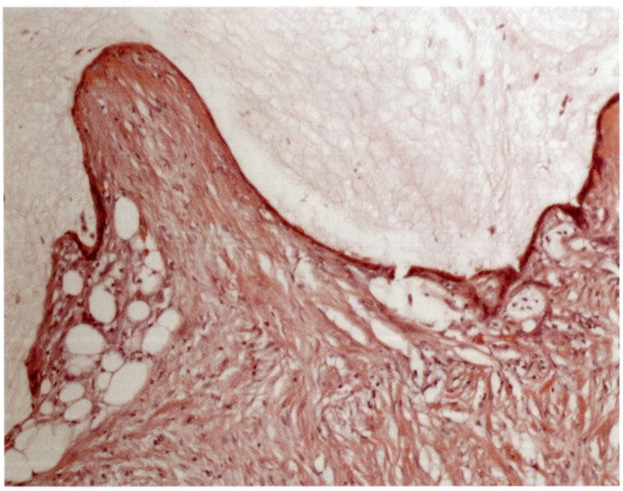

Figure 28.1: Histological features of recurrent tumor removed 7.17.95. Pools of mucus adjacent to flattened low-grade adenocarcinoma.

Pathology

The mass (7 cm in diameter) contained numerous cysts filled with "semisolid mucinous material." Histologically the wall of the cysts was lined with columnar epithelium with loss of polarity and hyperchromatic nuclei (Figure 28.1). The low-grade dysplasia and mucus formation suggested mucinous carcinoma and pseudomyxoma peritonei. Some of the isolated deposits showed mucin devoid of epithelial cells.

Operation (4.12.97)

Obstructive symptoms occurred 16 months after the operation, requiring further surgery. A metastatic mass of mucinous carcinoma, densely adherent to the left ureter, was removed. The liver was normal. No other deposits were present. Histologically, signet ring cells were identified within the tumor.

Operation (7.3.99)

A further recurrence in the left lower abdomen, 12 cm in size, was resected in continuity with 20 cm of ileum, the left ureter, and left kidney.

Operation (8.25.01)

Laparotomy was performed for a symptomatic recurrence, most of which was excised in a "debulking" procedure. This required excision of psoas muscle, a loop of ileum, and the ileorectal anastomosis. A new ileorectal anastomosis (IRA) was constructed.

Follow-Up

In March 2004, the patient was admitted to the hospital, suffering a massive rectal hemorrhage due to a vascular fistula between the external iliac artery and the small bowel. This was successfully controlled by the insertion of a vascular stent by interventional radiology. The patient succumbed to metastatic disease some months after this complication.

Comment

Okuno et al report that the incidence of mucoid colorectal cancer was 6.4% in a series of 540 patients.[1] The incidence of mucoid cancers arising in association with ulcerative colitis is higher: Mayer et al report an incidence of 37% (mucinous 25%, signet ring cancer 12%).[2] Umpleby et al[3] found such tumors were more common in the proximal colon. Compared to nonmucinous colorectal cancer, the mucinous type exhibit an increased risk of local spread, lymph node metastasis, and peritoneal dissemination.[1,3,4] The mucinous tumor may cause a widespread malignant mucinous ascites, which has been included in the classification of pseudomyxoma peritonei. Ronnett et al prefer the term peritoneal mucinous carcinomatosis (PMCA).[5] In the case described here, the recurrent mucoid tumors were less generalized. Debulking surgery, as advocated by Sugarbaker, et al[4] did achieve palliation. It is of interest that the first noted recurrence of the colitis cancer was 14 years after the colectomy. Over the ensuing 9 years, abdominal surgery was performed on 4 occasions, usually followed by relief of symptoms for approximately 2 years.

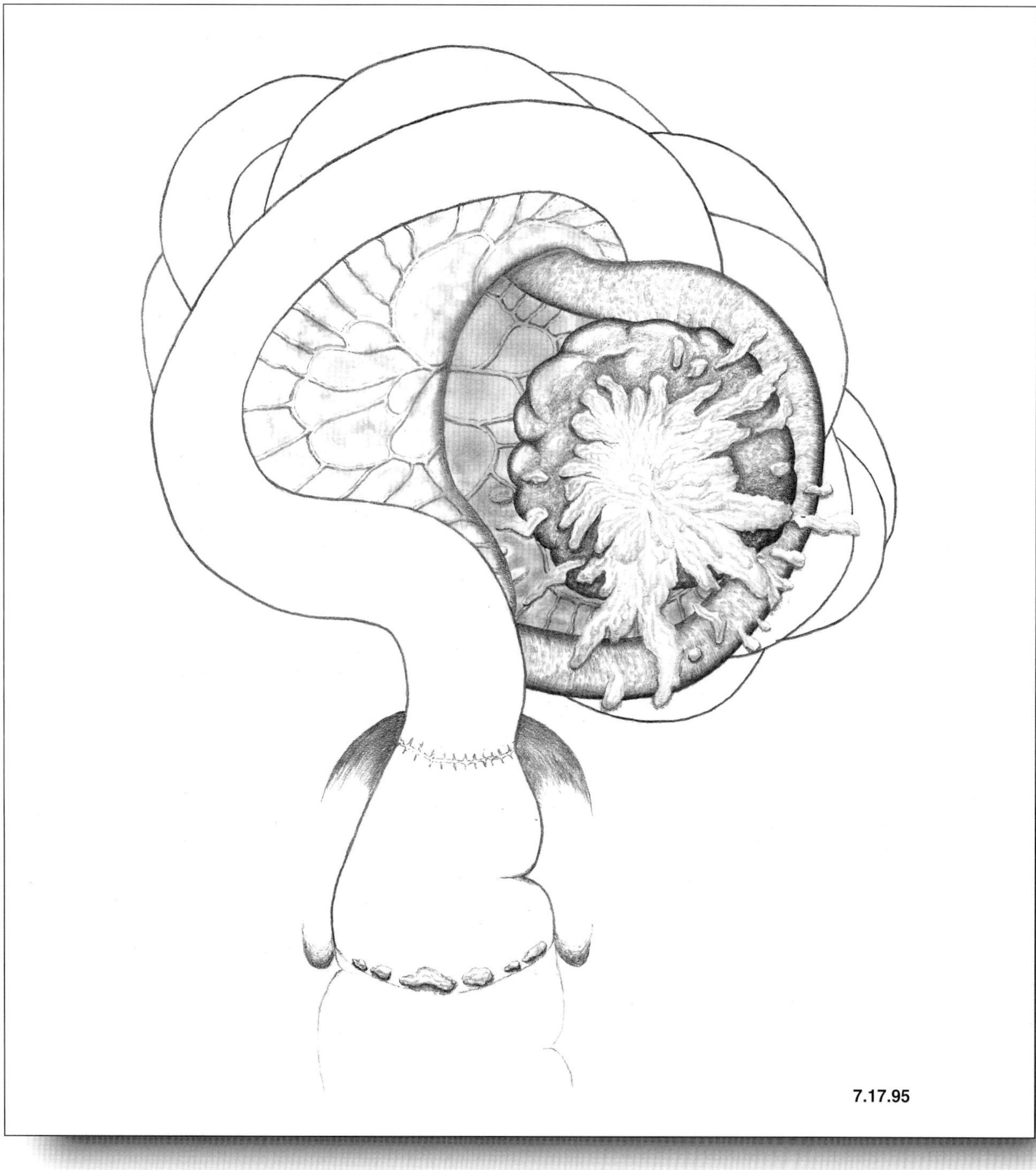

CASE

29 Anaplastic Colon Cancer

Male, 36 Years

History

The patient presented with a 2-year history of diarrhea and intermittent rectal bleeding. Colonoscopy was limited to 30 cm by a large polypoid mass thought to be carcinoma. Biopsies were inconclusive. There were 6 polyps in the rectum 10 mm–20 mm size. A barium enema confirmed these findings, suggesting there was infiltration by the large sigmoid lesion as well as additional small polyps in the descending colon (10) splenic flexure (1) and hepatic flexure (1).

Operation (8.22.85)

A large carcinoma of the mid distal sigmoid colon was present. It was 11 cm in length, with multiple nodules over its serosal aspect, and palpable mesenteric lymph nodes. There were no other metastases. The bowel was resected from proximal sigmoid to mid rectum.

Pathology

There was a malignant ulcer present, measuring 6 cm × 4 cm, associated with submucosal permeation of carcinoma producing thickened "folds" on the mucosal surface and extending over a distance of 11 cm. Small polyps (6) were also included in the resected specimen. Histological examination revealed undifferentiated carcinoma extending widely by permeation of submucosal lymphatics as well as deep penetration of the bowel wall, extending into the pericolic fat. Vascular invasion by carcinoma was a prominent feature histologically. There was heavy infiltration of the tumor by neutrophils. The serosal nodules were confirmed as carcinoma as well as metastases in a large mass of lymph nodes within the mesentery. (Dukes C:T_3 N_3 M_0). The presence of significant numbers of malignant serosal nodules made the staging of the pathology more difficult.

Follow-Up (2003)

Further polyps (60–70) were removed by colonoscopy over the subsequent 12 years. A large polyp (benign) in the ascending colon was removed by right hemicolectomy (9.10.97). At the last follow-up visit there was no evidence of metastatic disease.

Comment

The tumor exhibited features of both the scirrhous and lymphangiosis forms of linitis plastica, a classification proposed by Shirouzu et al.[1] The lymphatic permeations of the cancer in the submucosal layer of the colon produced remodelling of the mucosa around the malignant ulcer to form prominent mucosal folds characteristic of one of the morphological types of linitis plastica. The histological appearance can be anticipated by the naked eye findings. The resection in this patient was regarded as probably noncurative, in the presence of serosal nodules of carcinoma, and yet the patient remained free of recurrence for more than 18 years after operation.

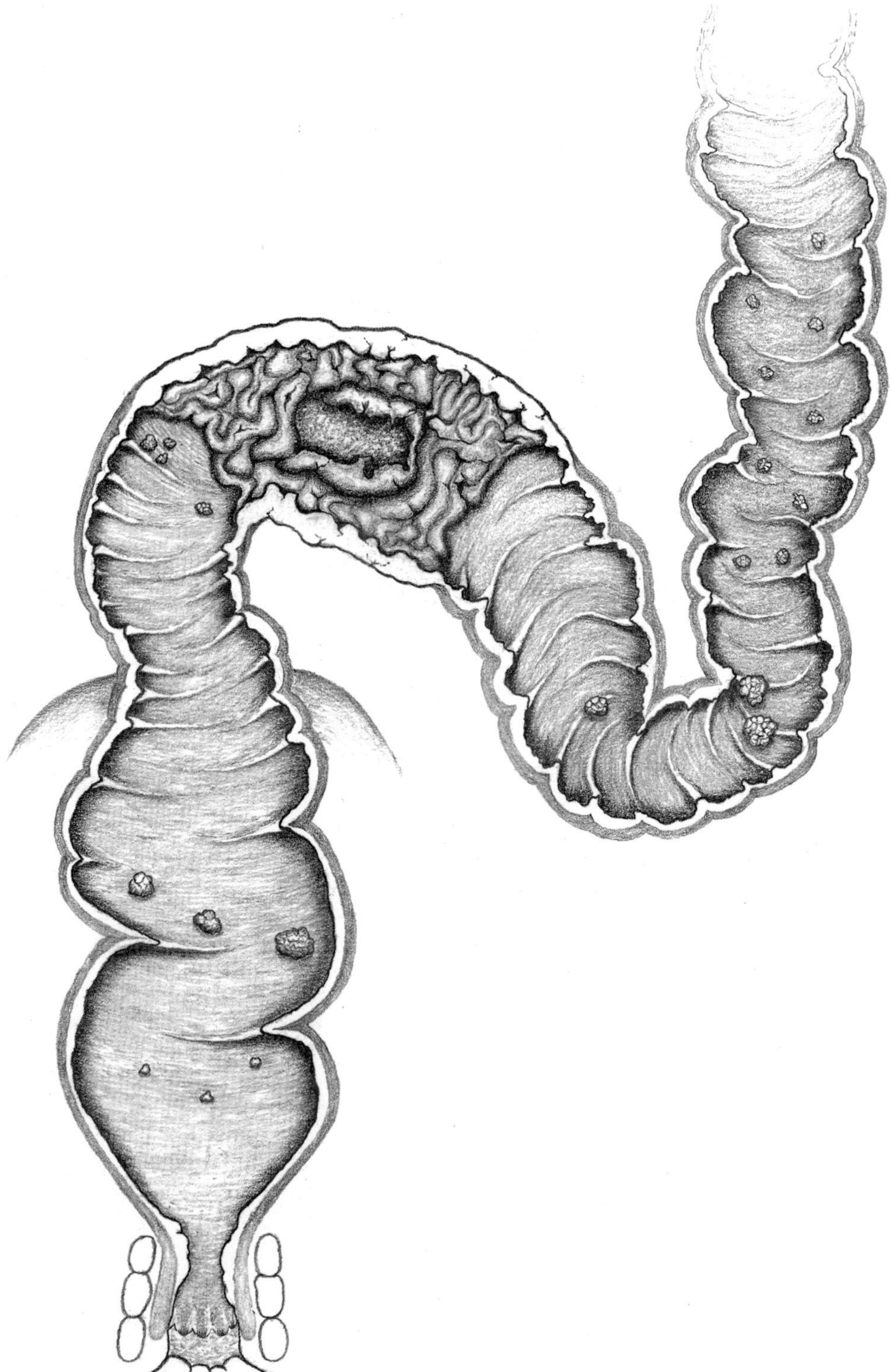

CASE

30 Linitis Plastica of the Colon and Rectum

Male, 32 Years

History

The patient complained of rectal bleeding, diarrhea, and lower abdominal discomfort for 2 months. There had been a weight loss of 35 lbs in 12 months. A nonmobile mass was present in the left lower abdomen. On rectal examination and sigmoidoscopy, abnormal mucosa was present that was not typical of adenocarcinoma. Crohn's Disease was considered prior to referral. A barium enema demonstrated a long stricture with "scalloped" margins involving rectum and sigmoid. Biopsy of "inflamed and edematous mucosa" at 10 cm revealed anaplastic carcinoma. Biopsy of an enlarged lymph node in the neck (Figure 30.1) showed anaplastic carcinoma with signet ring cells present. Other investigations revealed the patient was suffering from thyrotoxicosis, and therapy with carbimazole was commenced. Despite the ominous prognosis, operation was performed since the patient had constant rectal symptoms and requested that at least an exploratory laparotomy be undertaken.

Operation (12.23.69)

At operation, the rectum and distal sigmoid were converted into a firm "hosepipe-like" structure by diffuse spread of the tumor. There was extensive lymph node involvement that extended into the mesentery of the left colon. The distal limit of the submucosal spread appeared to be 5 cm from the anal verge. There was a 1.5 cm metastasis in the left lobe of the liver. Resection with a straight coloanal anastomosis and proximal colostomy was performed.

Pathology

Examination of the resected specimen indicated that the poorly differentiated tumor (Figure 30.2) arose in the rectum with diffuse submucosal, intramural, and extramural spread to produce the "tubular" morphology. Signet ring cells were prominent. The distal margin of the specimen was positive for carcinoma. Extensive lymph node metastases were confirmed.

Postoperative Course

Postoperative recovery was slow. Digital examination revealed a small subclinical defect in the anastomosis. The patient continued to lose weight and steadily deteriorated until he died 7 weeks after operation.

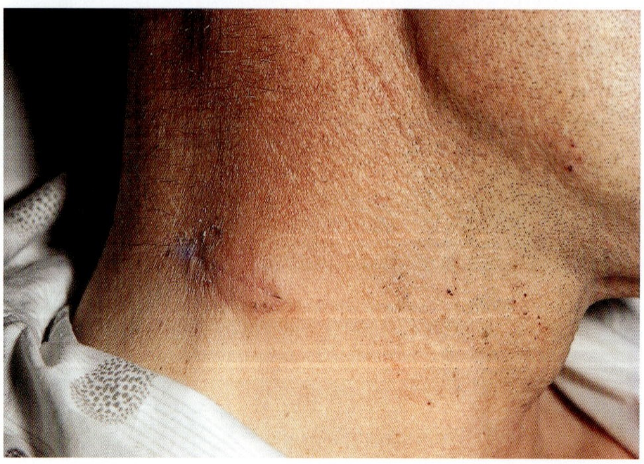

Figure 30.1: Cervical lymph node metastasis.

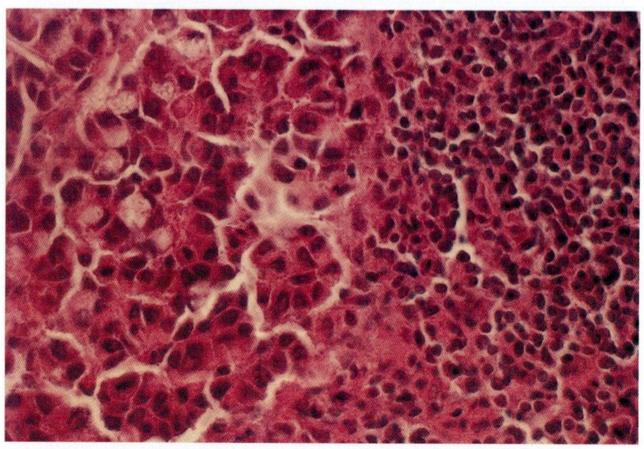

Figure 30.2: Colon: Anaplastic adenocarcinoma, including signet ring cells.

Comment

Signet ring colorectal cancer is rare and accounted for 0.7% of colorectal cancer reported by Nissan et al.[1] Linitis plastica is a morphological classification, and in these colorectal cancers, the incidence of signet ring histology is 16.6%.[2] The poor survival of patients with colorectal linitis plastica is well known.[1,3,4] This case was the most aggressive example encountered by the author. The operation did achieve relief from the distressing rectal symptoms, but resection with and end stoma or a palliative stoma alone would have been a more appropriate procedure. The patient's limited survival was never going to facilitate satisfactory function of a straight coloanal anastomosis after closure of the proximal colostomy.

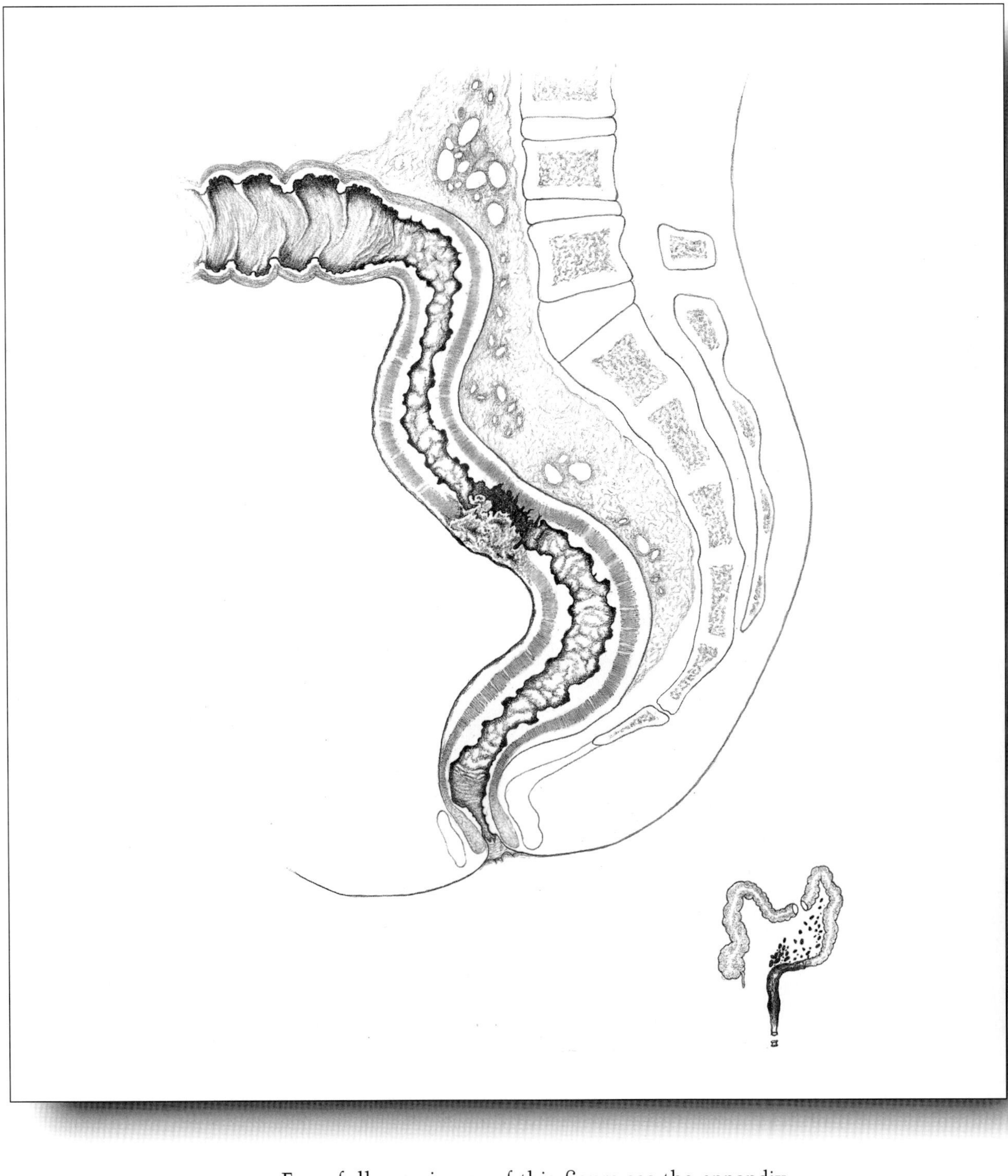

For a full-page image of this figure see the appendix.

CASE

31 Curative Resection of Rectal Cancer Despite Liver Metastases

Female, 55 Years

History

In January 1989 the patient was investigated for heavy rectal bleeding. A fungating carcinoma of the rectum was diagnosed 10 cm from the anal verge. The lumen at this level only just permitted examination by the colonoscope. Computerized tomography (CT) examination showed no evidence of perirectal spread, but both lobes of the liver appeared to contain numerous small metastases. The patient was informed that her life expectancy was approximately 12 months. A course of "palliative" radiotherapy (45Gy) was administered to the rectal tumour followed by a further treatment (6 Gy) 1 month later. Sigmoidoscopy 3 months after treatment revealed no visible tumor, but subsequently recurrence occurred. Further radiotherapy (8 Gy) and local excision with a urological resectoscope failed to control the lesion, and the patient was referred in July 1990.

Sigmoidoscopy revealed a stricture of the rectum at 10 cm, which would not permit the passage of the sigmoidoscope (17 mm). The tumor edge was visible. A further CT examination of the liver was associated with ultrasound (US) examination and fine needle aspiration. The liver lesions were now regarded as cysts (Figure 31.1). This diagnosis was supported by the lack of any increase in size since the initial CT (18 months previously).

Operation (8.13.90)

No metastatic disease was identified in the abdomen. The liver contained multiple benign cysts. The carcinoma was located in the intraperitoneal rectum, and there was no evidence of perirectal spread. An extended low anterior resection with a proximal loop ileostomy was performed. The anastomosis was subsequently measured at 7 cm. Recovery was uneventful.

Pathology

The tumor showed macroscopic evidence of tumor attenuation by radiotherapy. It was 30 mm in diameter with a thin, rolled margin and a flat contour.

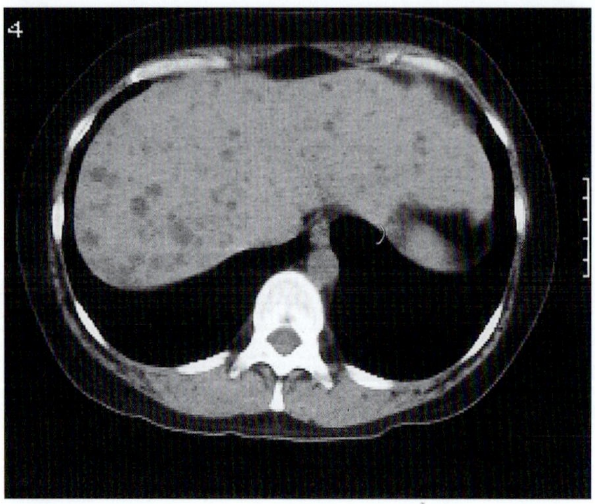

Figure 31.1: The review CT scan (7.30.90) shows the low density foci in the liver that were diagnosed as liver cysts at this examination.

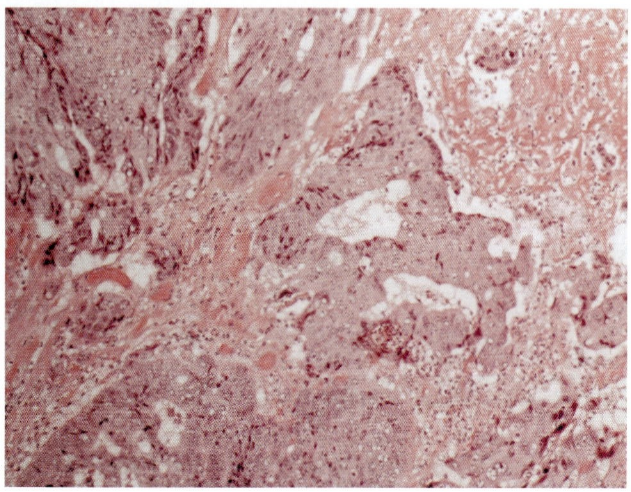

Figure 31.2: In this section, there are no obvious microscopic features of a radiotherapy effect on the carcinoma. Vessels elsewhere displayed endarteritis obliterans.

The base was covered by a yellow slough. There was thickening and edema around the lesion but no excessive fibrosis. There was narrowing of the lumen at the level of the tumor. Histologically the lesion was well differentiated and did not penetrate beyond the muscle layer of the rectum (Dukes A, T_2 N_0 M_0). There was minimal evidence of previous radiotherapy (Figure 31.2).

Operation (10.15.90)
Closure of loop ileostomy.

Follow-Up (2004)
The patient has remained free of recurrence or metachronous colorectal tumors for 13 years, 7 months.

Comment
The error in diagnosis was devastating for the patient, who already had a history of endogenous depression and lived with "palliative" care for 18 months. At the present time, by virtue of improved techniques, this radiological misdiagnosis is less likely. At operation, a generous distal margin (6 cm) for resection was selected to enable the anastomosis to be made in the lower third of the rectum, beyond the area of maximum radiation effect. The indication for the proximal loop ileostomy was the treatment with 59 Gy prior to operation. The high dose of radiotherapy, which became preoperative rather than palliative, may have significantly contributed to the local and systemic control of the malignancy.

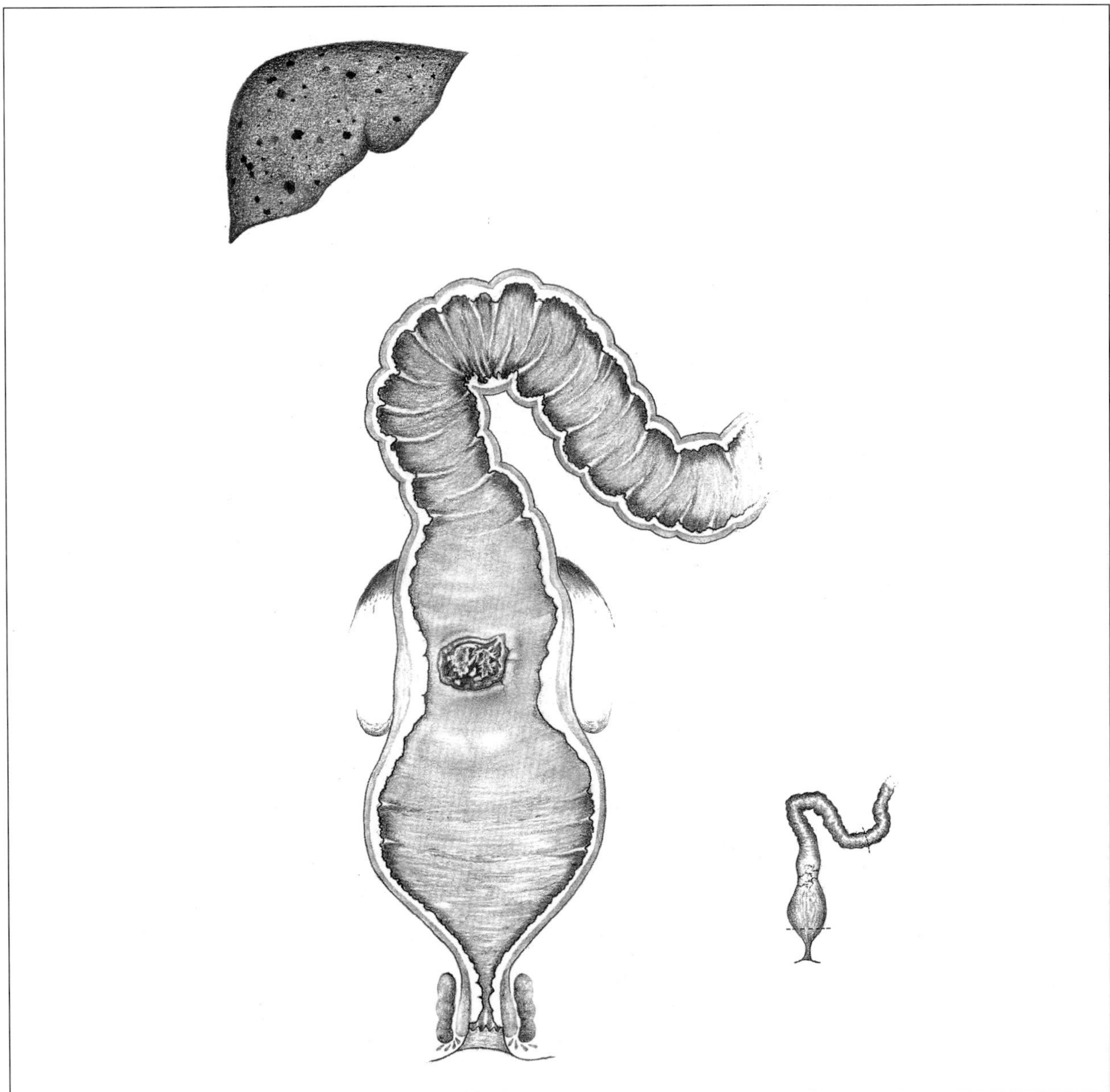

CASE

32 Small Sigmoid Cancer: "Mega" Lymph Nodc Metastasis

Male, 69 Years

History

The patient presented with a 4-month history of urinary symptoms (frequency and dysuria) associated with noncolicky abdominal pain. There were no bowel symptoms. On abdominal examination, there was a large, smooth suprapubic mass that reached the level of the umbilicus. A urologist made a diagnosis of urinary retention, but investigations were normal. A barium enema showed a distorted sigmoid colon "stretched" over the abdominal mass. Rigid sigmoidoscopy revealed 2 small polyps in the rectum.

Operation (11.29.66)

The mass was found to be a large spherical cystic mass within the sigmoid mesocolon, approximately 12 cm in diameter. It was intimately associated with the sigmoid colon and a loop of terminal ileum. Two lesions (1 soft, 1 firm) were palpable in the mid sigmoid colon. There was no evidence of other intraabdominal pathology. Resection of the sigmoid colon, mass, and 30 cm of terminal ileum was performed with 2 anastomoses.

Pathology

The lesions in the sigmoid colon were a pedunculated benign polyp and a small plaque-shaped adenocarcinoma 15 mm × 15 mm. The latter was not in continuity with the intramesenteric mass. The mass contained obvious tumor tissue which was friable and soft in consistency. There were areas of necrosis and liquefaction within the mass. Adenocarcinoma was confirmed histologically in the colon and mesenteric mass. (The extent of any infiltration of the resected ileum is not known).

Follow-Up

One year after the operation (11.14.67), the patient underwent laparotomy to investigate abdominal pain and anemia. Laparotomy revealed a large preaortic mass of metastatic nodes and a further large mass in the mesocolon. No resection was undertaken. The patient died of metastatic disease during the following year.

Comment

The pathology in this patient was of interest because the primary tumor was small, whereas the lymph node involvement was huge and associated with necrosis. The author has seen this type of "mega" lymph node pathology only twice in treating more than 2000 patients with colorectal cancer. Currently, the patient would be treated with postoperative adjuvant chemotherapy. The prognosis of a patient undergoing a curative operation for colorectal cancer may be directly related to the size of the largest metastatic lymph node.[1]

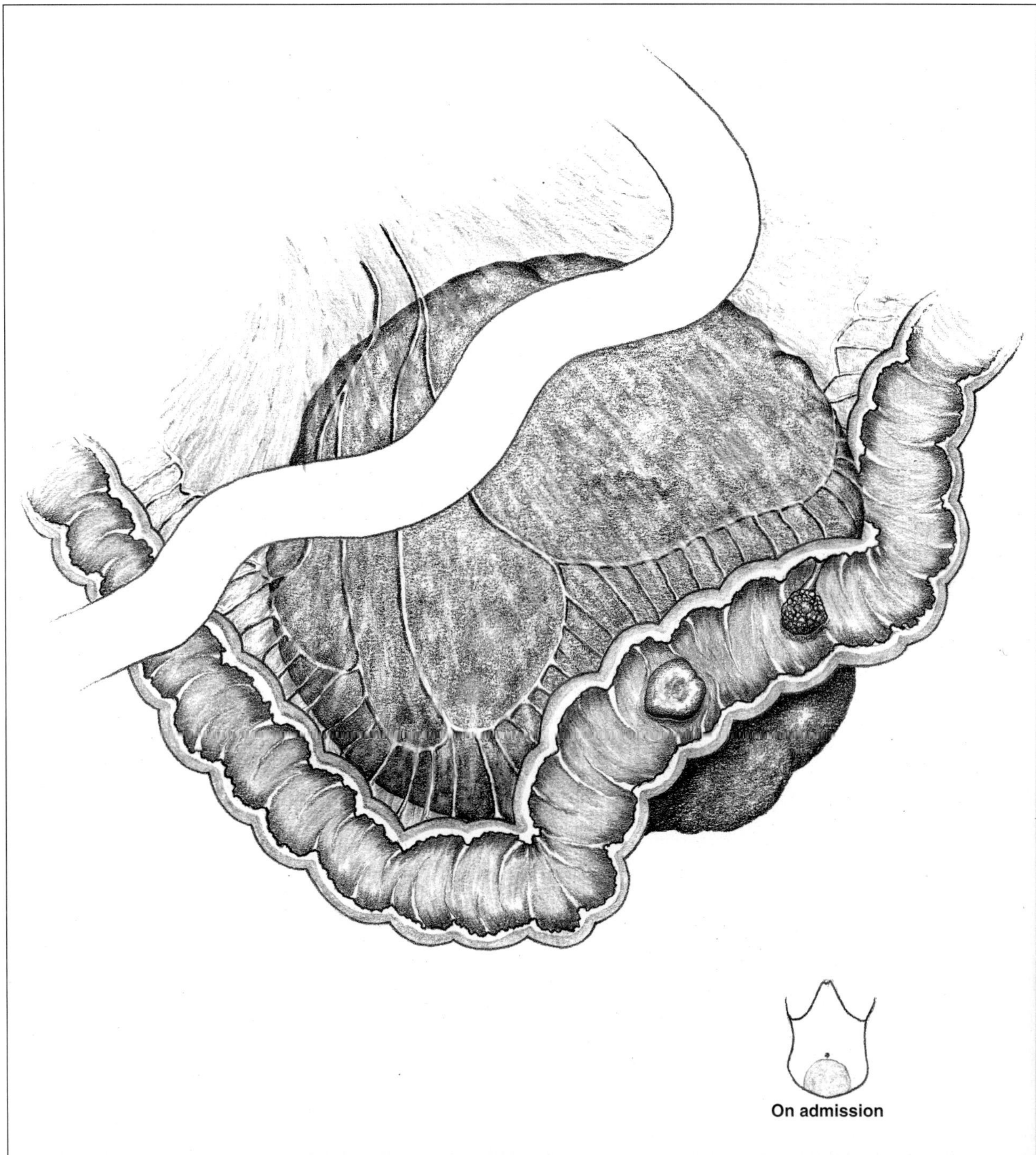
On admission

CASE

33 Rectal Cancer Infiltrating the Buttock Via an Anal Fistula

Male, 70 Years

History

For 2 months the patient had noticed an "abscess" in the right buttock associated with rectal bleeding, constipation, and loss of weight. There was a large rectal cancer found at the 7 cm level, and biopsy of ulcerating nodules on the surface of the buttock also revealed adenocarcinoma. The buttock mass measured 8 cm × 15 cm (Figure 33.1). Laparotomy and colostomy were performed. The surgeon considered the tumor to be nonresectable. The patient was referred for further opinion and management. Examination under anesthesia revealed a subepithelial cord of hard tissue extending from the distal edge of the rectal cancer into the buttock mass. The rectal lesion appeared fixed. Investigations revealed no evidence of other metastases. The patient was treated with two courses of 5 fluorouracil and Lomustine administered by regional perfusion via the right common iliac artery. Preoperative radiotherapy was considered but not given.

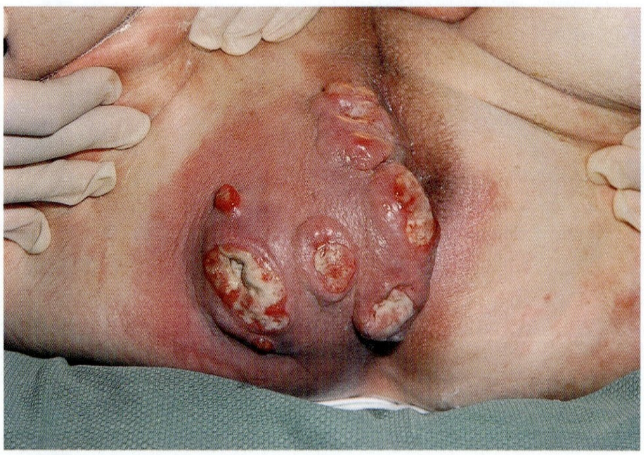

Figure 33.1: Appearance of the right buttock prior to intra-arterial perfusion with chemotherapy.

Operation (10.4.77)

Abdominoperineal excision (APE) of the rectum, including a wide excision of the buttock mass in continuity, was performed.

Pathology

Examination of the specimen revealed a large ulcerated and polypoid tumor encircling the rectum 6 cm above the dentate line. The "core" of malignant tissue connecting the primary tumor to the buttock mass did so via an anal fistula. The tumor in both areas was well differentiated adenocarcinoma. There were no metastases in the lymph nodes. The tumor had extended into the mesorectum. The margins of the pelvic dissection were not involved.

Follow-Up

An enlarged lymph node was noted in the right inguinal region 5 months after the APE. Block dissection was performed, revealing metastatic adenocarcinoma in 1 node. The patient remained free of metastases until he died of "natural causes" at age 82, 11 years and 9 months after the resection of the rectal cancer.

Comment

The initial presentation of this patient suggested a devastating malignancy with a poor prognosis. There was a reduction in the size of the buttock mass after regional chemotherapy. The combined treatment and the biology of the tumor were probably responsible for the long period of cancer-free survival.

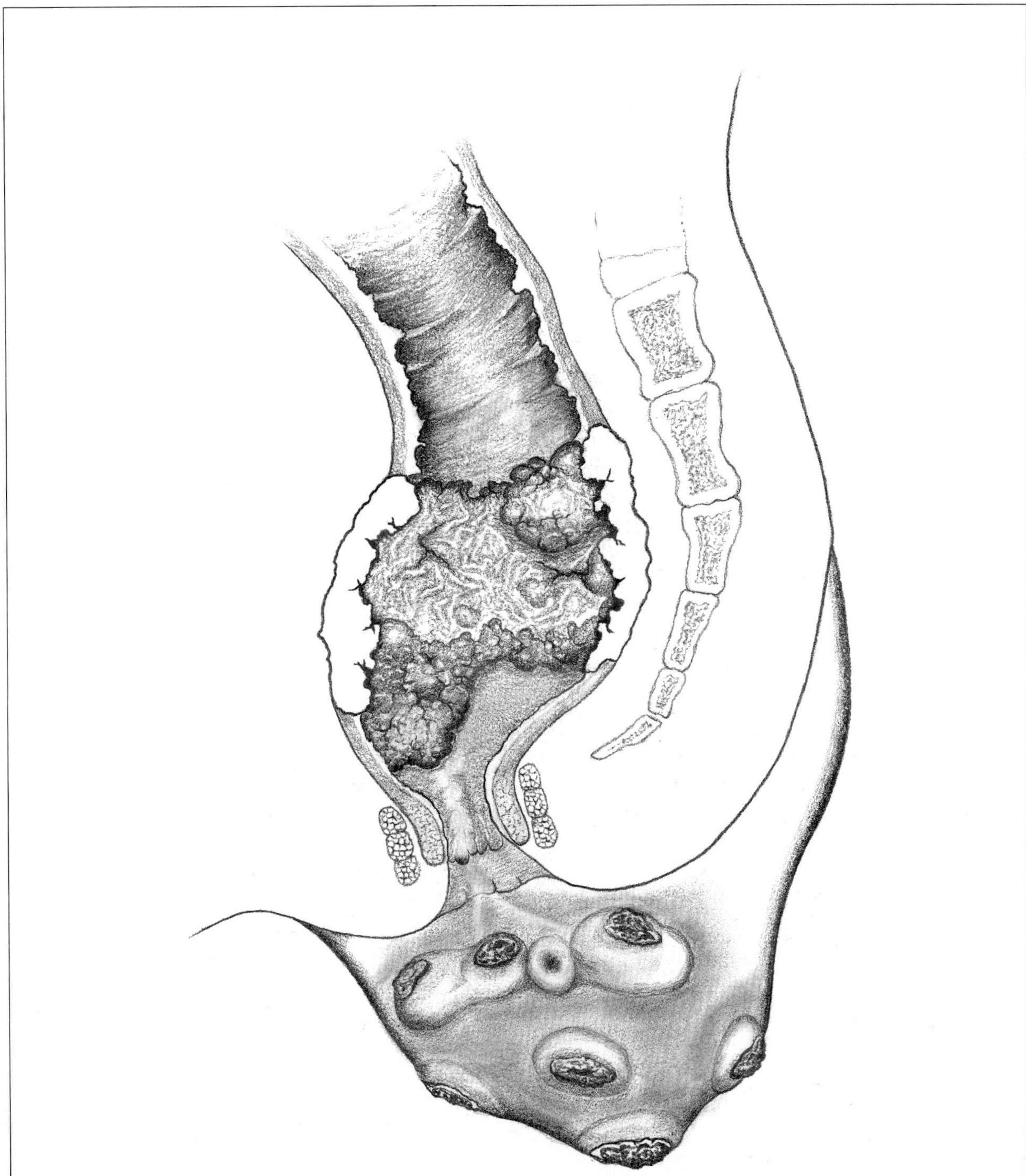

CASE

34 Lucky Local Recurrence

Female, 43 Years

History

In February 1976 the patient underwent a curative resection of a moderately well differentiated adenocarcinoma of the lower third of the sigmoid colon. The vascular ligation was immediately below the upper left colic artery. The distal margin of the tumor clearance was 5 cm. A 2-layer anastomosis was performed which was later measured at 13 cm from the anus. At operation, the uterus was noted to be enlarged and retroverted with a large fibroid on the upper part of the posterior surface. The carcinoma involved 2/3 of the lumen for a distance of 45 mm and "partly infiltrated" the muscularis propria. One mesenteric lymph node 2 cm from the colon contained adenocarcinoma, 12 other lymph nodes were negative (Dukes C, T_2 N_1 M_0). One year after operation, clinical examination and examination under anesthetic revealed a mass in the "pouch of Douglas" (PD), attached to the uterus and the wall of the bowel at the level of the anastomosis. Investigations for metastatic disease elsewhere were negative. [Computerized tomography (CT) and transrectal ultrasound (TRUS) assessment of the pelvis were not available for this patient in 1976].

Operation (3.14.77)

Laparotomy revealed many adhesions in the pelvis but no metastases in the remainder of the abdomen. The uterine fibroid and the left ovary obscured the recurrent tumor in the PD. An en bloc excision of the conglomerate mass included the uterus, both ovaries, and 18 cm of large bowel with a distal margin clearance of 4 cm of rectum. A colorectal anastomosis was performed with a single interrupted layer of dexon sutures.

Pathology

The recurrent tumor was 17 mm in diameter and was adjacent to the anterior aspect of the anastomosis. It was infiltrating the bowel wall immediately above the anastomosis where ulceration of the mucosa (10 mm in diameter) had occurred. There was malignant invasion of the left ovary. The uterus was attached to the recurrence by benign adhesions. The solitary mass of tumor was moderately well differentiated adenocarcinoma.

Follow-Up (2005)

The patient has attended regular follow-up investigations. There has been no recurrence of the carcinoma since the re-resection more than 28 years previously.

Comment

In a review by Abulafi and Williams, the local recurrence (LR) rate from colon cancer was found to be between 4.5% and 17.8%.[1] From the United Kingdom Large Bowel Cancer project, Phillips et al reported an LR rate from left colon cancer of 12%.[2] Local recurrence rates of 3.1% and 3.8% have been reported from specialist colorectal units.[3,4] This patient was fortunate that the LR was detected on rectal examination by an experienced colorectal surgeon during a routine follow-up visit. Interpretation of the clinical findings was made more difficult by the presence of the uterine fibroids. Carcinogenic embryonic antigen estimations were not performed routinely for this patient during 1976–1977. At the present time, endoluminal ultrasound would probably be the investigation of choice to assess the type of lesion described in this case. Its use in staging T_3 and T_4 primary rectal cancer is credited with a high degree of accuracy.[5] Robinson et al. concluded that magnetic resonance imaging (MRI) is an accurate technique for assessing locally recurrent disease.[6] This accuracy may be increased with the use of an endorectal probe with MRI examination. The prognosis may be adversely affected by the surgical technique employed in the original resection.[4] Read et al. suggest a wide excision of the mesentery should be performed, and, for left colon resections, a high vascular ligation is preferred.[4] The outcome has been related with significance to the number of lymph nodes identified in the mesentery of the resected specimen.[7,8] Re-resection with curative intent for local recurrence subsequent to colon cancer is possible in few patients.[9]

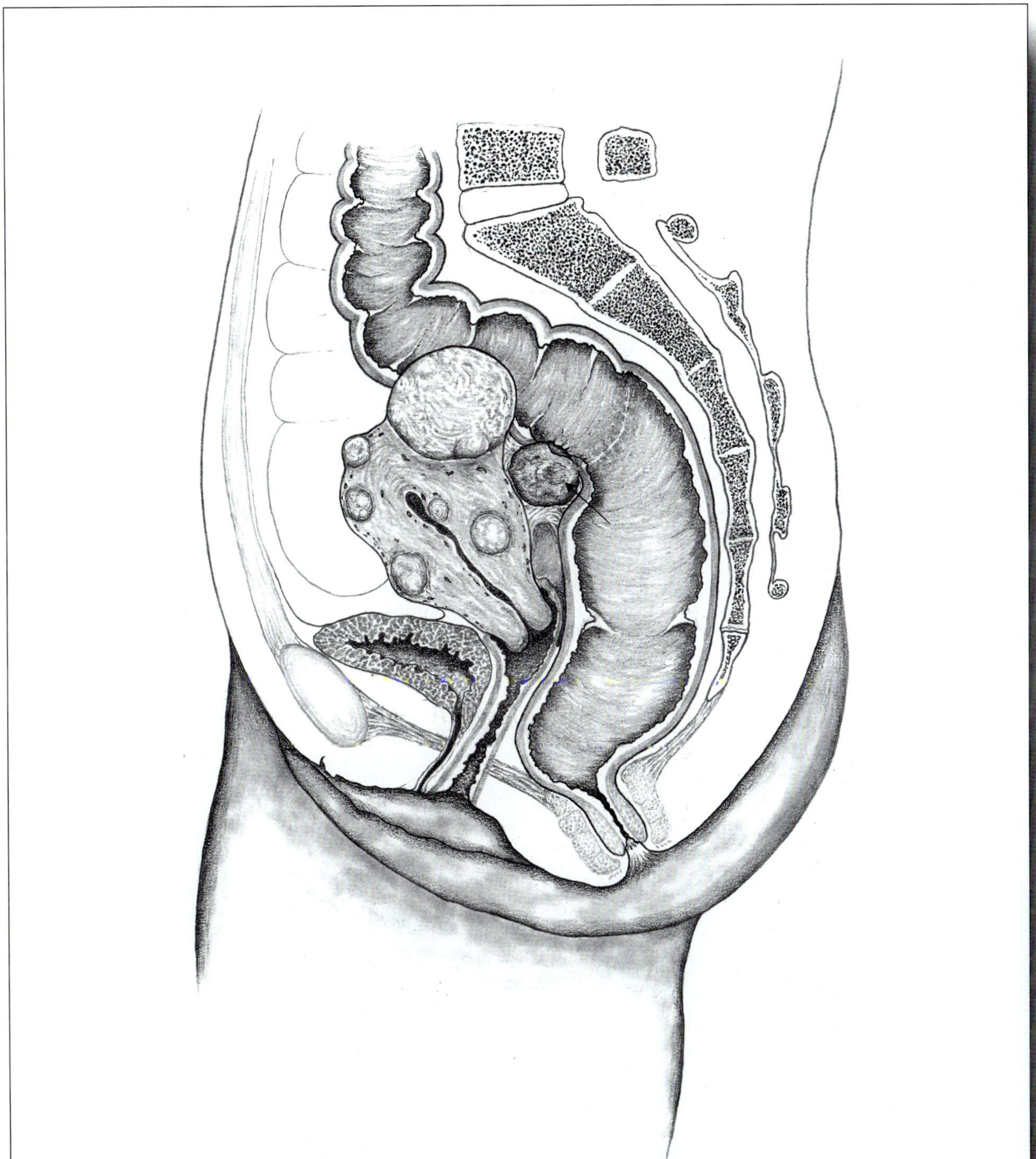

CASE

35 Thoraco-Abdominal Approach to Carcinoma of the Splenic Flexure

Male, 31 Years

History

The patient developed ulcerative colitis (UC) at the age of 14 years (1948) and was referred for a surgical opinion in 1966 with a history of UC for 17 years. He had recently noticed intermittent pain in the left lumbar region and pain under the left costal margin on deep inspiration. Sigmoidoscopy showed minimal active colitis. A barium enema demonstrated total colitis, a large polypoid lesion of the splenic flexure, and a stricture of the upper descending colon 9 cm in length regarded as malignant (Figure 35.1).

Operation (6.10.66)

Laparotomy revealed a large mass at the splenic flexure that was adherent to the diaphragm, the lower ribs, and spleen. There were no obvious intraabdominal metastases. Biopsy of an enlarged node at the origin of the inferior mesenteric artery (IMA) was negative for carcinoma. A thoraco-abdominal approach was then employed to enable further assessment and dissection of the mass. Resection was performed with en bloc removal of colon, spleen, tail of pancreas, portion of 3 ribs (11th, 10th, 12th), and the lateral aspect of the left diaphragm, as malignant invasion of these structures appeared to have occurred. The resected margin of the diaphragm was sutured to the chest wall at a higher level (Figure 35.2). The right colon resection was deferred, in view of the duration and complexity of the left colon resection. The postoperative recovery was satisfactory.

Pathology

The macroscopic appearance of the mucosa (featureless, fragile, and hyperemic) and the histological features were typical of chronic ulcerative colitis. The proximal carcinoma was 40 × 40 mm, localized to the colon wall (Dukes A, T_2 N_0 M_0). The distal tumor was annular, with marked narrowing of the lumen, and extended 55 mm along the colon. This

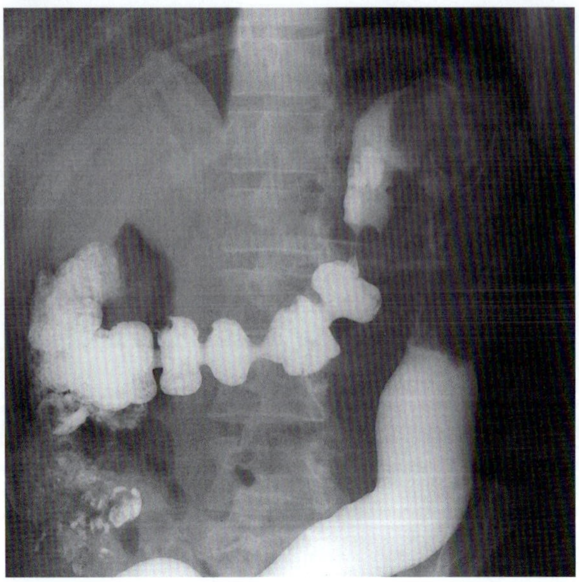

Figure 35.1: Two carcinomas at the splenic flexure demonstrated by barium enema.

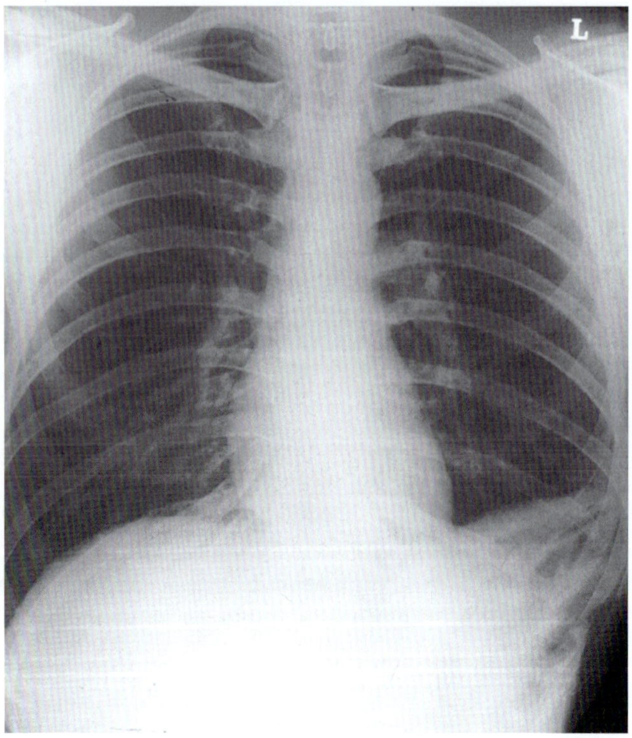

Figure 35.2: Chest x-ray 2 years after operation shows the position of the transposed left hemidiaphragm.

larger tumor had penetrated well beyond the muscle wall of the colon but was attached to the diaphragm and ribs by a prominent layer of fibrous tissue (Dukes B, T_3 N_0 M_0). Both tumors were well differentiated, with obvious mucoid formation in the distal lesion. There were 36 lymph nodes in the resected mesentery, none of which contained metastases on histological examination.

Operation (11.16.66)

The right colon and colostomy were resected. An end-to-end ileorectal anastomosis was performed, leaving 15 cm of rectum. Postoperative recovery was satisfactory.

Follow-Up (2005)

The patient has remained well for 39 years with no recurrence or further carcinoma of the large bowel. Regular sigmoidoscopy examinations show minimal inflammatory changes of the mucosa of the rectum without dysplasia. Bowel frequency is 5/24 hrs.

Comment

In 1964, 15 months prior to the diagnosis of multiple carcinomas, a follow-up contrast enema had shown no evidence of any lesion in the vicinity of the splenic flexure. He had known high risk factors for supervening malignancy: the colitis commencing at an early age and symptom duration of 17 years. Lennard-Jones has assessed the risk as 12% in patients with a history of 10–25 years.[1] Mayer, reporting on 39 patients with ulcerative colitis cancer, found 18% of the patients had a history of less than 8 years.[2] The nature of the patient's symptoms and the size of the larger tumor on x-ray suggested that local extension in this "remote" region of the abdomen could be significant. This was confirmed at laparotomy via an upper left paramedian incision. The thoracoabdominal incision through the bed of the seventh rib provided optimal access to the most difficult part of the operation. There is little doubt that without this exposure the pathology would have been regarded as nonresectable. In the author's series of 2093 patients with colorectal cancer, there were 47 splenic flexure lesions. The thoracoabdominal approach was employed in 4 patients. Landman et al. report from the Cleveland Clinic that, in 5 multivisceral resections of splenic flexure cancers, some part of the diaphragm was included in the en bloc excision.[3] Attachment to other viscera is not always due to malignancy as there is frequently an inflammatory reaction around the tumor. Contiguous malignant infiltration has been reported in 44%,[4] 48%,[3] and 52%[5] of multivisceral resections. At operation it can be impossible for the surgeon to define a safe plane of dissection to avoid violation of the tumor clearance, which results in increased local recurrence[6] and decreased survival.[7] Currently, preoperative computer tomography (CT) and/or magnetic resonance imaging (MRI) examinations may be of assistance, although the distinction between fibrous tissue and malignant infiltration can still be difficult. The patient's long term survival has been associated with regular follow up examinations of the residual 13 cm of rectum. Although patients who develop ulcerative colitis cancer tend to have a higher incidence of Dukes C and D tumors, Johnson et al. found there was not a significant difference in the 5 year cancer-specific survival of curative operations compared with noncolitic colorectal cancer.[8] The only other reference found describing the thoracoabdominal approach for splenic flexure cancer was that of Walfisch and Stern.[9]

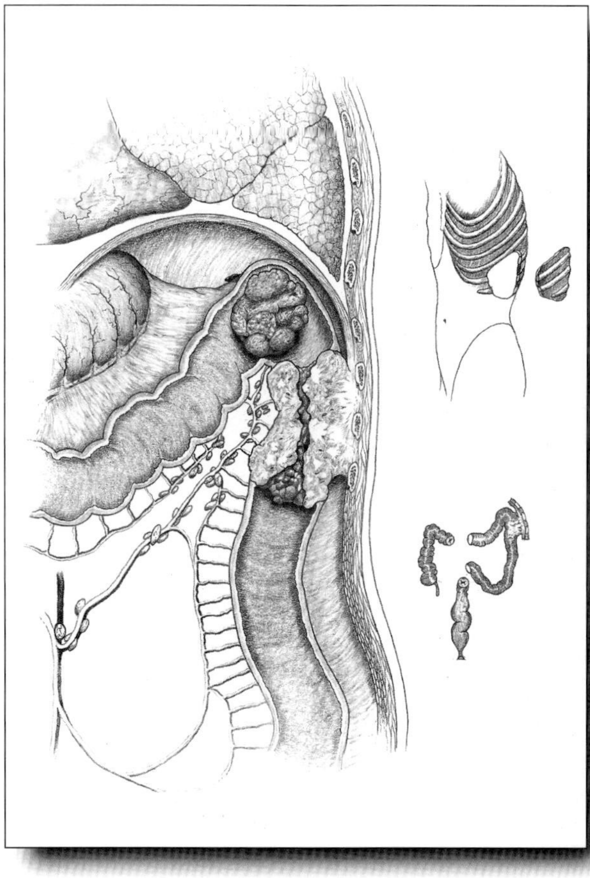

For a full-page image of this figure see the appendix.

PART V Diverticular Disease

CASE

36 Was It Diverticulitis?

Female, 63 Years

History

In August 1994 the patient was admitted to the hospital with severe pain and tenderness in the left iliac fossa accompanied by fever and vomiting. A pelvic ultrasound suggested a possible left-sided pelvic mass. Laparoscopy by a gynecologist revealed normal ovaries and "extensive diverticular disease." Antibiotics were administered and the symptoms settled. A subsequent barium enema confirmed the diagnosis of sigmoid diverticular disease. Nine months later, a series of similar episodes occurred over a period of 12 weeks, resulting in a further admission to hospital for 7 days. Elective operation was advised for recurring diverticulitis.

Operation (8.11.95)

There was marked diverticular disease involving the sigmoid colon but no focus of diverticulitis was identified. The remainder of the colon and small bowel were normal. Both ovaries were normal. The large bowel was resected between the sigmoid descending junction and the upper third of the rectum. The anastomosis was completed with a circular stapler. Two diverticula in the mid descending colon were inverted.

Pathology

No evidence of active inflammation was found on examination. Marked diverticulosis was present with associated thickening of the muscularis propria. The mucosal folds were prominent and distorted, consistent with long standing diverticular disease.

Follow-Up (2004)

One year after operation, examination revealed a stenosis of the anastomosis (at 10 cm). There were no associated symptoms, and a 17 mm diameter sigmoidoscope passed beyond the stenosis without difficulty. This degree of stenosis was not treated. The patient has been free of gastrointestinal symptoms for 9 years.

Comment

Morson reported that, in a series of 173 patients with symptomatic diverticular disease treated by resection at St Mark's Hospital, no evidence of inflammation was found in 32.4% of the specimens.[1] The patients had been treated during a period when various radiological criteria of inflammation, since proven incorrect, were accepted. The incidence of noninflammatory diverticular disease found after resection is infrequently reported. In the author's series of 206 patients managed by elective open resection, the incidence was 12.1%.[2] In a series of 162 laparoscopic resections reported by Le Moine et al., the incidence was 56.2%.[3] The selection criteria for operation will greatly affect this incidence. These patients present with no evidence of complications on clinical examination or investigation but have a convincing history characterized by chronic left iliac fossa pain or "attacks of diverticulitis." The possible explanations for the absence of inflammation on pathological examination are: (i) resolution of an inflammatory focus beyond detection; (ii) the symptoms are due to dysfunction of the colon affected by the diverticular disease; and (iii) the patient's symptoms are due to irritable bowel syndrome in the presence of incidental diverticular disease.

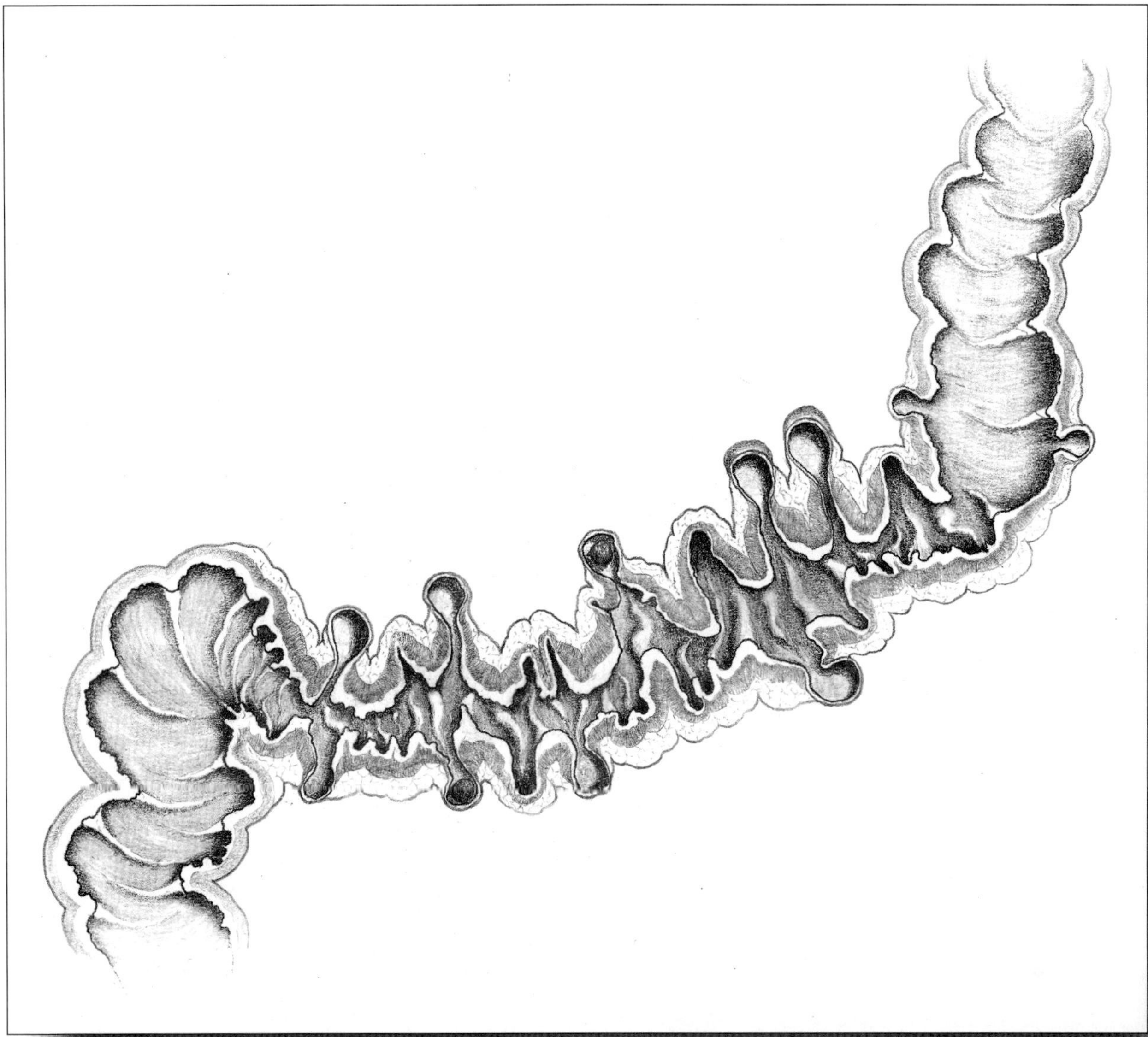

CASE

37 Large Pseudopolyp of the Sigmoid Colon

Male, 59 Years

History

The patient was referred after an urgent laparotomy during which a transverse colostomy was performed for an inflammatory mass in the lower sigmoid and rectum. Subsequent colonoscopy was limited to the distal sigmoid, where a 10-mm polyp was removed (villous adenoma). Anterograde colonoscopy via the colostomy revealed marked narrowing of the sigmoid colon due to diverticular disease and a large polyp with a broad pedicle which could not be snared with safety.

Operation (2.23.1995)

High anterior resection.

Pathology

Chronic inflammation, muscle thickening, and redundant mucosa were present in the sigmoid colon due to diverticular disease. Several areas of redundant mucosa showed intense hyperemia. In the center of the specimen, there was a large "polyp" 40mm in width, described by the pathologist as a "semicircular flap of mucosa." Microscopic examination of the polyp revealed numerous thick-walled blood vessels in the mucosa and submucosa with no evidence of adenoma.

Operation (6.9.1995)

The transverse colostomy was closed.

Follow-Up (2001)

At 5 years and 9 months there were no further gastrointestinal symptoms, and colonoscopy was normal.

Comment

The interest in this patient is the unusual large pseudopolyp that had formed from the redundant mucosa within the sigmoid diverticular disease. This entity has been described as "polypoid prolapsing mucosal folds"[1] and "crescentic fold disease,"[2] the latter representing the early stage of this pathology. The histological appearances are identical to those seen in mucosal prolapse of the rectum.[1] The changes are presumably due to traction and subsequent prolapse of the mucosa, which initially appears as hyperemic patches. Kelly found this abnormality in 7% of resected specimens.[1] Figures 37.1 and 37.2 (from a different patient) show two forms of the pathology.

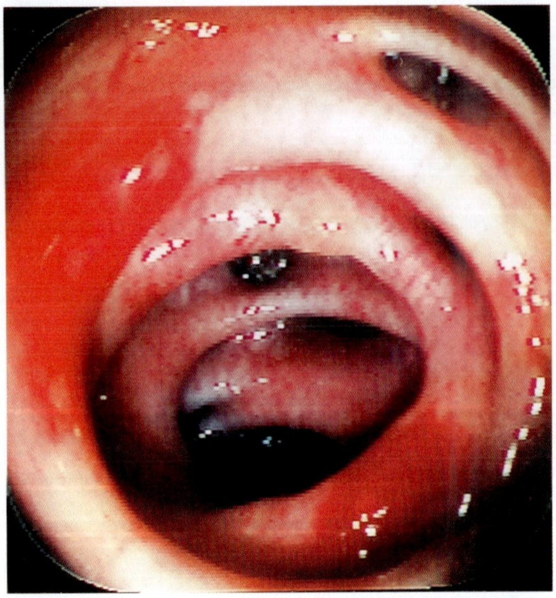

Figure 37.1: Hyperemic patches in chronic diverticular disease ("crescentic" fold disease) from a different patient.

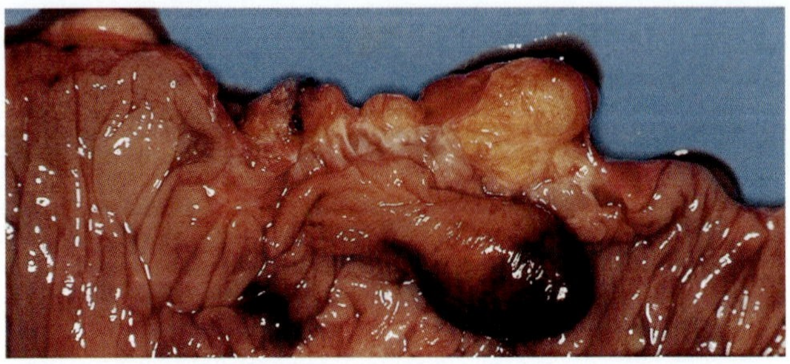

Figure 37.2: Example of a further stage of the pathology (pseudopolyp) from same patient shown in Figure 37.1.

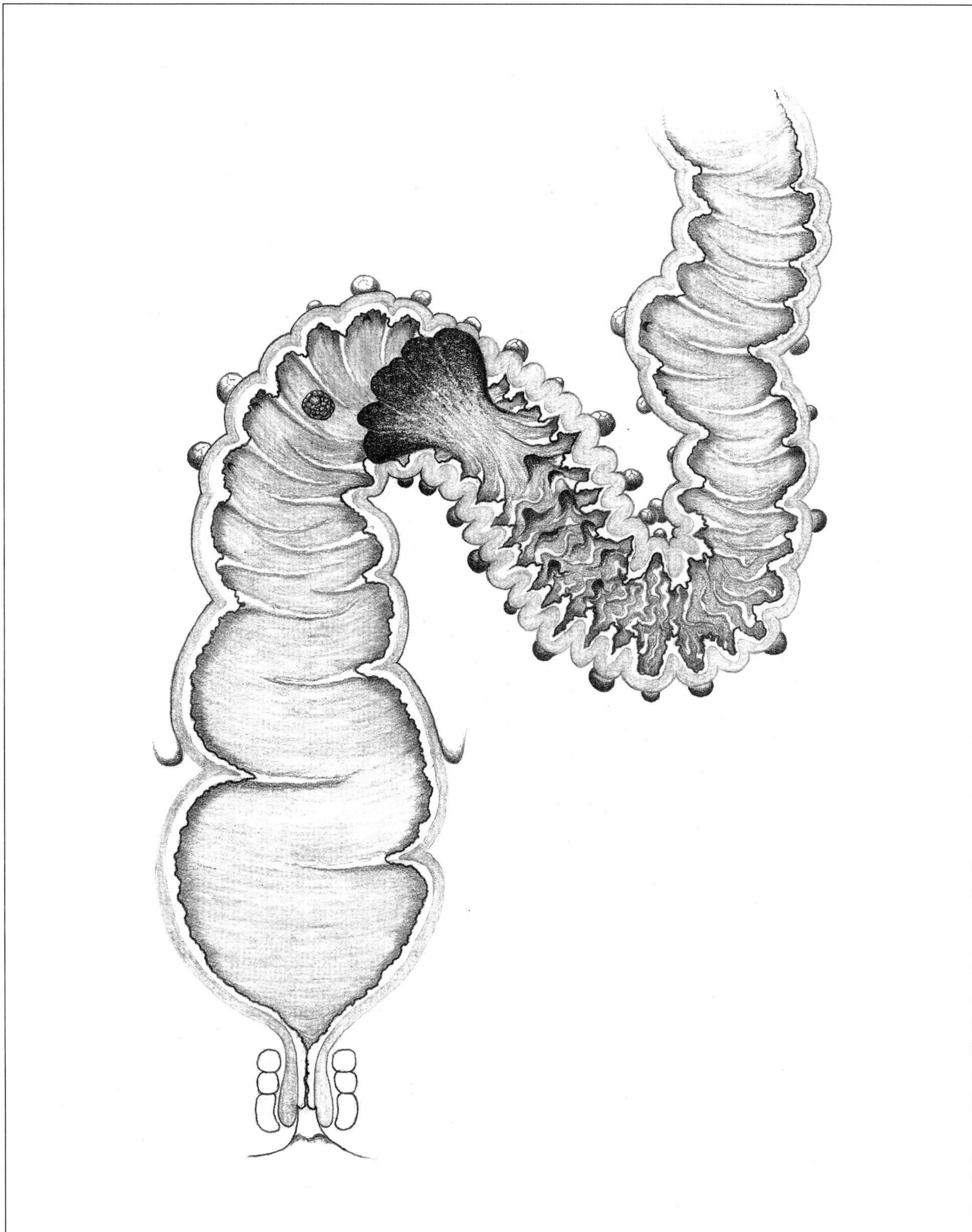

CASE

38 Which Operation for Acute Diverticulitis with Peritonitis?

Male, 56 Years

History

One year prior to emergency admission to the hospital, the patient had an attack of abdominal pain that was diagnosed as diverticulitis. At the time of this urgent admission, he complained of left iliac fossa pain, vomiting, and diarrhea. There was lower abdominal tenderness maximal on the left. A computerized tomography (CT) examination showed diffuse induration surrounding the sigmoid colon with bubbles of gas beyond the lumen. Some free fluid was present but no loculated collection suitable for catheter drainage. Over a period of 4 days, there was no significant improvement and operation was advised.

Operation (5.25.98)

There was a focus of acute diverticulitis in the sigmoid colon which had perforated into the sigmoid mesentery forming an abscess which burst as soon as the sigmoid colon was handled. There was minor contamination of the operative field by the leaking purulent fluid. There were adhesions and collections of yellow gelatinous fibrin near the perforation, between loops of small bowel, and in the right subphrenic spaces. Most of the sigmoid colon was resected without anastomosis. The peritoneal cavity was copiously irrigated with saline, and suction drains were placed in the right subphrenic spaces.

Pathology

Examination confirmed the diagnosis of diverticulitis with extensive acute inflammation and the presence of a mesenteric abscess.

Postoperative

Recovery from operation was uncomplicated. Sigmoidoscopy and colonoscopy were performed and found to be normal, and the patient was scheduled for Stage 2 surgery.

Operation (11.23.98)

Reversal of the Hartmann operation was performed with a stapled anastomosis in the mid rectum. The immediate postoperative recovery was satisfactory, but readmission was required for a bleeding duodenal ulcer. This was managed by laparotomy and suture of the bleeding vessel. Since then the patient has remained free of gastrointestinal symptoms (2005).

Comment

This patient's acute diverticulitis, present for approximately a week prior to laparotomy, caused a fibrinous peritonitis. Free perforation (via the mesenteric abscess) was imminent as evidenced by the disruption of the abscess as soon as mobilization of the colon was commenced. This event persuaded the surgeon to perform a Hartmann procedure instead of resection and immediate anastomosis, which in retrospect was probably overly conservative. The patient was otherwise healthy with no comorbidity, and there was no fecal peritonitis. There has been increasing evidence that anastomotic integrity is not jeopardized by the presence of peritonitis.[1,2] The literature currently supports that immediate anastomosis is safe if the patient's general state will allow the longer procedure.[3,4] The Hartmann reversal operation in this patient was complicated by upper gastrointestinal bleeding requiring major surgery, underlining the fact that this operation has the potential for significant complications. Despite this criticism, the Hartmann operation may still be the safest option in an elderly patient with comorbidity and gross peritoneal sepsis.

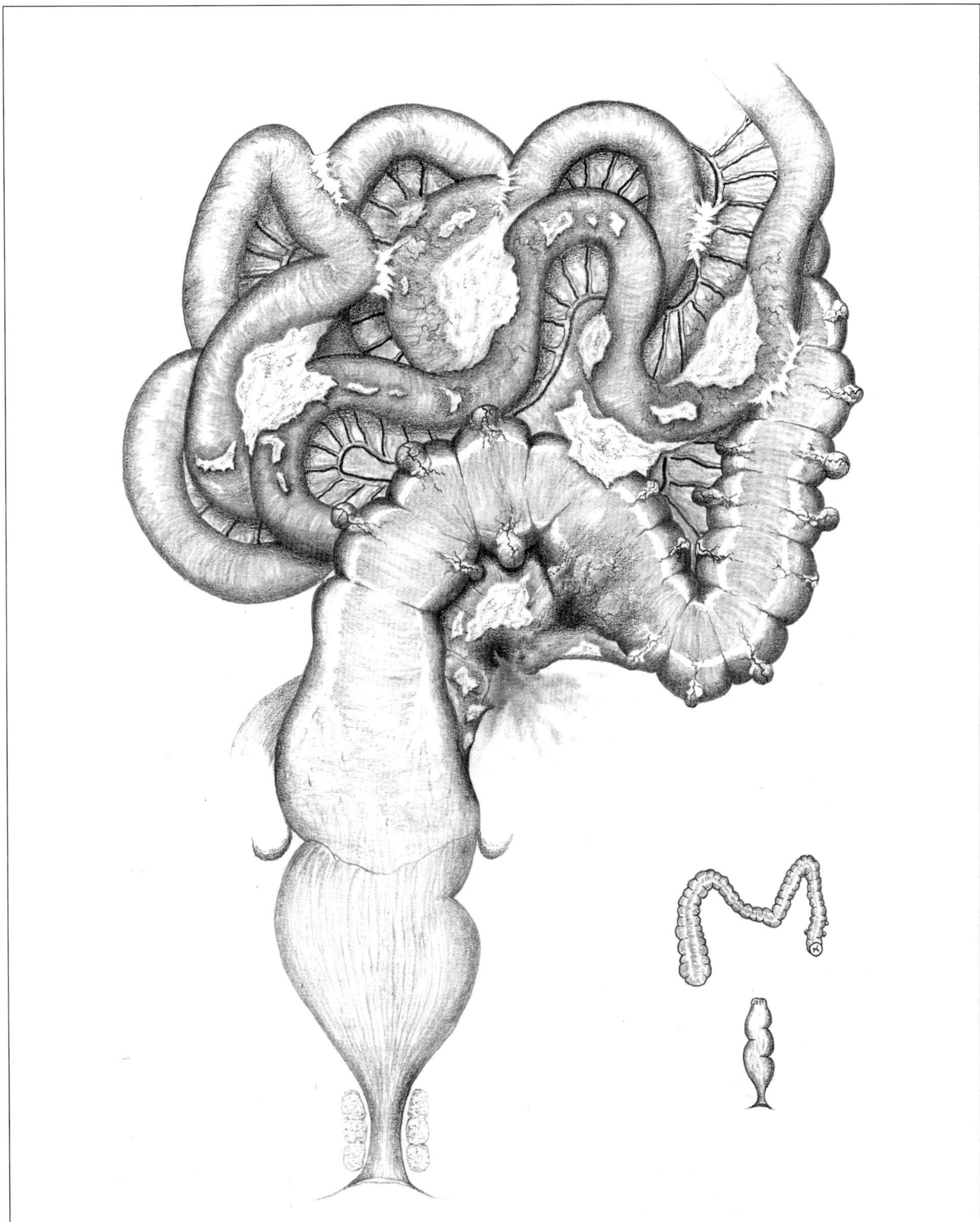

CASE

39 Waiting to Die

Female, 67 Years

History

In 1977 the patient underwent laparotomy for a suspected carcinoma of the sigmoid colon. The surgeon found a large fixed mass firmly adherent to the pelvic structures, which he considered to be inoperable. A left-sided loop colostomy was performed. The patient was subsequently informed that her disease was incurable cancer. After a 5-year period, by which time no deterioration in her health had occurred, the patient was referred for a second opinion. Clinical examination revealed a pelvic mass. Flexible sigmoidoscopy was possible only to 25 cm, at which level no malignancy was identified. Review of the barium enema films performed prior to the laparotomy in 1977 showed a stricture of the sigmoid with mucosal continuity throughout (Figure 39.1). The diagnosis was now considered to be diverticulitis.

Operation (11.5.82)

Laparotomy revealed a large hard mass in the sigmoid colon, which itself was kinked and adherent to the uterus, left fallopian tube, and left ovary.

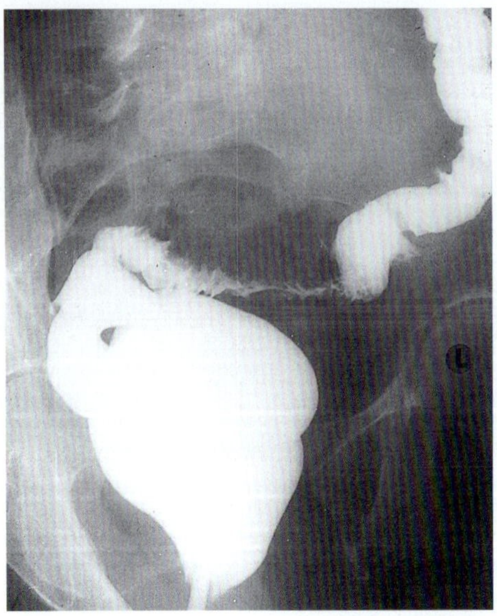

Figure 39.1: The barium enema demonstrates typical mucosal continuity within the diverticular stricture.

On the basis of the morphology of the mass, it was difficult to exclude carcinoma as the primary pathology. There was no evidence of intraabdominal metastases. The surgical approach, however, was guided by the interpretation of the barium enema of 1977. A low anterior resection was performed with removal of the colostomy. The uterus was separated from the mass, but the left adnexal structures, involved in tough adhesions, were removed "en bloc" with the sigmoid colon. To avoid damage to vital structures on the left brim of the pelvis, intramuscular dissection of the colon at that point left a "patch" of colon musculature protecting the left ureter and iliac vessels from dissection trauma.[1] Cholecystectomy was performed for a gallstone.

Pathology

The serosal surface of the colon showed chronic inflammatory changes with an increase in the pericolic adipose tissue. Muscular thickening was present in the strictured segment associated with a chronic inflammatory infiltration. The wall of the colon was 11 mm in thickness. There was no focus of suppuration within the specimen. The mucosa was intact but compressed and redundant within the stricture. The findings were consistent with the diagnosis of phlegmonous diverticulitis.[2]

Follow-Up (2004)

The patient's recovery was delayed due to a severe wound infection that appeared after discharge from the hospital. In the immediate and early postoperative period, the patient was euphoric having been "delivered" from a terminal malignancy. This was followed by a longer but temporary period of profound depression. The patient has experienced no further significant bowel trouble and, at the age of 89 years, was in reasonable health.

Comment

Although the barium enema examination is not usually the strategic investigation to differentiate diverticular disease and carcinoma of the sigmoid colon, it can be very helpful. If the stricture shows a mucosal pattern within it, then malignant disease is unlikely. Other features (less reliable), which support diverticular disease, are a tapered transition at the proximal and distal limits of the stricture and a lengthy disease segment.[3] If the diseased segment of sigmoid colon can be negotiated with the colonoscope, then this is the preferred investigation. The degree of stricturing and the axial distortion of the colon may obstruct endoscopy. In these circumstances, a small caliber endoscope may be successful. Computerized tomography (CT) is regarded as an important investigation if acute diverticulitis is suspected, but its role in the assessment of longstanding disease is less clear. This patient's barium enema was a classic example of diverticulitis incorrectly interpreted and incompletely investigated, which caused her the anguish of waiting to die for 5 years.

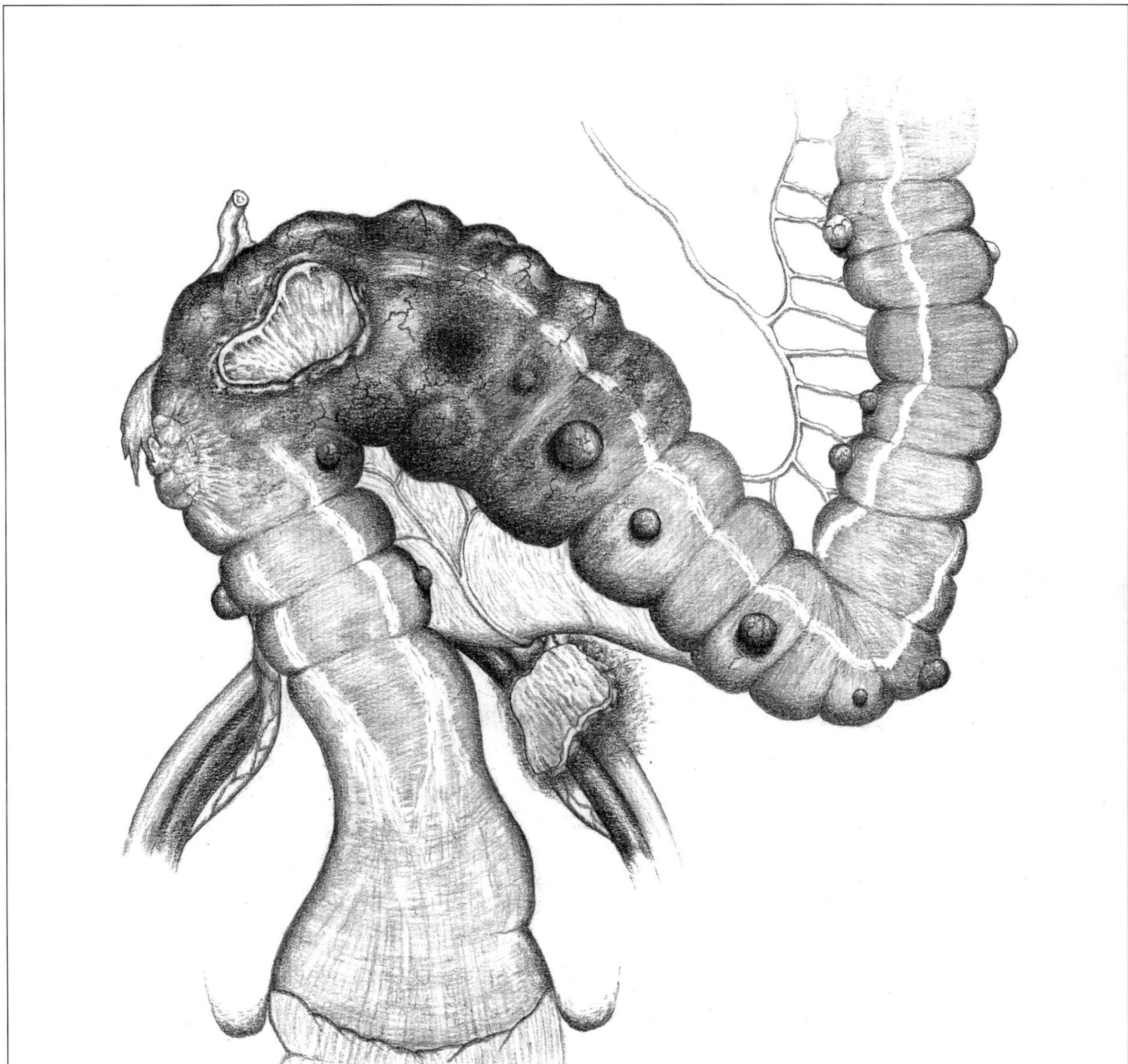

CASE

40 Distal Abscesses and Diverticular Disease

Male, 56 Years

History

The patient presented with a 1-month history of lower abdominal pain and narrow frequent stools. Previous, less severe attacks had been diagnosed as diverticulitis, which had responded to antibiotic treatment. There was abdominal tenderness in the suprapubic region. Rectal examination revealed a fixed, hard mass involving the anterior pelvis. Flexible sigmoidoscopy was not possible beyond 20 cm due to marked narrowing of the lumen. A barium enema demonstrated a stricture of the sigmoid colon consistent with diverticular disease. There was no significant concern regarding the possibility of carcinoma.

Operation (8.3.89)

The mid third of the sigmoid colon was the site of an inflammatory mass adherent to the bladder with an intervening chronic abscess. As the sigmoid colon was mobilized from the pelvis, a further abscess was apparent between the rectum and the seminal vesicles. To reach healthy bowel wall for anastomosis, further distal dissection was required, revealing a third abscess between the rectum and the prostate. There was no abscess track connecting these 3 abscesses. The chronic inflammatory tissue between the rectum and the anterior structures was dense and fibrous. The bowel was resected from the lower descending colon to the lower third of the rectum. The rectal wall was friable and denuded of muscle anteriorly and, therefore, not ideal for anastomosis. The colon was lavaged between the site for a transverse colostomy and the divided descending colon. An end-to-end anastomosis was performed with a double stapling technique. The anterior part of the "doughnut" was thin. The anastomosis, a short distance above the pelvic floor, was too low to insert supporting sutures. A transverse colostomy was performed to protect a precarious anastomosis. Suction drains were placed in the anterior pelvis to diminish the possibility of continuing sepsis from the "inflammatory nests" on the bladder, seminal vesicles, and prostate.

Pathology

The resected bowel measured 35 cm in length. There was a 9 cm segment of chronically inflamed colon in the middle of the specimen. The wall of the colon in this area was markedly thickened with muscular hypertrophy and fibrosis, causing stricture formation. The serosal surface was inflamed and puckered. Within the inflamed segment, a diverticulum containing pus was identified as the primary focus of the diverticulitis. The mucosa showed no specific features.

Postoperative Course

This was satisfactory, and contrast enema examination of the anastomosis prior to the patient's discharge from the hospital showed no evidence of anastomotic leak.

Operation (10.17.89)

The transverse colostomy was closed.

Comment

The pericolic and perirectal abscesses were not in continuity, and while multiple abscesses can complicate chronic diverticulitis, such discontinuous, deep, and anterior extraperitoneal abscesses are unusual. An ultralow anterior resection was necessary to obtain distal bowel for anastomosis that was unaffected by secondary contiguous inflammation. Even so, the rectal wall was less than satisfactory. The proximal stoma combined with colon lavage was an essential precaution.

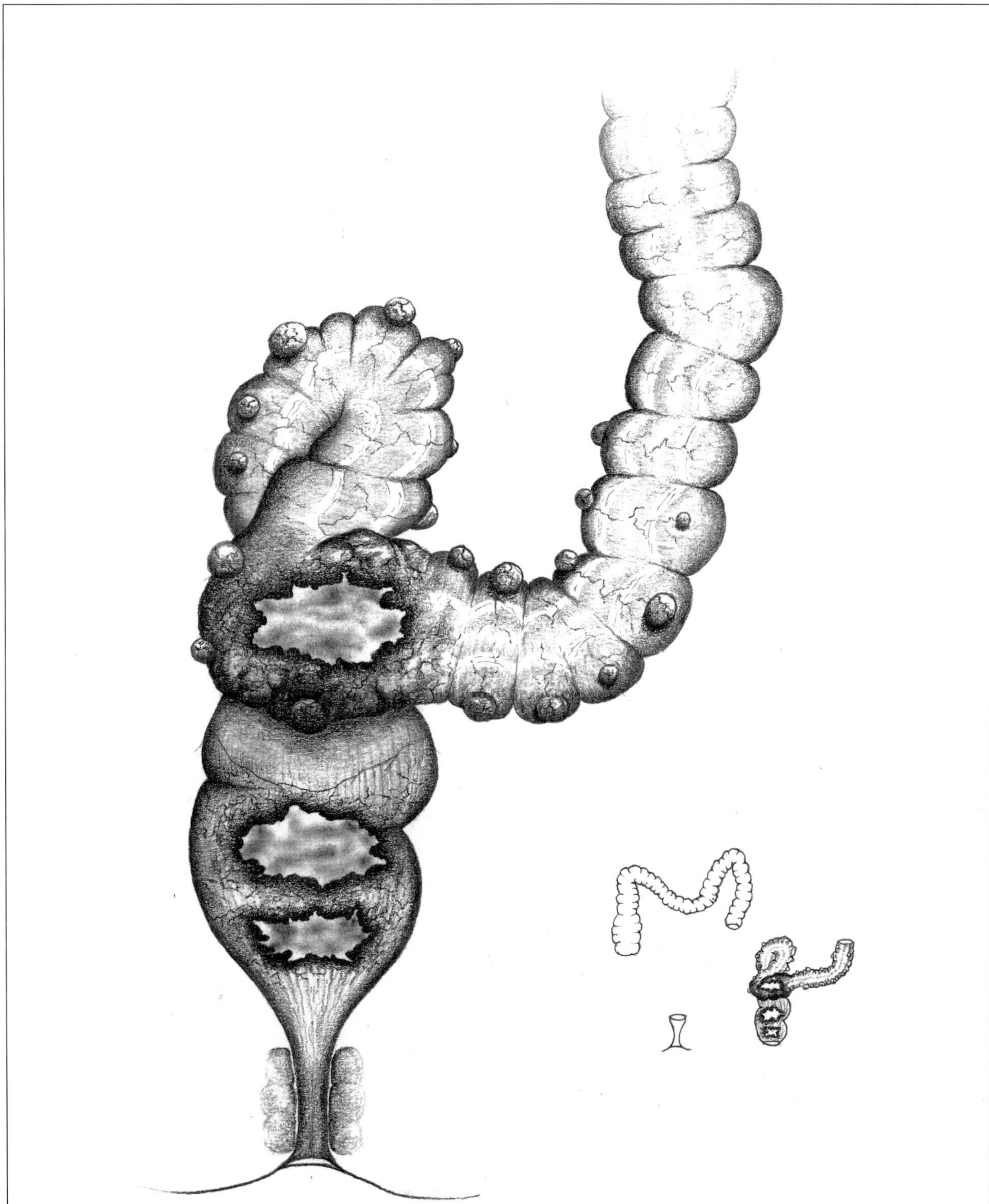

CASE

41 Coloperineal Fistula

Male, 53 Years

History

The patient complained of attacks of lower abdominal pain for 7 years. An intermittently discharging abscess in the right ischiorectal fossa had been present for 1 year (Figure 41.1). The referring doctor had been able to pass a probe into the abscess for a depth of 12 cm. A sinogram demonstrated a connection with the sigmoid colon in which there was extensive diverticular disease. Rectal examination revealed marked induration anteriorly and laterally around the rectum at the level of the prostate. Rigid sigmoidoscopy revealed no pathology to 16 cm. A barium enema confirmed the findings of the sinogram (Figure 41.2).

Operation (5.29.75)

The sigmoid colon was indurated and fixed to the pelvic floor by marked fibrosis. A proximal loop ileostomy was performed. Over the next 7 months, the patient stated he "hadn't felt so well in years." There was some diminution in the perirectal induration.

Operation (2.17.76)

The sigmoid colon was dissected free from the recto vesical fossa. The fistula was demonstrated passing distally between seminal vesicles, prostate, and rectum. This area was not dissected. There was no abscess associated with the fistula. Following resection, the proximal colon was anastomosed to the intraperitoneal rectum by hand suture. Postoperative contrast studies demonstrated a radiological anastomotic leak (AL).

Operation (2.15.77)

Closure of the ileostomy was delayed by the presence of the AL and persistent sequestrated barium in the presacral space related to contrast studies of the anastomosis.

Follow-Up (1980)

The patient's last documented follow up was 4 years, 10 months after ileostomy closure. There were no bowel symptoms.

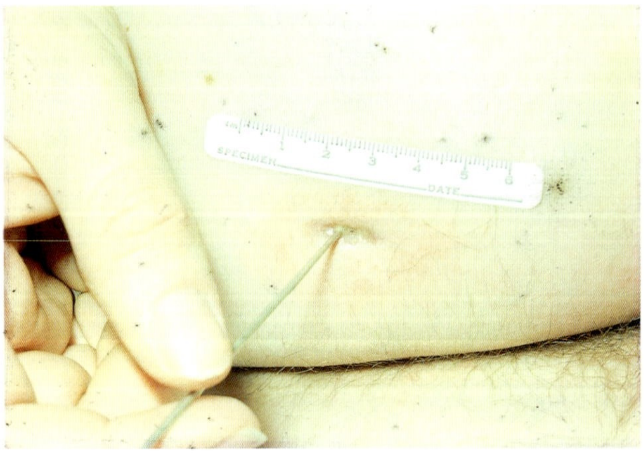

Figure 41.1: External opening of fistula onto right buttock.

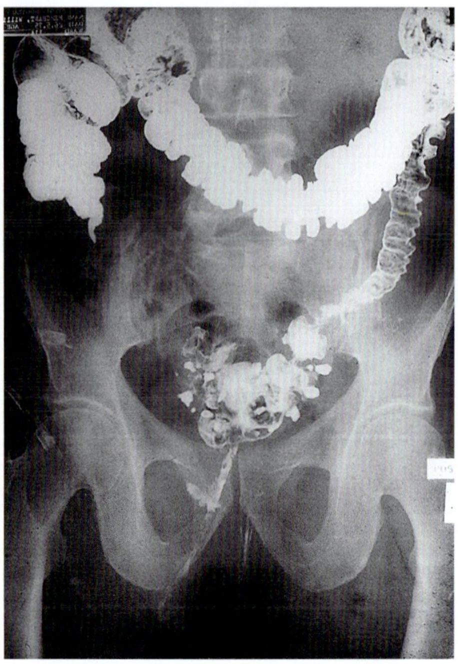

Figure 41.2: Fistula track and diverticular disease seen on barium enema.

Comment

In the author's series of fistulae due to diverticulitis, this is the only coloperineal fistula encountered. A report from the Cleveland Clinic by Fazio et al. included 93 patients with colocutaneous fistulae.[1] Only 5 developed spontaneously, and no coloperineal fistula was reported. Parks and Gordon reported 4 cases of sigmoid perineal fistula due to diverticulitis, stating that no local perianal treatment is required, since the fistulae heal once the source of the infection is resected.[2] The operation probably could have been managed in 2 stages rather than 3. There was, however, improvement with the patient's general health and some diminution of the pelvic reaction as a result of the preliminary ileostomy.

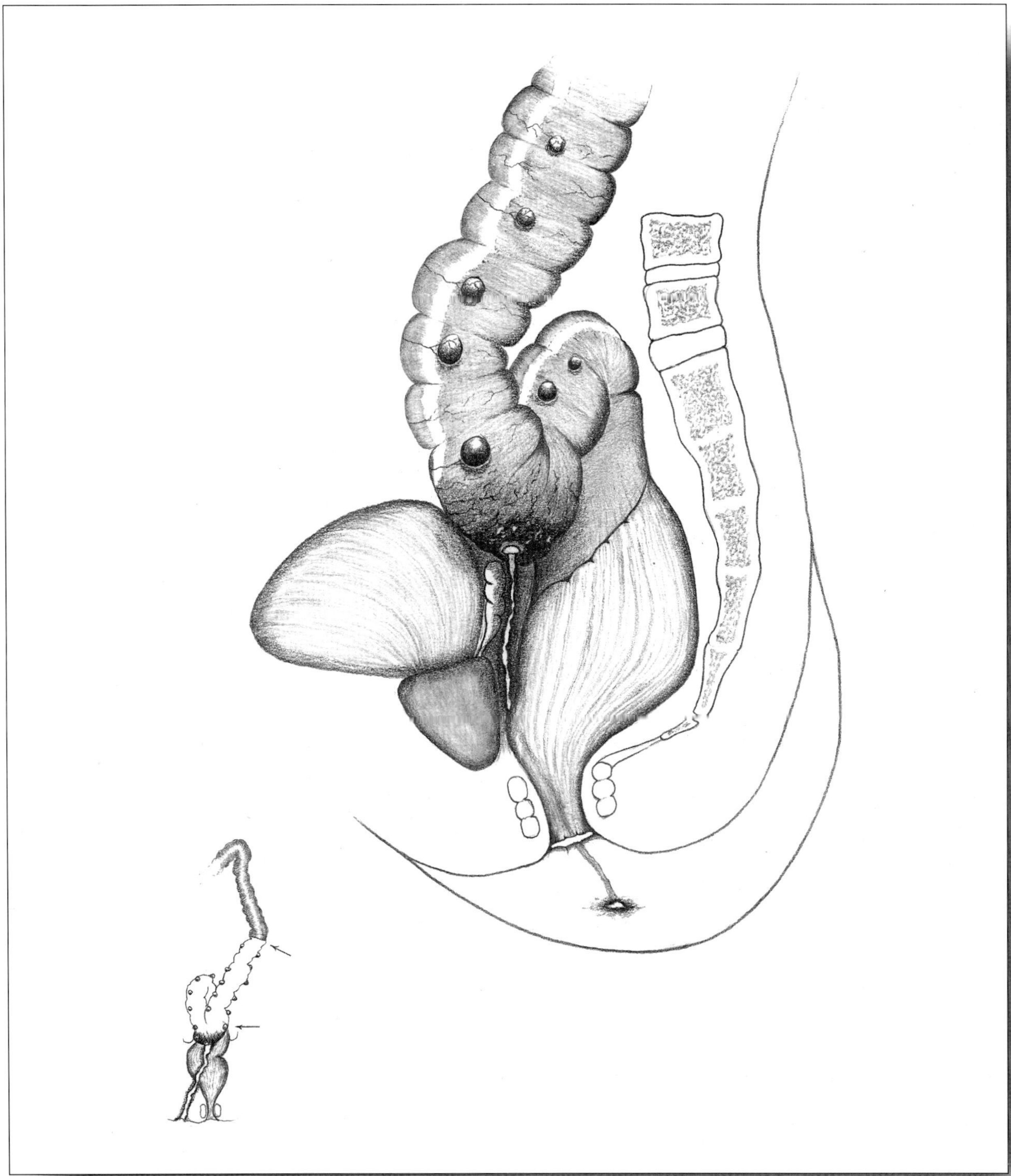

CASE

42 Diverticulitis: Extensive Abscess in the Mesorectum

Male, 66 Years

History

Lower abdominal pain had been present for 2 months, with an increased frequency of bowel action. At times the stools were loose. During this period there had been a fever treated with antibiotics. There was tenderness in the left iliac fossa. No pelvic mass was apparent on rectal examination. Limited colonoscopy revealed diverticular disease of the sigmoid colon with marked narrowing of the lumen, which prevented further advancement of the instrument.

Operation (12.23.91)

There was a large inflammatory mass involving the rectosigmoid and upper third of the rectum. Carcinoma could not be excluded. The left colon showed evidence of chronic obstruction. The proximal colon was distended, in particular, the cecum was markedly affected with dehiscence of the seromuscular layer. A low anterior resection (a circular stapler anastomosis) and a loop ileostomy were performed. Postoperative recovery was slow but uneventful.

Pathology Examination

The opened specimen demonstrated diverticular disease with a stricture and redundant "polypoidal" mucosa. A diverticulum was identified communicating with a complex serpiginous abscess in a markedly thickened mesorectum. Histological examination showed nonspecific inflammatory changes consistent with diverticulitis.

Operation (2.3.92)

Closure of loop ileostomy.

Follow-Up (1996)

Subsequent colonoscopy revealed no mucosal abnormality of the colon. The patient was known to be in good health 5 years after the bowel resection.

Comment

The clinical features underestimated the extent of the pathology found at operation. The abscess in the mesentery of the sigmoid and mesorectum was complex and would have tracked further if resection had been avoided. An abscess in the mesorectum as distal as in this example is unusual. Although complicated, the disease was still localized to the large bowel and its mesentery, which greatly reduced the risk of postoperative morbidity.

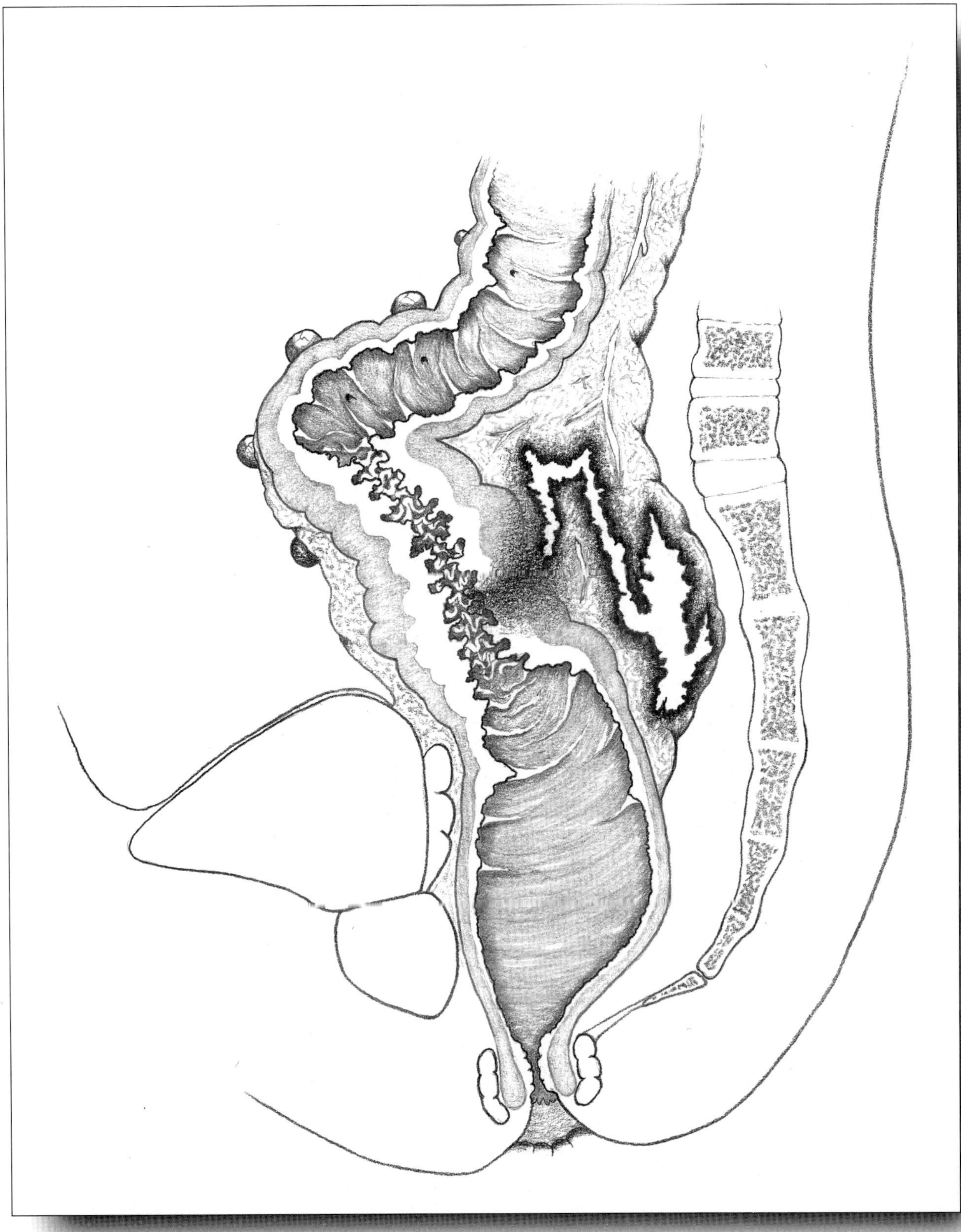

CASE

43 Diverticulitis: Colovesical Fistula

Female, 85 Years

History

The patient presented with a 5-week history of urinary frequency, hematuria (clots), and probable pneumaturia. Constipation had been present over the same period. An intravenous pyelogram revealed an extravesical mass on the upper left aspect of the bladder. A colonoscopy confirmed diverticular disease of the sigmoid colon where the lumen was narrowed and the mucosa hyperemic and edematous. A cystoscopy examination confirmed a mass bulging into the upper left wall of the bladder and covered with hyperemic mucosa. A fistula opening was not identified. Operation was advised, mindful of the fact that the patient's husband had died some years previously after a resection for diverticular disease.

Operation (7.28.97)

Catheters were placed in both ureters. Laparotomy revealed a mass in the mid proximal third of the sigmoid colon adherent to the left side of the bladder, which was indurated at that site. Digital dissection separated the colon and bladder to reveal a small chronic perforation in the colon that had been in communication with an abscess in the wall of the bladder. The sigmoid colon and upper rectum were resected and an anastomosis performed with a circular stapler. The abscess cavity in the wall of the bladder was curetted and suction irrigation drains placed into the defect. No communication between the abscess and the lumen of the bladder was identified.

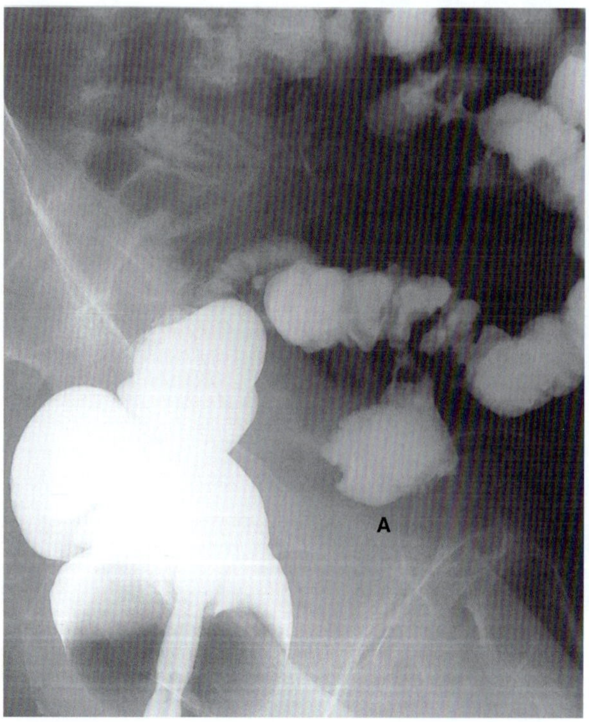

Figure 43.1: Barium enema shows significant extravasation of barium into an abscess cavity (A).

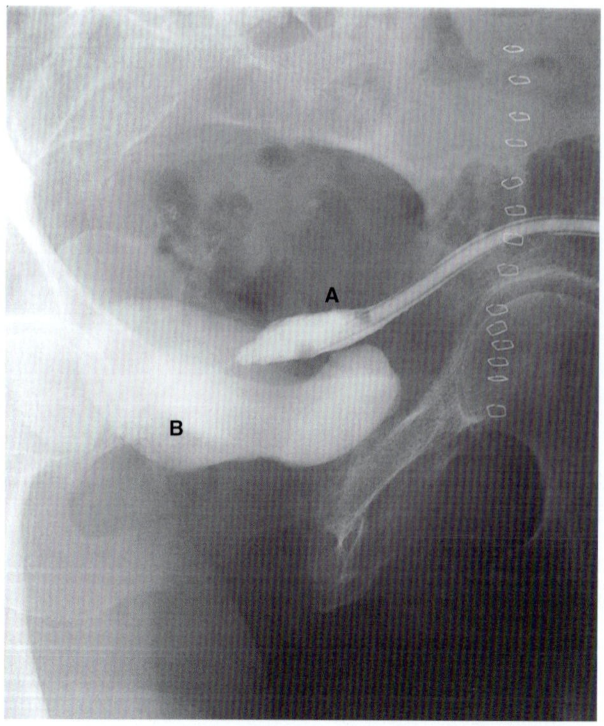

Figure 43.2: Sinogram (day 11) showing significant contraction of abscess cavity (A) and communication with bladder lumen (B).

Pathology
The resected colon showed changes of chronic diverticular disease. In addition to the site of the chronic perforation, there were several diverticula showing evidence of focal inflammatory changes.

Postoperative Course
On the 10th postoperative day, a limited gastrograffin enema showed no evidence of a leak from the anastomosis. On the 11th postoperative day, a sinogram showed contraction of the bladder wall abscess and a communication with the lumen of the bladder (Figure 43.2). On the 16th postoperative day, a sinogram showed resolution of the abscess space and no communication with the bladder. The drain was removed.

Follow-Up (2005)
The patient developed dementia within a year of the operation and, at the age of 92, requires full-time care. There has been no recurrence of gastrointestinal symptoms.

Comment
The diverticular abscess was clearly demonstrated by the barium enema (Figure 43.1) but not by the colonoscopy which, however, was essential to exclude carcinoma. In the assessment of colovesical fistula (CVF), a computerized tomography (CT) examination (not performed in this case) is credited with an accuracy of more than 90%.[1] At operation, the track of the fistula into the lumen of the bladder was not demonstrable. It can be identified in 2/3 of patients with a CVF due to diverticular disease.[2] The one-stage resection, even in the presence of an abscess, is currently recommended for elective operation for CVF.[1,3] The prolonged suction drainage of the abscess site was instigated to reduce the risk of delayed pelvic sepsis.[4] The communication with the bladder was demonstrated on the postoperative sinogram (Figure 43.2).

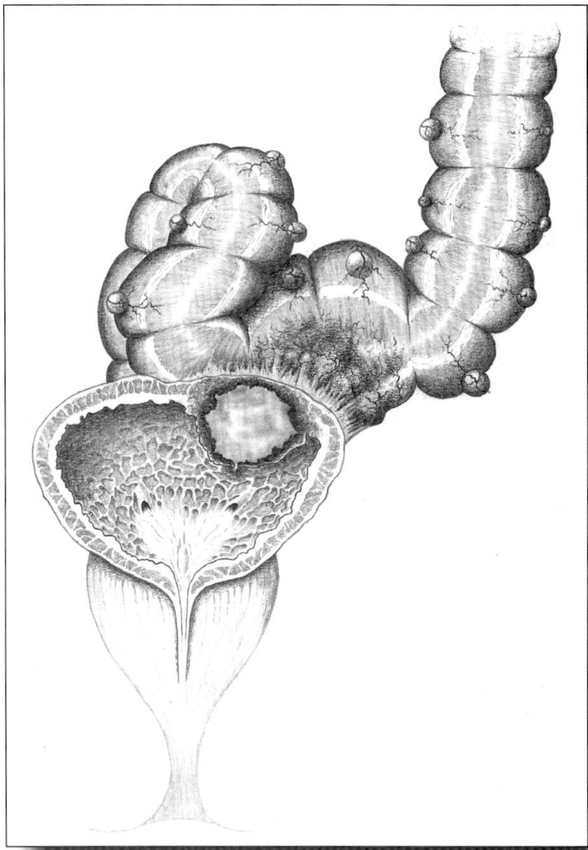

For a full-page image of this figure see the appendix.

CASE

44 Dissecting Diverticulitis

Male, 83 Years

History

The patient, whose health problems included ischemic heart disease and atrial fibrillation, presented with an episode of rectal bleeding that occurred over a 2-day period. A barium enema showed "extensive diverticular disease involving the sigmoid colon, where there is a parallel sinus track 7 cm in length, inferior to the narrowed sigmoid lumen" (Figure 44.1). Colonoscopy was only possible to 33 cm, where a stricture prevented further access to the colon. There were no endoscopic features at that level to suggest malignancy. Surgical treatment was advised for the complicated diverticular disease and the possibility of an occult colon cancer.

Operation (3.14.88)

The sigmoid colon showed features of well established inflammation with induration of the bowel wall, hyperemic serosa, fatty infiltration of the pericolic tissue, and adhesions to the adjacent structures, in particular, the bladder. There was no pathology in the colon proximal to the sigmoid. The bowel was resected from the sigmoid descending junction to the upper third of the rectum with anastomosis.

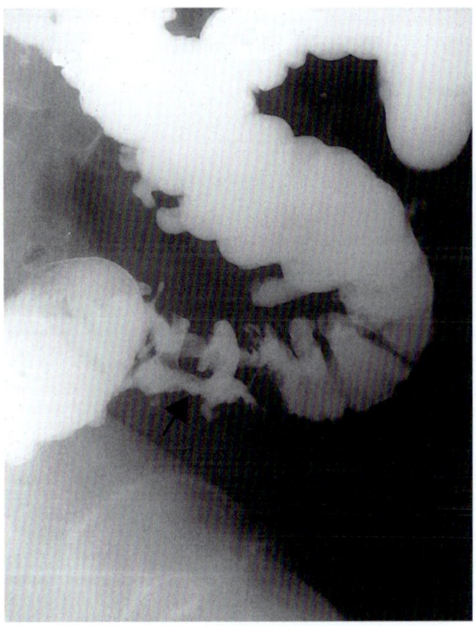

Figure 44.1: The barium enema demonstrates the longitudinal abscess parallel to the bowel (arrow).

Pathology

Chronic diverticulitis was confirmed. The stricture, 9 cm in length, was due to muscle thickening, fibrosis and a chronic abscess. The mucosa within the stricture was edematous and redundant due to the axial shortening of the bowel. The long abscess was immediately external to the muscularis propria but had not penetrated the peritoneum covering the colon. The site of a perforated diverticulum within the abscess was clearly identified.

Further Progress

Postoperative retention of urine required a transurethral prostatectomy. Histological examination of the prostatic tissue revealed carcinoma. In view of the patient's age, no therapy was recommended. The patient was last examined 7 months after the bowel resection. The anastomosis at 13 cm was satisfactory There were no bowel symptoms.

Comment

The presentation with a brief episode of minor rectal bleeding was not typical of chronic inflammatory diverticular disease. The inflammatory process, well advanced, was "silent" clinically, and, in the presence of an impassable stricture, raised the possibility of carcinoma. The abscess track was extramural and subperitoneal along the axis of the bowel so that the infection remained localized within the peritoneal compartment surrounding the colon. The term "dissecting diverticulitis" is suggested as a suitable description for this unusual manifestation of diverticulitis.

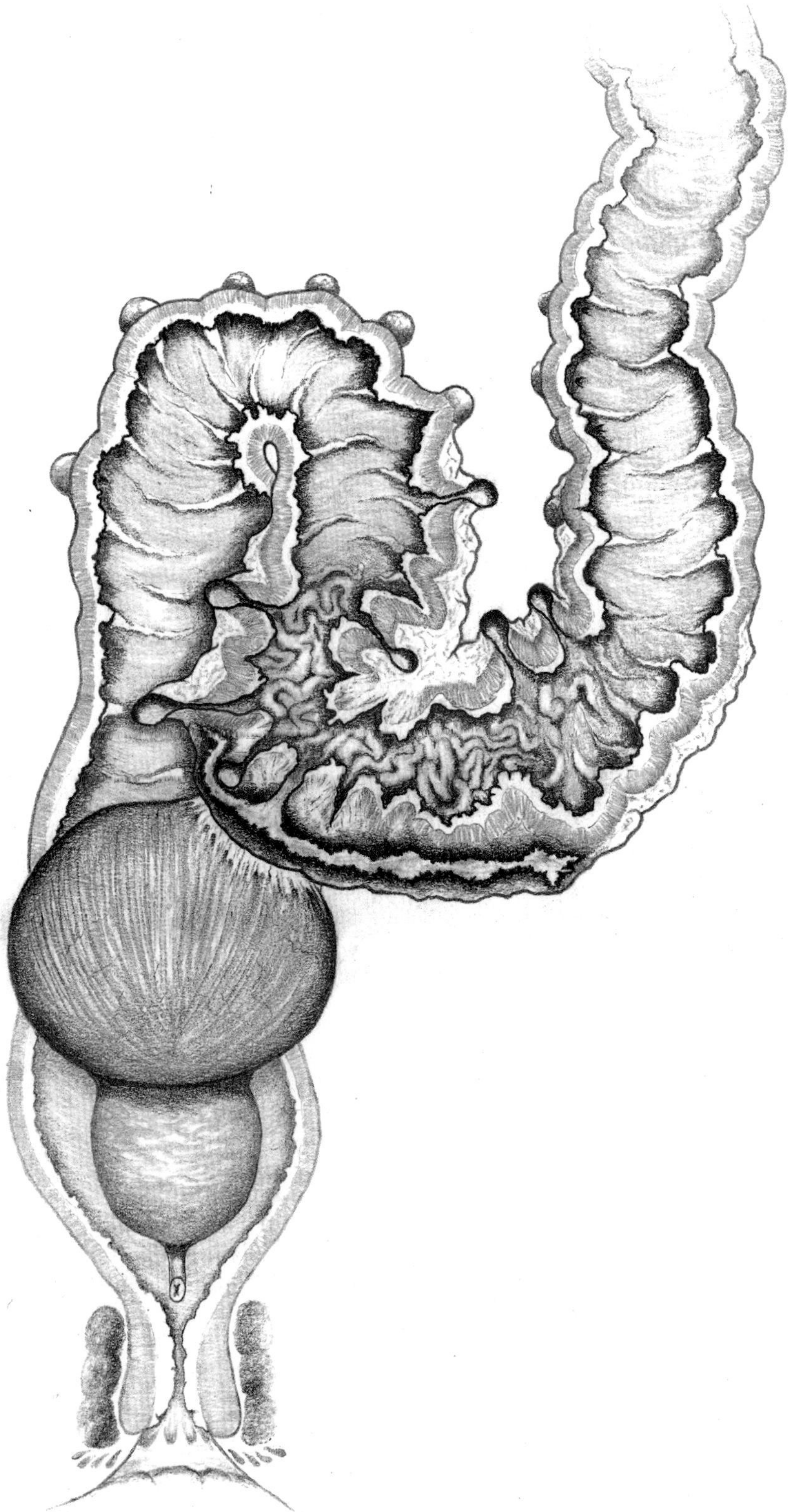

CASE

45 Annular Extramural Dissecting Diverticulitis

Female, 67 Years

History

The patient had undergone laparotomy for a "diverticular abscess" 16 years previously, but details were not available. The present illness commenced with pain in the left iliac fossa 6 weeks previously and was accompanied by diarrhea and abdominal distention. A tender mass was present in the left iliac fossa (LIF) that was also palpable on rectal examination. The pelvic floor was subtle on palpation, indicating it was not involved. Colonoscopy was limited by a stricture in the sigmoid colon. There was no endoscopic evidence of malignancy. A limited barium enema demonstrated a stricture of the mid sigmoid colon with obstruction proximal to it (Figure 45.1). There was mucosal continuity within the stricture, suggesting it was inflammatory.

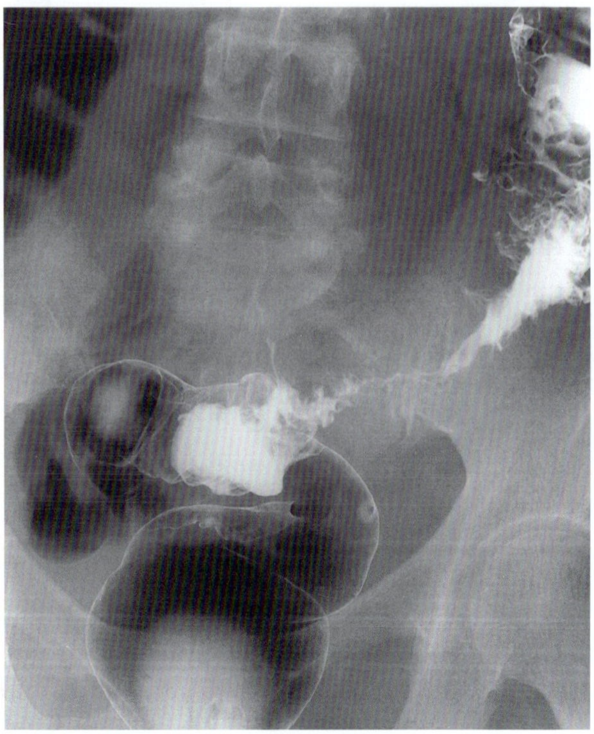

Figure 45.1: The barium enema demonstrates the stricture, with mucosal continuity.

Operation (4.2.84)

A large inflammatory mass was present in the mid third of the sigmoid colon "prolapsed" into the pelvis and adherent to adjacent structures. There was no pericolic abscess present. The large bowel was dilated due to the obstruction. There were many diverticula in the left colon and splenic flexure with areas of induration in the latter. The bowel was resected from mid rectum to distal transverse colon, and, after retrograde irrigation of the colon from the proximal level of resection, the anastomosis was constructed with a circular stapler. Although the circulation in the marginal vessels appeared adequate, much of the colon exhibited a cyanotic discoloration. This was thought to be a manifestation of the colon obstruction accompanied by significant edema of the bowel wall. A loop ileostomy was performed.

Postoperative Course

A cautious sigmoidoscopy 24 hours after operation revealed that the colon at the anastomosis (8 cm) was a good color although markedly edematous. A limited contrast enema prior to the patient's discharge from hospital demonstrated the anastomosis to be intact.

Pathology

The stricture was due to a severe focus of diverticulitis that had formed an extramural encircling abscess at the level of the perforated diverticulum. There was marked fibrosis associated with the abscess as well as muscular thickening and redundancy of the mucosa. In the vicinity of the splenic flexure, 4 foci of localized diverticulitis were identified.

Operation (6.15.84)

The loop ileostomy was closed 7 weeks after the resection.

Follow-Up (2004)

No further bowel trouble has occurred in a 20-year follow up period.

Comment

The onset of diverticulitis of the colon may be relatively silent and more like malignant disease. The established pathology in this patient suggested the inflammatory process had been present for longer than the history of 6 weeks. The annular abscess had dissected around the colon in the extramural plane. This configuration has been noted in 1% of the author's series of elective resections for diverticular disease.[1] Multiple foci have been present in 16.6% of 208 primary (no previous resection) operations and 5 foci in 0.5%.[1] The poor circulation of the colon was attributed to the acute on chronic obstructive pathology in the bowel wall. If misinterpreted, it could persuade the surgeon to resect an excessive length of colon. The postoperative sigmoidoscopy on the first postoperative day was a reassuring investigation.

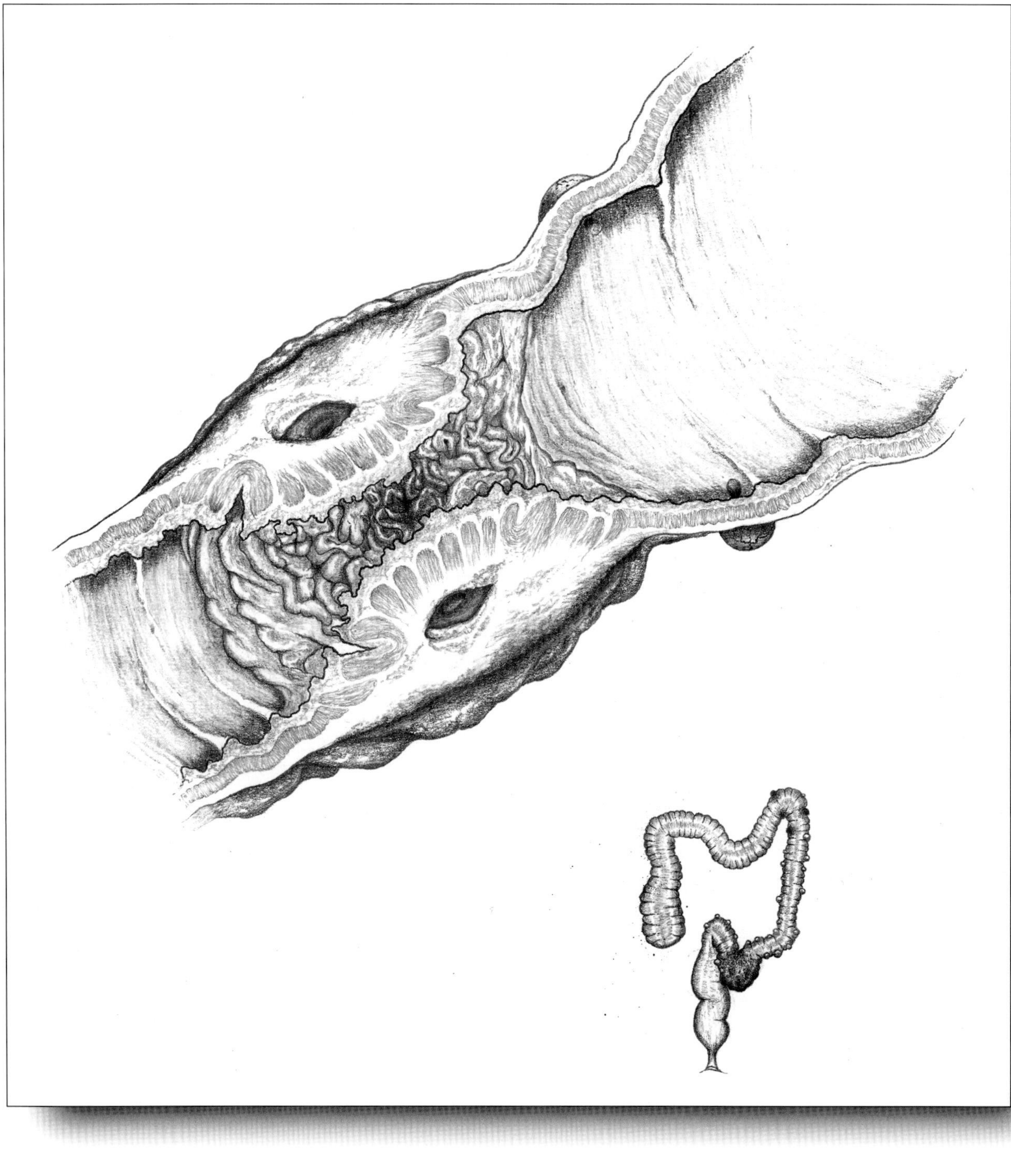

CASE

46 Giant Diverticulum

Female, 71 Years

History

The patient had noticed left-sided abdominal discomfort, night sweats, and a discharge of pale green mucus from the rectum for 2 months. Pelvic examination revealed a soft cystic mass in the pelvis. On flexible sigmoidoscopy, there was purulent material in the sigmoid colon and rectum and diverticular disease was noted. A barium enema examination reported diverticular disease with narrowing in the sigmoid colon most likely due to benign disease (Figure 46.1). Examination under anesthesia revealed a soft fluctuant mass in the pelvis and left iliac fossa that appeared to soften during examination. A diagnosis was made of pelvic abscess due to diverticulitis.

Operation (5.19.75)

There was a large cystic swelling attached to the mid sigmoid colon with chronic inflammatory changes on the surface. The swelling extended into the pelvis. Diverticular disease was present in the sigmoid colon. Resection of the sigmoid colon with anastomosis was performed.

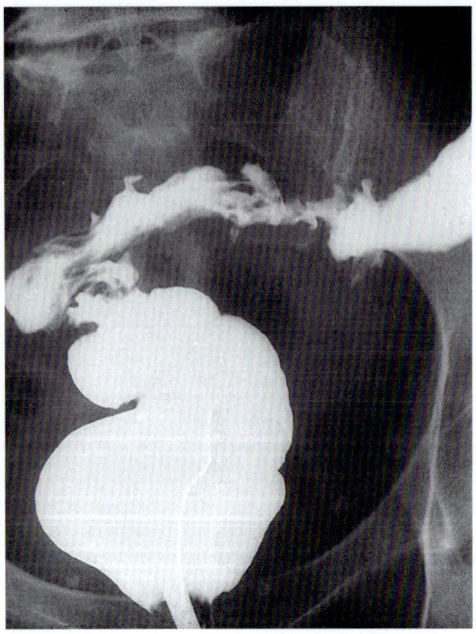

Figure 46.1: The barium enema failed to demonstrate the giant diverticulum.

Pathology

A cystic swelling 10 cm in diameter was attached to the colon. On section, its wall was 0.4 cm in depth. There was a communication with the lumen of the colon (Figure 46.2). There was purulent material within the "cyst," the lining of which showed changes of chronic inflammation. Histological examination of the wall of the cyst revealed dense vascular collagen tissue with 1 focus of colonic epithelium.

Comment

The giant diverticulum presented as a pelvic abscess. The lesion had formed a "sac of pus" within the pelvis. There was no radiological evidence of the lesion, which contrasts with the large gas-filled cyst on abdominal x-ray that can be present.[1,2,3,4] In the immediate preoperative period, the patient's night sweats ceased, undoubtedly due to the spontaneous discharge of pus into the lumen of the colon. Choong et al. reports 4 patients treated by diverticulectomy (2), initial diverticulectomy and subsequent sigmoid resection (1), and sigmoid resection (1) with successful outcome.[4] In reviewing the literature, they suggest that patients with few normal elements of bowel wall in the diverticulum be classified as Type I, whereas those with all layers of the bowel wall be classified as Type II and are related to colonic duplication. Patients with the thin-walled diverticulum, as occurred in this patient, are presumably the type that might be treated by diverticulectomy.

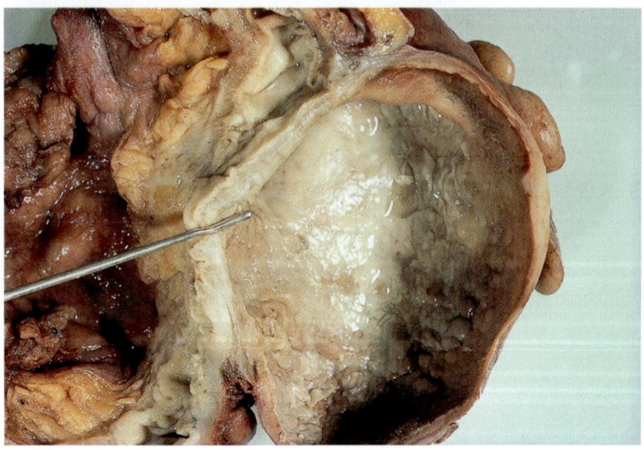

Figure 46.2: The communication between the colon and the thin-walled diverticulum.

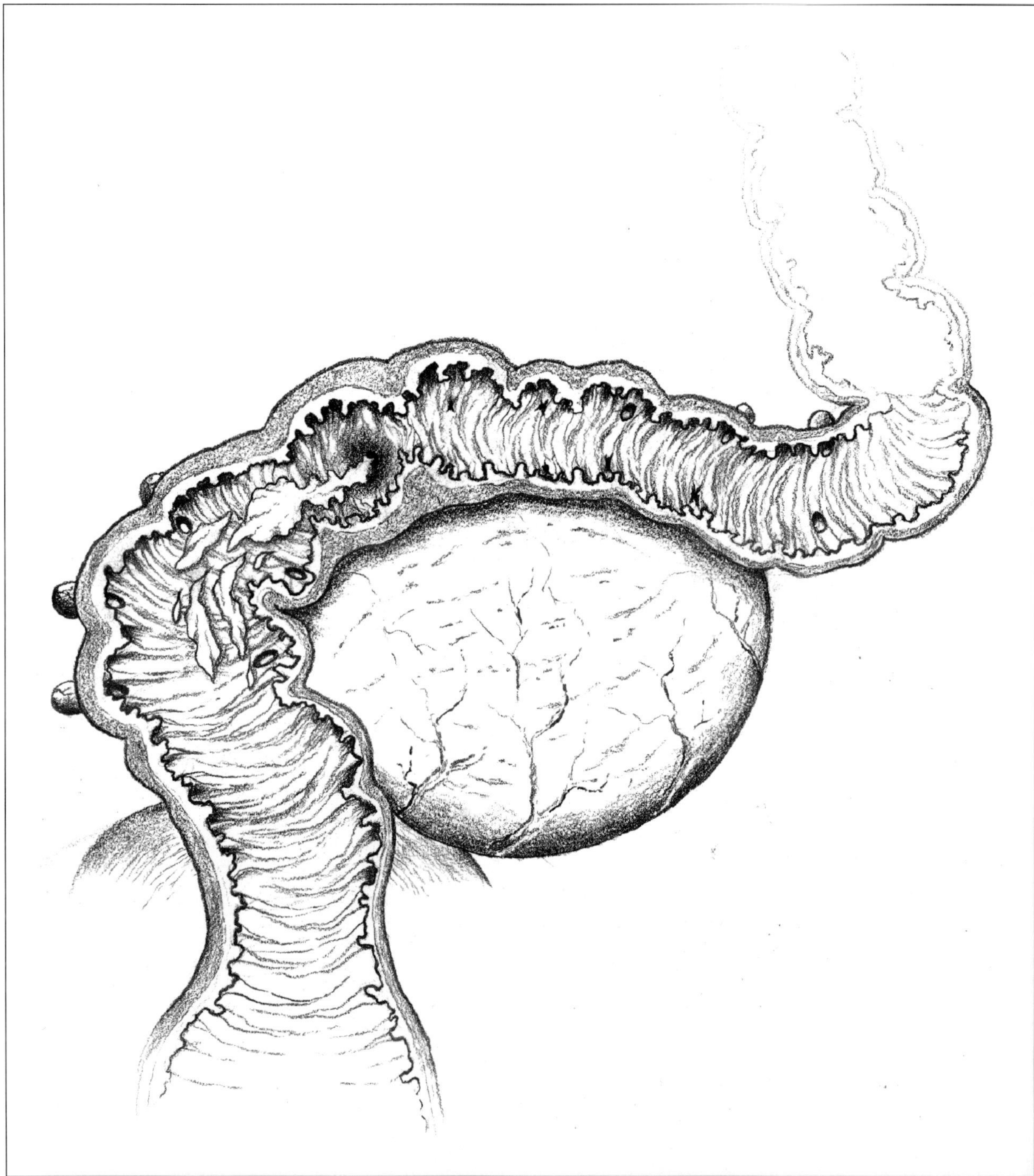

CASE

47 Giant Diverticulum

Male, 71 Years

History

The patient complained of pain and tenderness in the left iliac fossa for 10 days. There had been rigors during 1 night in this period. There was no disturbance of bowel function. Clinical examination was normal. A barium enema showed well marked diverticular disease in the sigmoid colon and an associated "giant cyst" containing fecal residue (Figure 47.1). Colonoscopy to the hepatic flexure revealed no stricture of the sigmoid colon or mucosal pathology.

Operation (6.10.82)

There was a large cystic swelling within the mesentery of the sigmoid colon which was attached to the bladder by an intervening small, chronic abscess. Changes of chronic diverticular disease were apparent. The sigmoid colon and upper rectum were resected with anastomosis.

Pathology

The 20 cm length of colon contained extensive diverticulosis with a large diverticulum that had a thick (1 cm) fibrous wall. The cavity of the lesion measured 4.5 cm in diameter and was packed with "ribbon like" material, presumably vegetable food residue that was not examined histologically. It was lined by chronic inflammatory tissue, and colonic mucosa was present in some areas. Communication with the lumen of the sigmoid colon was identified.

Comment

A giant diverticulum may be apparent on an abdominal x-ray as a large, gas-filled cyst (Figure 47.2). Choong et al report that this is present in most patients,[1] although it was not so in this patient or in Case 46. The incidence of giant diverticulum in the author's series of elective resection for diverticular disease was 2/208 (1%).[2] The condition requires

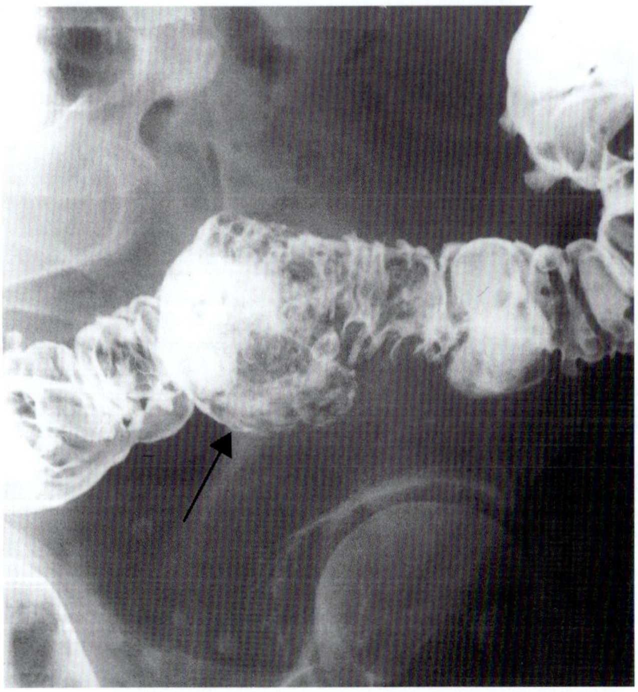

Figure 47.1: The barium enema demonstrates the diverticulum (arrow).

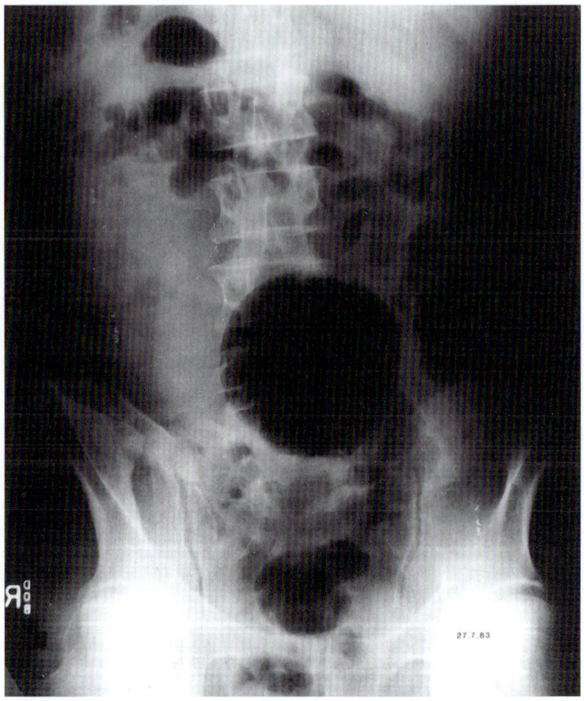

Figure 47.2: A giant diverticulum may present as a gas-filled "cyst" on plain x-ray of the abdomen (courtesy of Prof. E.L. Bokey). Different patient.

surgical treatment, because of the potential complications of infection, torsion, and perforation.[3] The latter two complications would seem unlikely in this case with a very thick-walled diverticulum and a broad attachment to the wall of the sigmoid colon. Diverticulectomy was not considered for this patient.

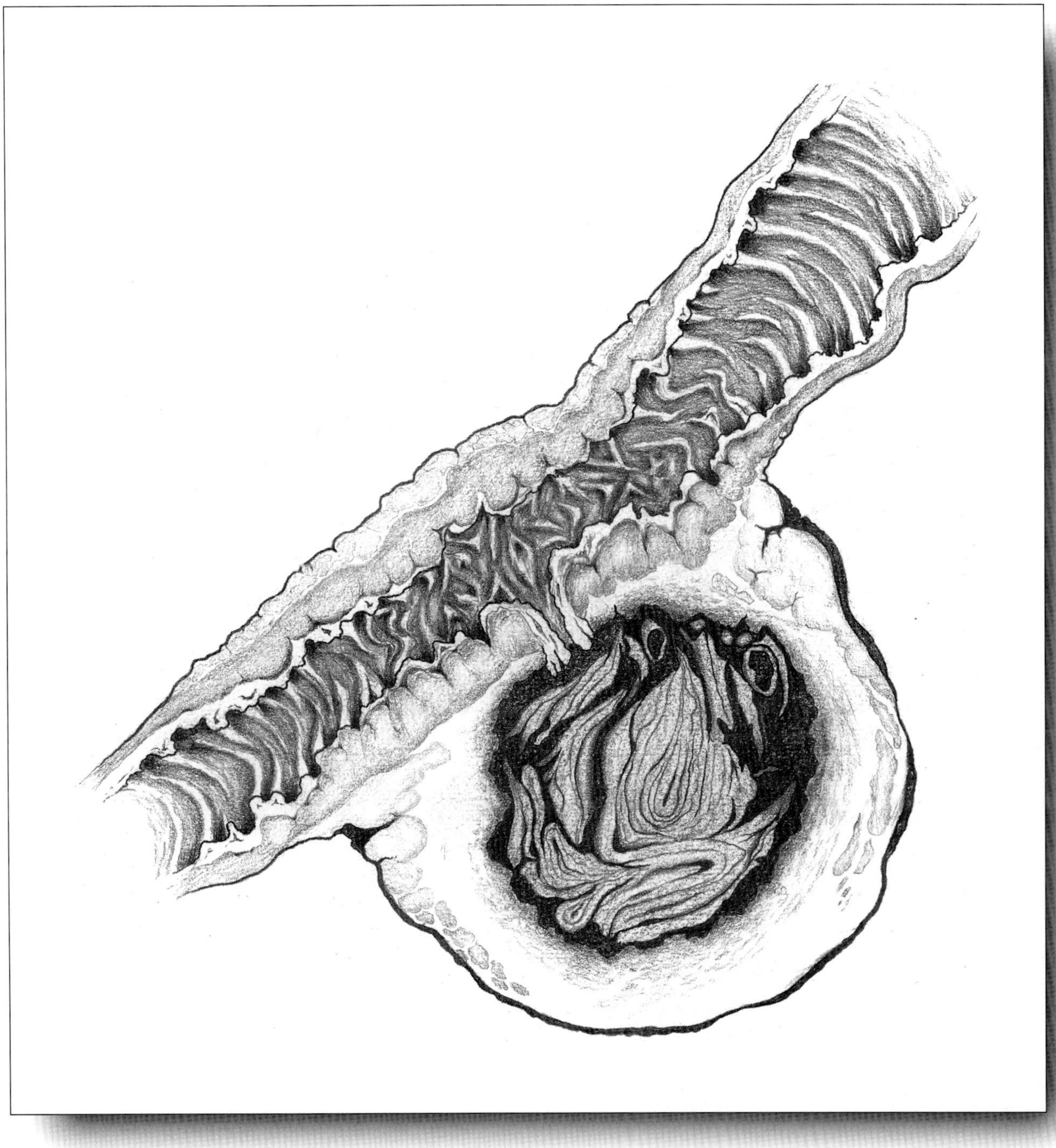

CASE

48 Diverticulitis: Large Bowel Obstruction

Female, 66 Years

History

Recurrent diverticulitis had been diagnosed 15 years previously, and mild episodes, always responding to antibiotic therapy, continued during this period. The patient presented with a 4-week history of lower abdominal colicky pain, constipation, and rectal bleeding on 1 occasion. A firm pelvic mass was present on rectal examination. A short colonoscopy was performed with the small caliber panendoscope, and a tight sigmoid stricture was negotiated, establishing the diagnosis of sigmoid diverticulitis. A cautious contrast enema showed dilatation of the colon above the stricture and no pathology in the proximal colon (Figure 48.1). Within a few weeks, the patient developed further severe pain, nausea, and vomiting. Operation was expedited.

Operation (6.24.94)

Laparotomy revealed marked dilatation of the colon above the pathology in the mid sigmoid colon. The wall of the colon was thickened, indicative of long-standing obstruction. The colon was deflated with a cannula and irrigated clear of feces. The bowel was resected from upper descending colon to lower third of the rectum, and a hand sutured anastomosis was performed. The operation was completed with a loop ileostomy.

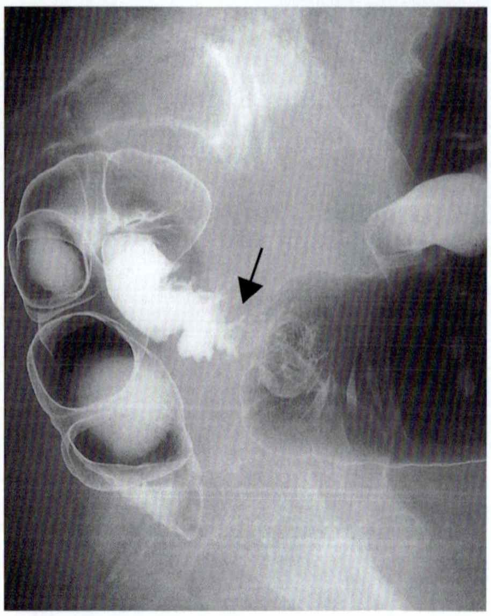

Figure 48.1: A barium enema demonstrates the diverticular stricture (arrow) and dilated colon.

Pathology

Examination confirmed the diagnosis of chronic diverticulitis with stricture formation at which point the thickness of the bowel wall measured 15 mm. There was an abscess within the strictured area, and the mucosa immediately proximal to the stricture was cyanotic, edematous, and ulcerated. Histologically these ulcers revealed no specific features; several diverticula in the sigmoid colon showed early abscess formation.

Operation (8.15.94)

The postoperative recovery was satisfactory. The ileostomy was closed 7 weeks after the resection.

Follow-Up

No further bowel problems occurred. Six months after operation, the patient was found to have a high grade transitional cell carcinoma of the bladder. Radical surgery was performed, but the patient died of metastatic disease 2 years later.

Comment

Surprisingly, chronic diverticular disease does not often present with the degree of acute obstruction seen in this case. The abscess (extramural) in the strictured segment may have precipitated the presenting obstruction. The multiple sites of early abscesses in diverticula is also uncommon. The mucosal ulceration may have been stercoral in origin. This mucosal pathology is sometimes seen in the vicinity of an obstructing left-sided carcinoma. It may be related to an alteration in the integrity of the mucosal defense system. The technical difficulties and potential risks caused by the presence of the dilated and thickened colon with its fecal content were overcome by intraoperative colonic irrigation.

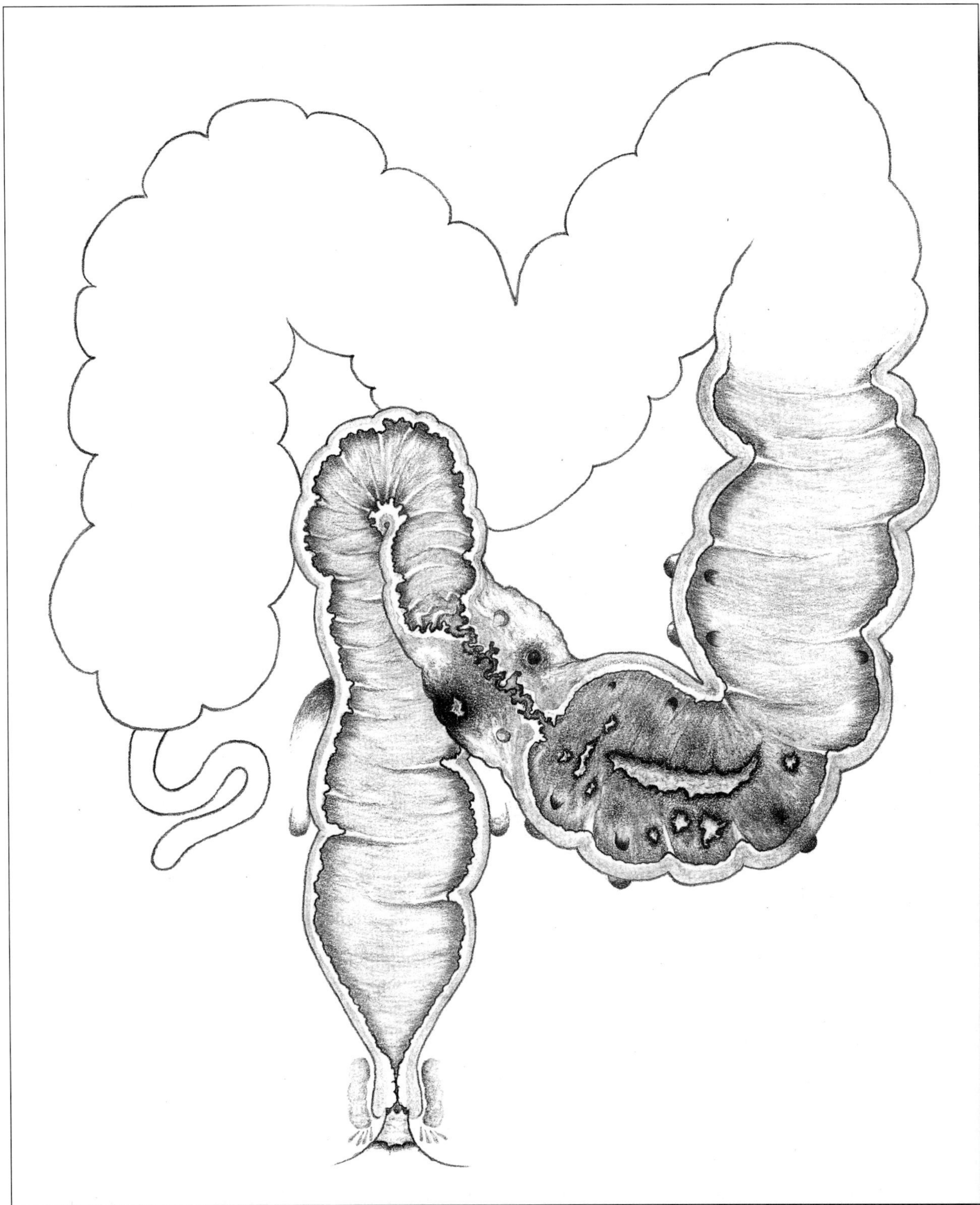

PART VI Inflammatory Bowel Disease

CASE

49 Ulceration in Crohn's Disease of the Small Bowel

The composite diagram illustrates some of the morphological types of ulceration that may be seen in small bowel Crohn's disease. Although a number of these ulcer types may appear in a patient in a contiguous segment or in skip lesions, one would not expect to see the full spectrum of ulceration in any one patient.

1. Small aphthous ulcers are the initial ulcerative lesion. They may be the only lesions or be adjacent to more severely affected bowel.
2. Slit-like fissure ulcers in otherwise normal mucosa.
3. Edema accentuates the "cobblestone" effect caused by transverse extensions of the linear ulcers. Some of the ulcers are covered with a fibrinous exudate.
4. Deep parallel ulcers adjacent to near normal mucosa. The linear ulceration is usually located on the mesenteric side of the lumen.
5. Extensive linear ulceration with more loss of mucosa isolating mucosal islands. This chronic disease is associated with thickening of all layers of the bowel wall and, as fibrosis predominates, a long stricture will form.
6. Recent ulceration that is solitary, deep, and situated in normal mucosa. Such a lesion can be the only focus of Crohn's disease present in the intestinal tract.
7. Healed ulceration that is covered with atrophic mucosa and is associated with loss of mucosal features and fibrosis.
8. Acute foci of ulceration surrounded by normal mucosa. The histological diagnosis of Crohn's disease may be difficult in this stage of the disease.
9. Acute severe and extensive ulceration usually affects only the terminal ileum in association with the fulminant form of acute Crohn's colitis. The mucosa is "shredded" by the severe inflammatory process, exposing the underlying muscle.

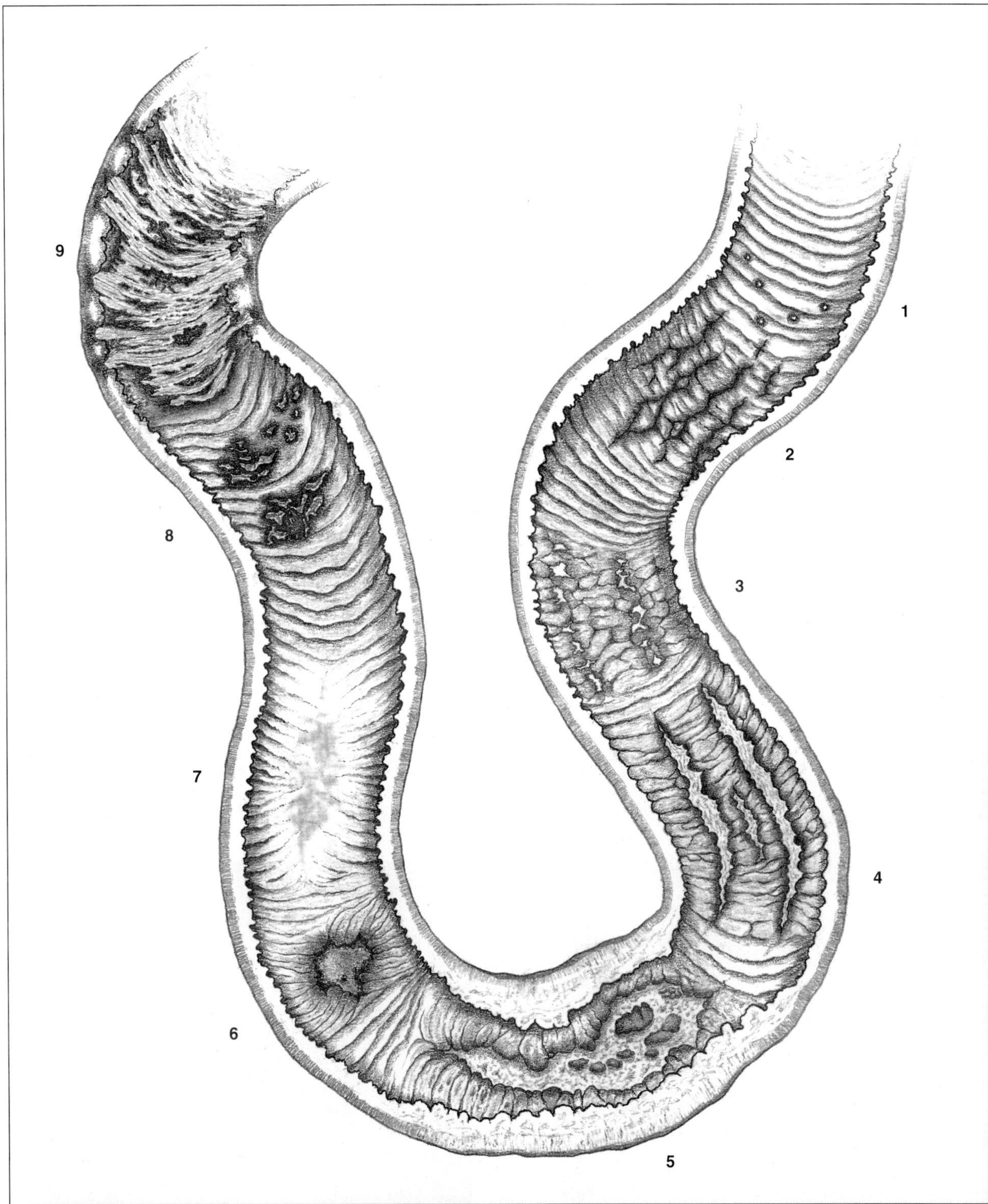
9
1
2
8
3
7
4
6
5

CASE

50 Recurrent Crohn's Disease

Female, 51 Years

History

1971 At 25 years of age **resection** of Crohn's disease of the ileum. Severe diarrhea continued despite medical treatment.

1978 **Resection of terminal ileum** (40 cm) for recurrent Crohn's disease (Figure 50.1). Severe diarrhea continued (14–15/day, 3–4 night). Figure 50.1 shows the involvement of the terminal ileum.

1981 **Resection of right colon** (25 cm) **and ileum** (40 cm) for recurrent Crohn's disease associated with large inflammatory mass. Diarrhea continued (8/day, 0/night).

1996 X-ray and colonoscopy evidence of recurrent disease with marked stricture formation (Figure 50.2).

1997 The patient remained debilitated with diarrhea (12–15/day), abdominal pain, and fever. **Resection of ileum** (26 cm) **and ascending colon** (6 cm) was performed for advanced Crohn's disease with stricture formation causing chronic obstruction. Remaining small bowel measured 115 cm.

1998 **Pyelotomy** for renal calculus and infection.

2000 (June) Diarrhea (12/day), anovaginal fistula with minor symptoms, managed conservatively.

2000 (October) Patient described her health as "good" with minimal symptoms from the anovaginal fistula. No further follow-up is available.

Comment

The case illustrates the relentless natural history of Crohn's disease over a 30-year period. The four resections failed to relieve the most troublesome symptom (diarrhea). Medical therapy was not helpful. The patient could not tolerate steroids which caused debilitating candidiasis. Until the last examination in October 2000, the patient preferred to manage without anti-inflammatory drug therapy.

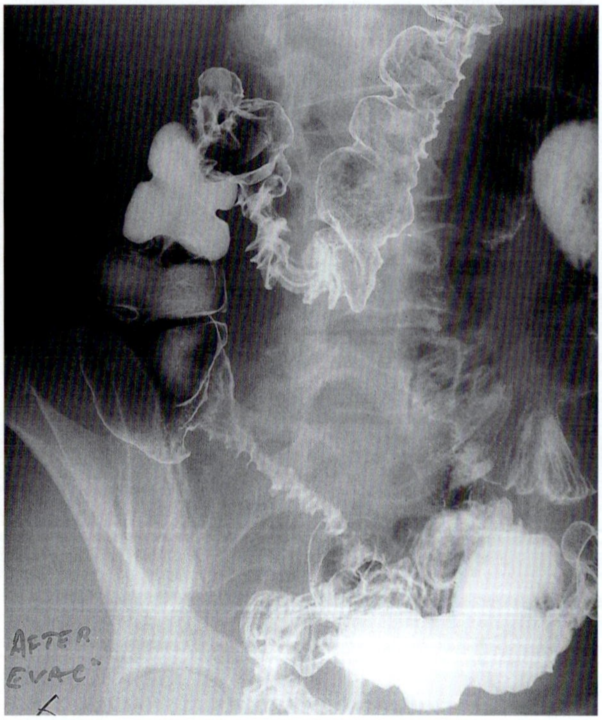

Figure 50.1: Recurrence in terminal ileum in 1978 after first resection.

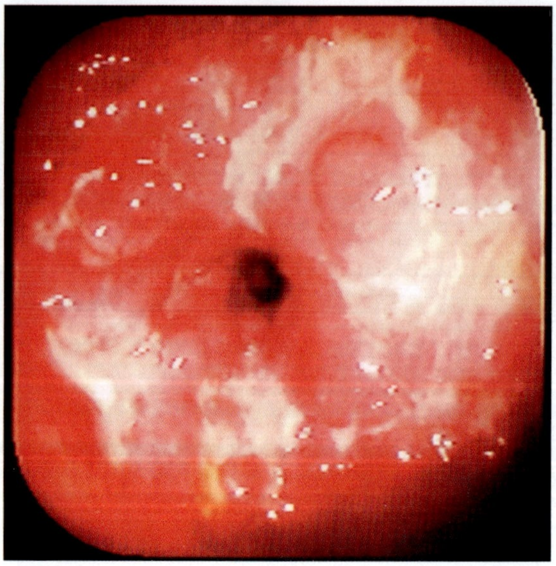

Figure 50.2: Colonoscopy (1996) showing recurrent Crohn's disease and anastomotic stricture.

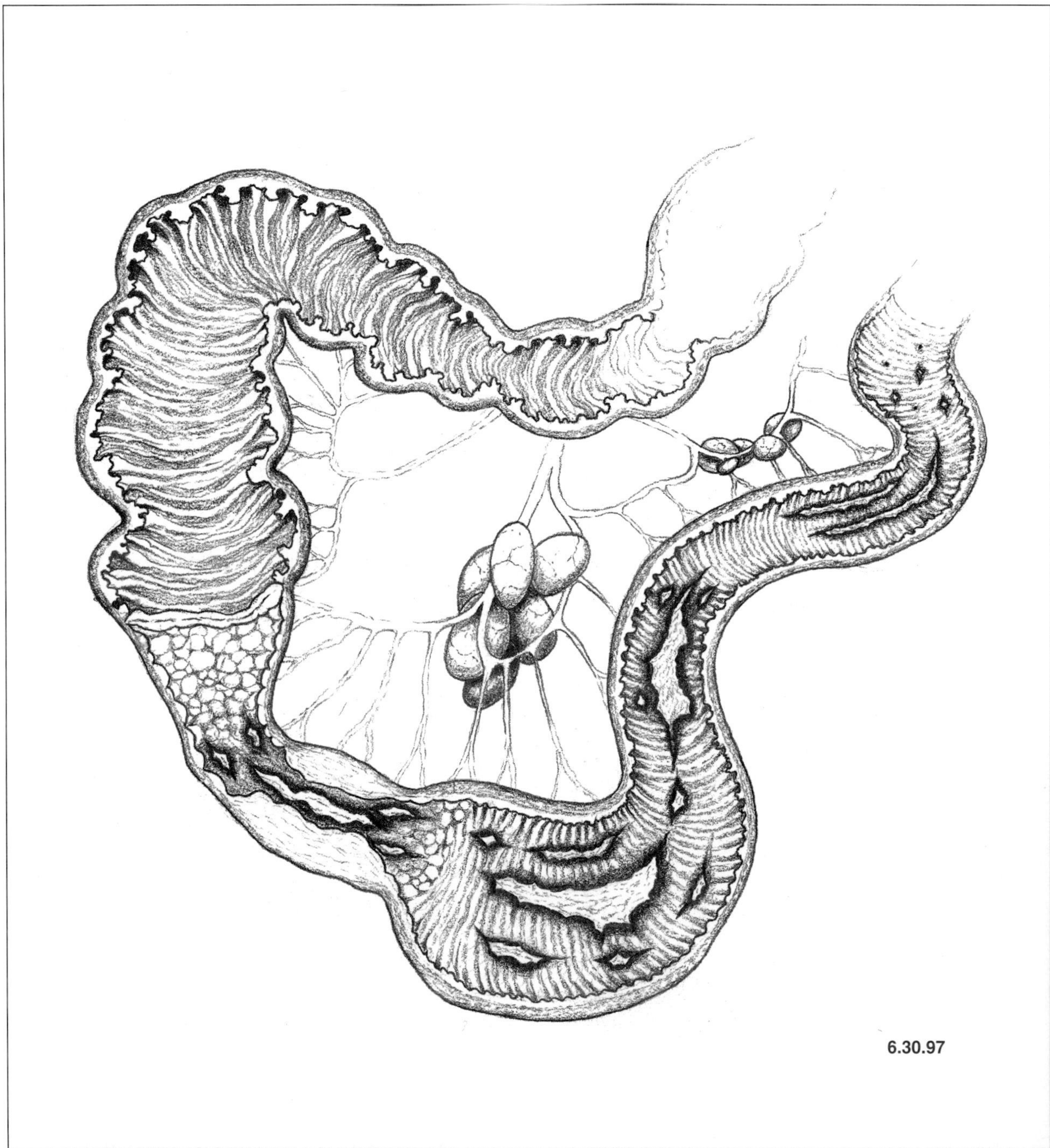
6.30.97

CASE

51 Crohn's Disease: Strictures of Ascending Colon and Doudenum

Female, 34 Years

History

Crohn's disease of the ascending colon was diagnosed in 1984. The symptoms of abdominal pain and diarrhea were relieved by treatment with prednisolone and sulfasalazine. Five years later, the patient was suffering from episodes of severe abdominal pain, and investigations revealed a long stricture of the ileum and ascending colon (Figure 51.1) associated with a large right-sided abdominal mass.

Operation (5.25.89)

A large mass involving the right colon was firmly adherent to the anterior abdominal wall and 15 cm of the adjacent terminal ileum, which was also affected by the inflammatory process. There were no

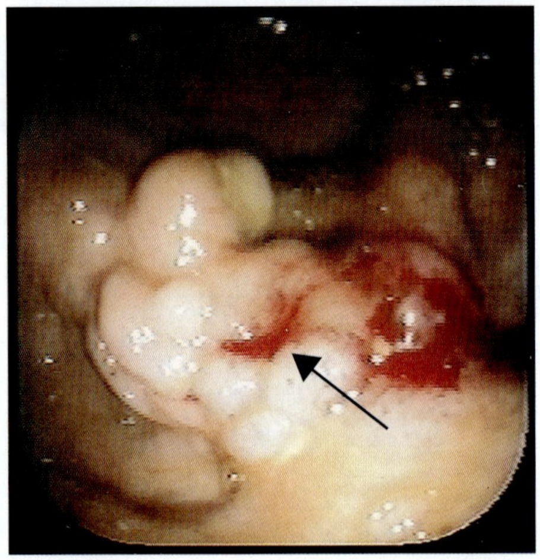

Figure 51.2: Recurrent disease with stenosis of the ileocolic anastomosis indicated by the arrow: March 2000.

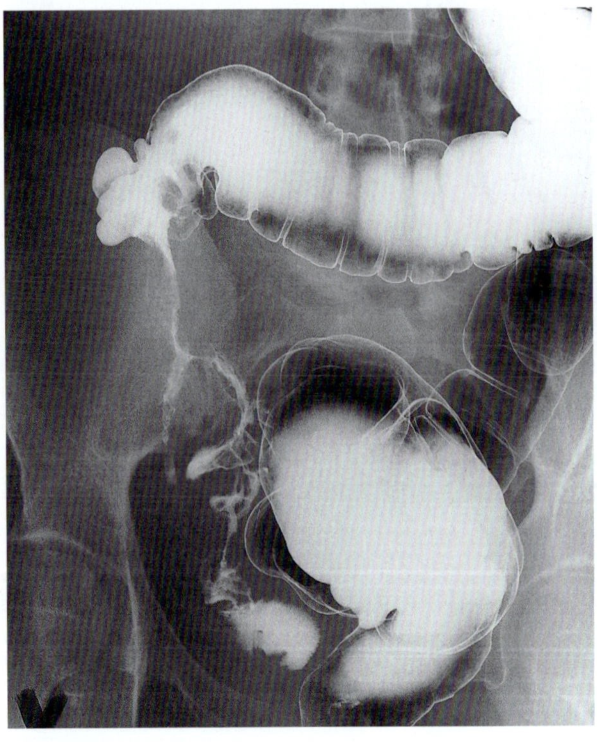

Figure 51.1: Demonstrating stricture and spasm of the terminal ileum and ascending colon prior to right hemicolectomy in 1989.

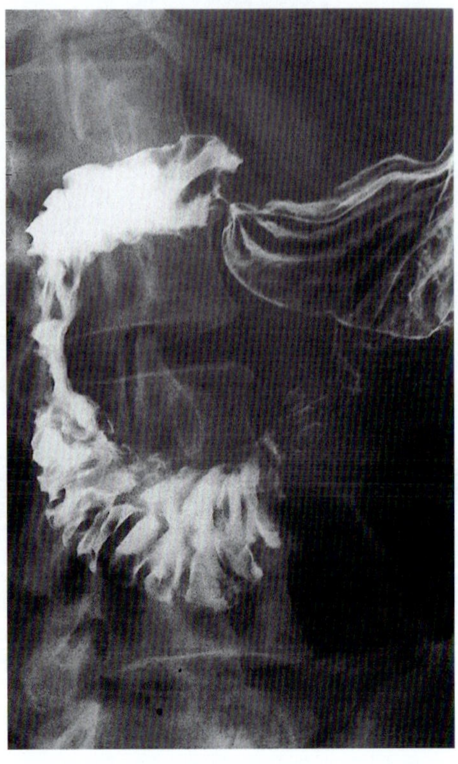

Figure 51.3: The stricture D2 persists with a further narrowed segment in D3: May 2004.

apparent "skip" areas affected in the remainder of the gastrointestinal tract. A right hemicolectomy with 20 cm of ileum was performed.

Pathology

The mass measured 10 × 11 cm and was mainly due to gross thickening of polypoid mucosa, muscle wall, and pericolic fat in the ascending colon. The mucosal surface within the stricture was atrophic, with scars due to previous ulceration. The appendix was markedly distended due to proximal obstruction of its lumen. There were 4 ulcers in the ileum, the largest of which extended for 9 cm along the mucosa. Prominent enlarged mesenteric nodes were present. The histological changes were consistent with Crohn's disease. Two typical granulomas were found in a lymph node.

Follow-Up (2004)

At colonoscopy (11.30.89), a dysplastic villous adenoma (0.9 cm) of the sigmoid colon was removed. Further colonoscopies were normal until 10 years and 6 months after resection when a stenosis of the anastomosis was diagnosed (Figure 51.2). A small bowel x-ray series demonstrated a stricture of the second part of the duodenum (0.6 cm in diameter). This was confirmed on panendoscopy, which revealed associated inflammation and ulceration. Biopsies showed inflammation not diagnostic of Crohn's disease although this diagnosis was accepted. The patient was treated with prednisolone for 5 months. Azathioprine and mesalazine were commenced in 2000 and are current therapy. The stricture in the second part of the duodenum has been treated at intervals with balloon dilatation. Now 15 years since operation, x-rays show persistence of the stricture in the second part of the duodenum and a moderate narrowing in the third part of the duodenum (Figure 51.3). Colonoscopy demonstrates persistence of the ileocolic anastomotic stricture. The patient has infrequent bouts of distention and reflux sometimes accompanied by vomiting.

Comment

The right hemicolectomy specimen showed active Crohn's disease in addition to resolved inflammation, which caused a mass, stricture, and pseudopolyps. The duodenal disease has persisted with the development of a second stricture. The patient's symptoms at present are not troublesome enough to justify surgical intervention. The incidence of duodenal involvement in patients with Crohn's disease is uncommon. Yamamoto et al have reported an incidence of 5% in a series of patients from Birmingham UK.[1]

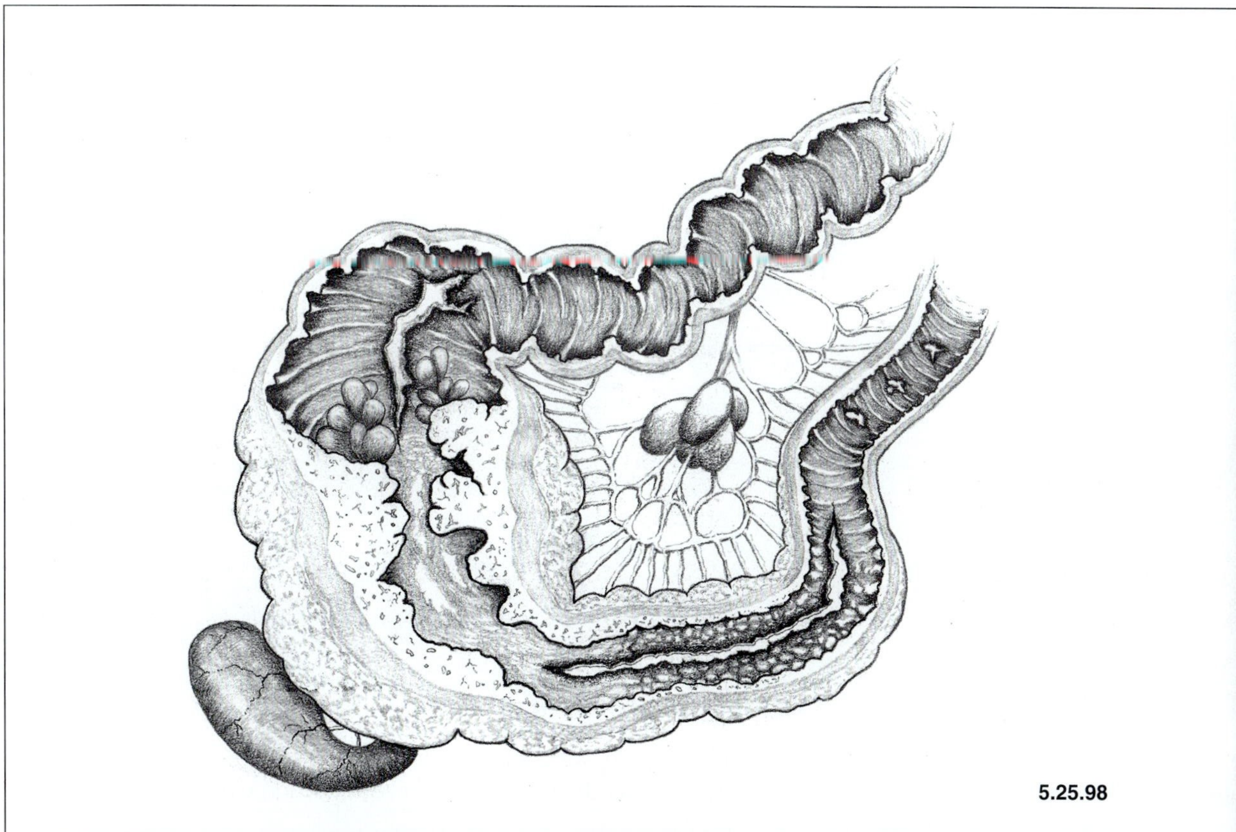

For a full-page image of this figure see the appendix.

CASE

52 The Appendix, Fistulae, and Pseudopolyps in Crohn's Disease

Female, 12 Years

History

In 1982 at the age of 9 years, the patient underwent appendectomy for persistent pain in the right iliac fossa. The distal two-thirds of the appendix was described as abnormal with slight enlargement and a vascular reaction on the serosal surface. The terminal 10cm of the ileum was thickened and hyperemic with some fibrin on its surface. The cecum appeared normal. The ileocecal lymph nodes were enlarged. Histological examination of the appendix showed mild nonspecific inflammation. In 1985, the patient was referred with an enterocutaneous fistula that had recently appeared in the appendectomy scar. There was a mass in the right iliac fossa and radiological investigation demonstrated a stricture of the terminal ileum.

Operation (10.25.85)

A phlegmonous mass involved the ileum and cecum and was attached to the anterior abdominal wall at the site of an ileocutaneous fistula. The terminal ileum was thickened and the ileum immediately proximal to it dilated, indicating chronic obstruction. There were enlarged mesenteric lymph nodes in the ileocecal region. The wall of the cecum and ascending colon was thickened and a palpable mass was within the cecum. No other pathology was detected. A right hemicolectomy was performed, which resected 20cm of ileum and 25cm of colon. The anastomosis was performed with a single interrupted layer of polyglactin 910 (vicryl) sutures.

Pathology

The terminal 6–7cm of ileum was markedly thickened, forming a tight stricture at the ileocecal junction. The mucosa was chronically inflamed, atrophic in appearance, and there were several small superficial ulcers present. There were 2 mucosal "bridges" present in the terminal ileum. The mucosa of the cecum and ascending colon also showed evidence of previous inflammation, now quiescent, with an atrophic appearance and healed ulceration. The more remarkable finding was a large mass of pseudopolyps in the cecum originating from the ileocecal junction. Immediately inferior to the polyps was an ileocecal fistula, which was distal to the site of origin of the ileocutaneous fistula.

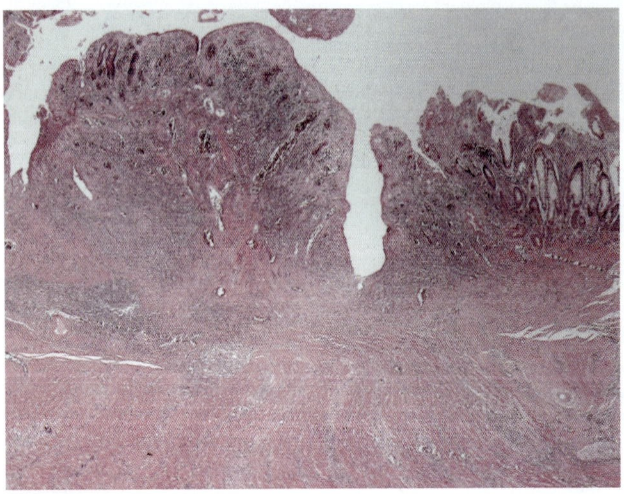

Figure 52.1: The ileum shows marked ulceration, fissure, and transmural inflammation.

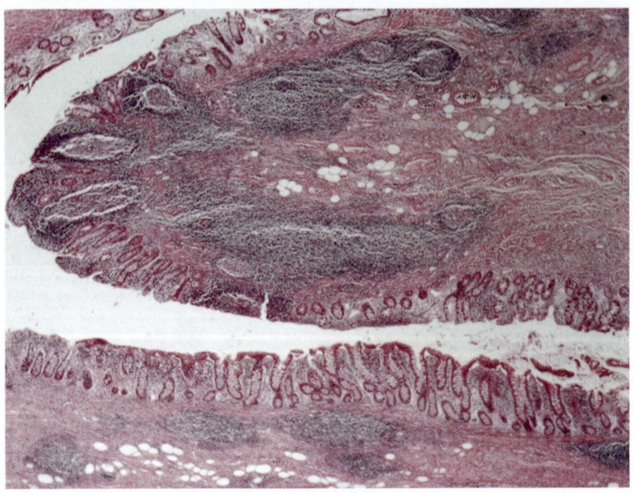

Figure 52.2: A pseudopolyp from the ileocecal junction showing a prominent lymphoid infiltrate. The architecture of the submucosa shows a traction effect.

Histologically, the mucosal changes in the pseudopolyps and ulcers showed nonspecific inflammation and fibrosis. The histological features in the bowel wall were consistent with Crohn's disease (Figure 52.1).

Follow-Up (2005)

Recovery from operation was satisfactory. There has been no further recurrence of the disease, 20 years since the ileocolic resection.

Comment

In the presence of Crohn's disease of the terminal ileum, involvement of the appendix is common. Keighley and Williams report an incidence of 24%.[1] They also state acute appendicitis in Crohn's disease as "exceedingly uncommon."[1] If operating for symptoms of acute appendicitis, many surgeons would perform appendectomy, in the presence of terminal ileitis, if the cecum were normal. Enterocutaneous and internal fistulae are recognized complications after appendectomy in the presence of Crohn's ileitis, the site of origin of the fistula being the terminal ileum[1,2] and not the appendiceal stump, as illustrated in this case report. Simonowitz et al. reviewed 20 patients who required bowel resection after incidental appendectomy in the presence of Crohn's ileitis. If the history was less than 7 days, minimal problems occurred during follow up. If the history exceeded 7 days duration, there was a 28% incidence of enterocutaneous fistula and a 44% incidence of cutaneous sinus.[2] The pseudopolyps in this patient were unusually large, and this may have been due to chronic intussusception of the polyps at the ileocecal junction (Figure 52.2). Although the ileocecal pseudopolyps appeared multiple, the lesion may qualify as an example of a giant inflammatory polyp in Crohn's disease.[3]

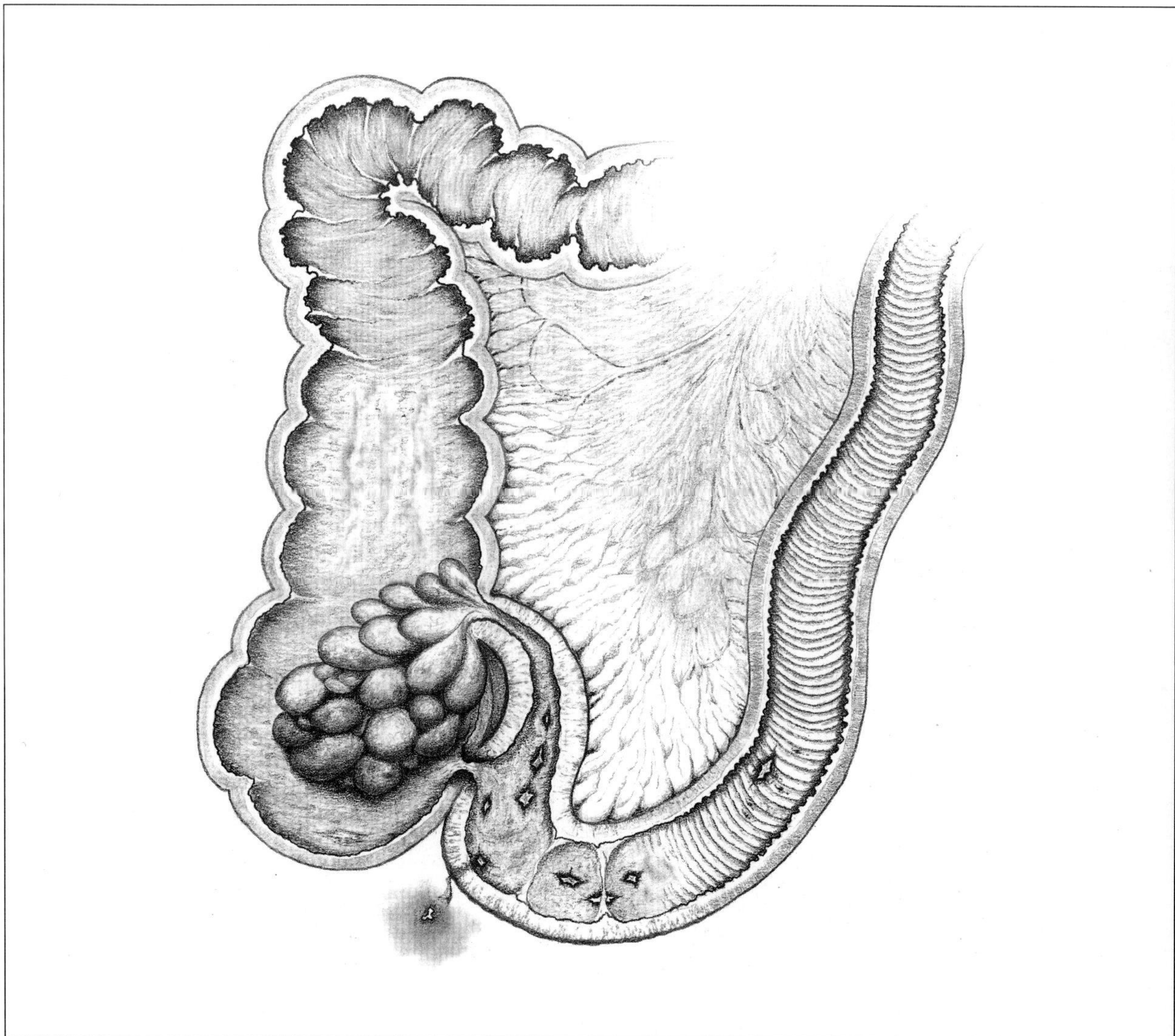

For a full-page image of this figure see the appendix.

CASE 53 A "Shamrock" Deformity Due to Crohn's Disease

Male, 52 Years

History

The patient was referred for possible surgical treatment in August 1988 with a 12-year history of Crohn's disease. He had been unwell for 12 months, with an increase in chronic diarrhea, particularly at night (×5). A barium enema showed a "disorganized" colon with shortening, sacculation, and strictures. A colonoscopy was possible only to 30 cm (stricture). An anal stricture was present, the mucosa in the mid upper rectum appeared normal, and proximal to this pseudopolyp formation was present. At this time, the patient was unwilling to undergo operation. In March 1992, clinical features of chronic large bowel obstruction were obvious. Investigations of the bowel lumen were limited by an impassible stricture at 30 cm, and a supervening carcinoma could not be excluded (Figure 53.1).

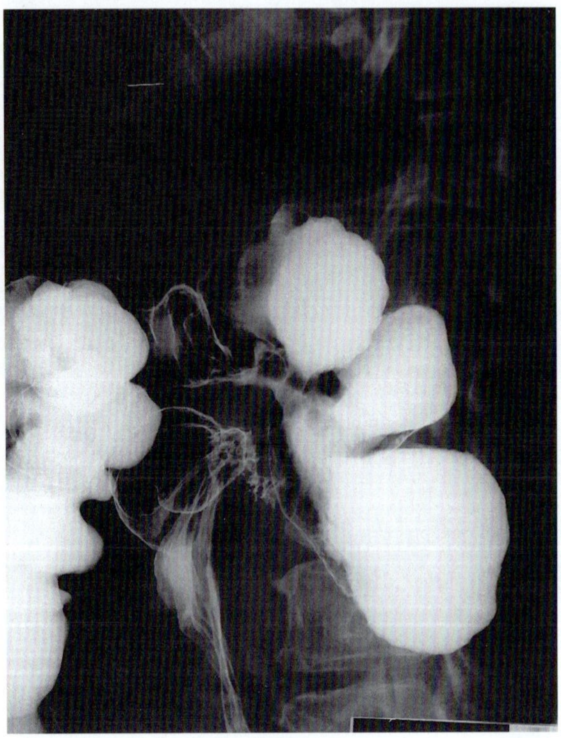

Figure 53.1: The barium enema (1992) shows the degree of bowel deformity at the splenic flexure.

Operation (2.18.93)

The transverse, descending, and sigmoid colon were grossly abnormal with shortening, thickened bowel wall, fat wrapping, and serosal inflammation. The splenic flexure was a conglomerate mass of sacculation, stricture, and colocolic fistula. The lower sigmoid colon appeared normal. There was no evidence of small bowel disease. Abdominal colectomy and ileosigmoid anastomosis were performed (end-to-end with single layer interrupted suture). Three centimeters of ileum was included in the resection.

Pathology

The opened colon revealed a bizarre distortion at the splenic flexure with 3 sacculations forming a "shamrock" deformity, two strictures, and a colocolic fistula. In the transverse colon, there were 2 areas of grouped filiform strands forming bridges across the lumen. The proximal colon showed changes of atrophic, chronically inflamed mucosa. Distal to the strictures, the inflammation of the mucosa was more marked with ulceration and "cobblestone" mucosa. Histological examination showed chronic transmural inflammation with multiple granulomata typical of Crohn's disease. The attached ileum was normal. There was no evidence of carcinoma in the strictures.

Follow-Up (2004)

The patient remains asymptomatic at 68 years of age, 11 years and 4 months following his resection. Bowel frequency is: 2–3 per day; 0 at night. Current medication is sulphasalazine 2 g daily (prescribed by his family practitioner).

Comment

The long duration of colitis was responsible for the severe malformation at the splenic flexure. The contraction of fibrosis related to extended linear ulceration, causing less-affected bowel to "pouch" or sacculate. In the past, there must have been a severe exacerbation of colitis to form the pseudopolyp filiform "bridges" in the transverse colon. This case demonstrates the difficulty of excluding carcinoma in a patient with Crohn's disease in the presence of an impassable stricture. The colon stricture in long standing Crohn's disease was the indication for surgical intervention in this patient, whose symptoms were minimal.

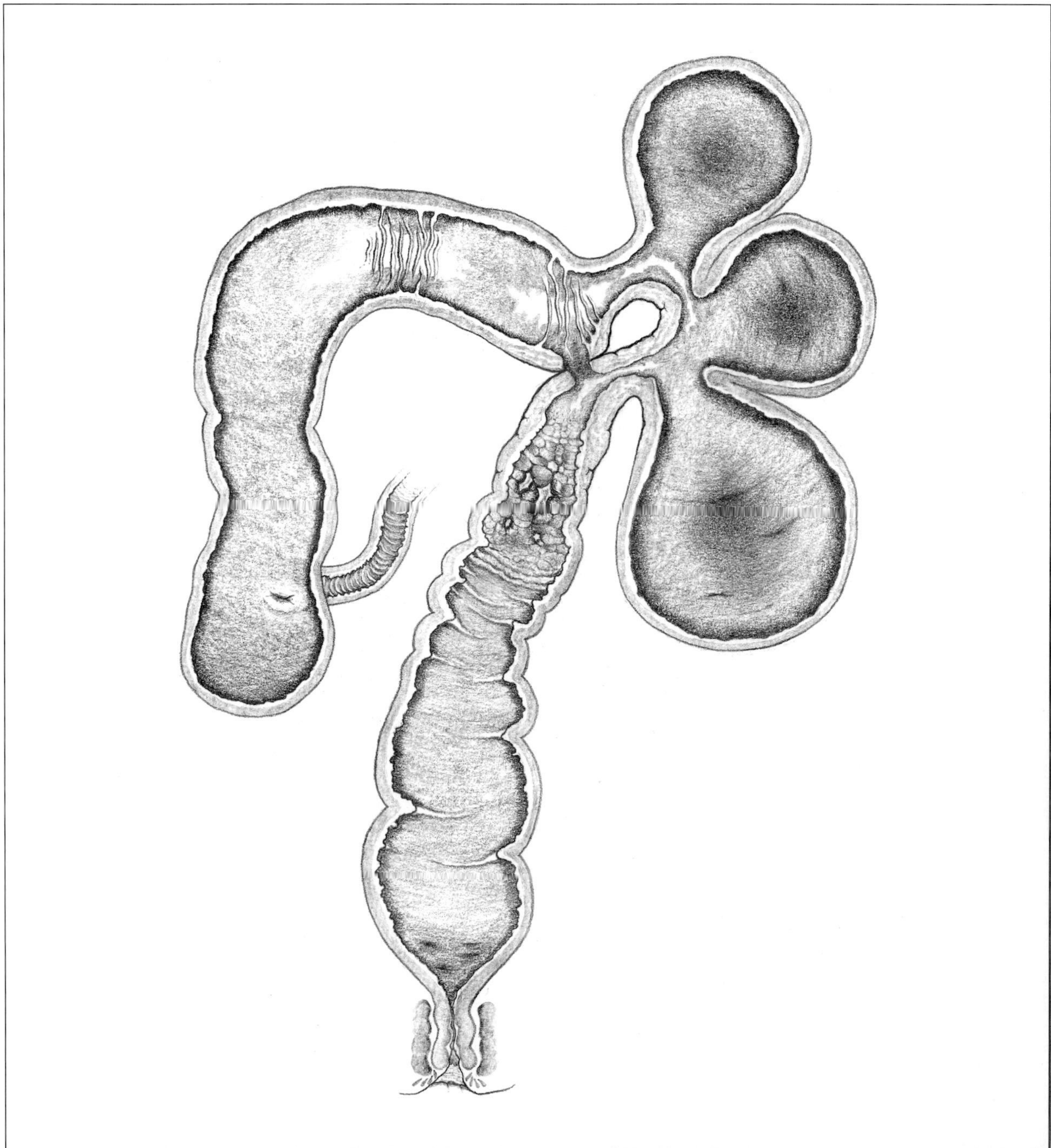

CASE

54 A Short "Hose Pipe" Colon: Crohn's Disease

Female, 22 Years (Part 1)

History

Crohn's colitis was diagnosed in 1979 at the age of 14 years. It manifested clinically with chronic diarrhea and multiple perineal fistulae, which responded for some years to maintenance therapy with prednisolone. In 1982, a contrast barium enema showed a remarkably shortened colon with sacculation of the transverse colon, "cobblestone" mucosa, incompetent ileocecal valve, and a long stricture of the left colon (Figure 54.1). In 1987, the patient presented with a mass and enterocutaneous fistula in the right iliac fossa. She was markedly small for her age (17 years) with no evidence of sexual development. The perineal disease was quiescent, an anal stricture was present, and the perineum deeply scarred from previous active fistulae. Colonoscopy revealed a shortened colon, (ileocecal valve at 50 cm) with a contracted lumen, areas of pseudopolyps, and typical ulceration of Crohn's disease. X-rays of the small bowel demonstrated a severely distorted terminal ileum, with "cobblestone" mucosa. After a further period of ill health supervened with fevers, weakness, and weight loss, the patient and family agreed to major surgical treatment.

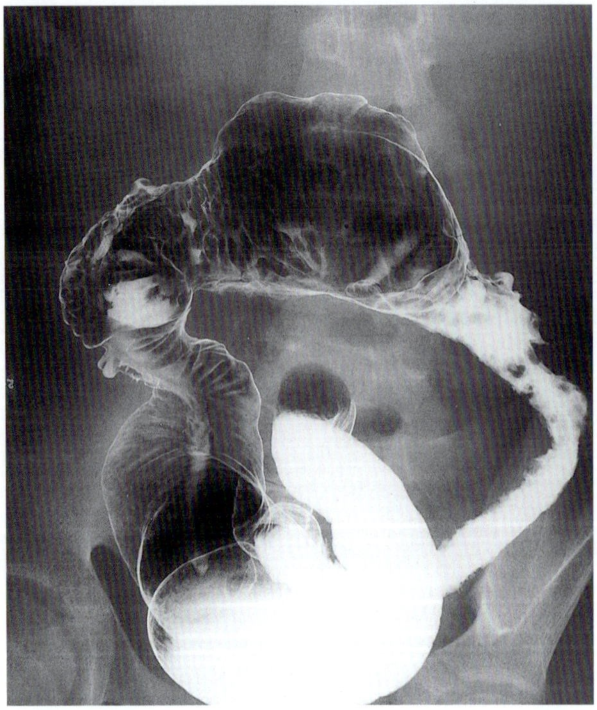

Figure 54.1: The barium enema demonstrates the marked shortening of the colon (1982).

Operation (12.14.87)

The terminal ileum showed changes typical of Crohn's disease on its peritoneal aspect, was attached to the anterior abdominal wall, and associated with a subcutaneous abscess and 3 external openings of a fistula. There were no skip areas of Crohn's disease affecting the small bowel. The colon was shortened and thickened with pouch-like dilatation of the transverse colon. Proctocolectomy was performed. A pedicle of greater omentum was transposed to the pelvis.

Pathology

The bowel was thickened, rigid, and contracted throughout its length. There was a stricture in the distal transverse colon. The "sacculation" of the transverse colon was a prominent feature of the opened specimen in which were active ulcers. The activity of the disease varied with more acute inflammatory disease, affecting the terminal ileum, transverse colon, splenic flexure, and rectum. Elsewhere, linear scars indicated the areas of previous ulceration. There was a long, narrow, healed ulcer scar present in the left colon and rectum. There was no normal mucosa present. The ileocecal junction was difficult to identify, and in this area there were several large smooth pseudopolyps. The anal canal was distorted by scar tissue and stricture. Histologically, the bowel wall was affected by transmural acute and chronic inflammation consistent with Crohn's disease but without granuloma formation.

Follow-Up

Within 5 weeks, the patient reported she was a "new person" enjoying good health. Four weeks later, pyoderma gangrenosum appeared adjacent to the ileostomy. This healed in 4 months with local treatment. For further follow up, see Case 55.

Comment

This patient's normal growth and sexual development was retarded by the onset of Crohn's disease at an early age and the continuous steroid therapy. Three years after the diagnosis was established, a barium enema demonstrated the "pouch" deformity of the transverse colon. After a clinical duration of 8 years, the chronic inflammatory process had produced marked deformity throughout the colon, which was a rigid and significantly shortened "hose pipe."

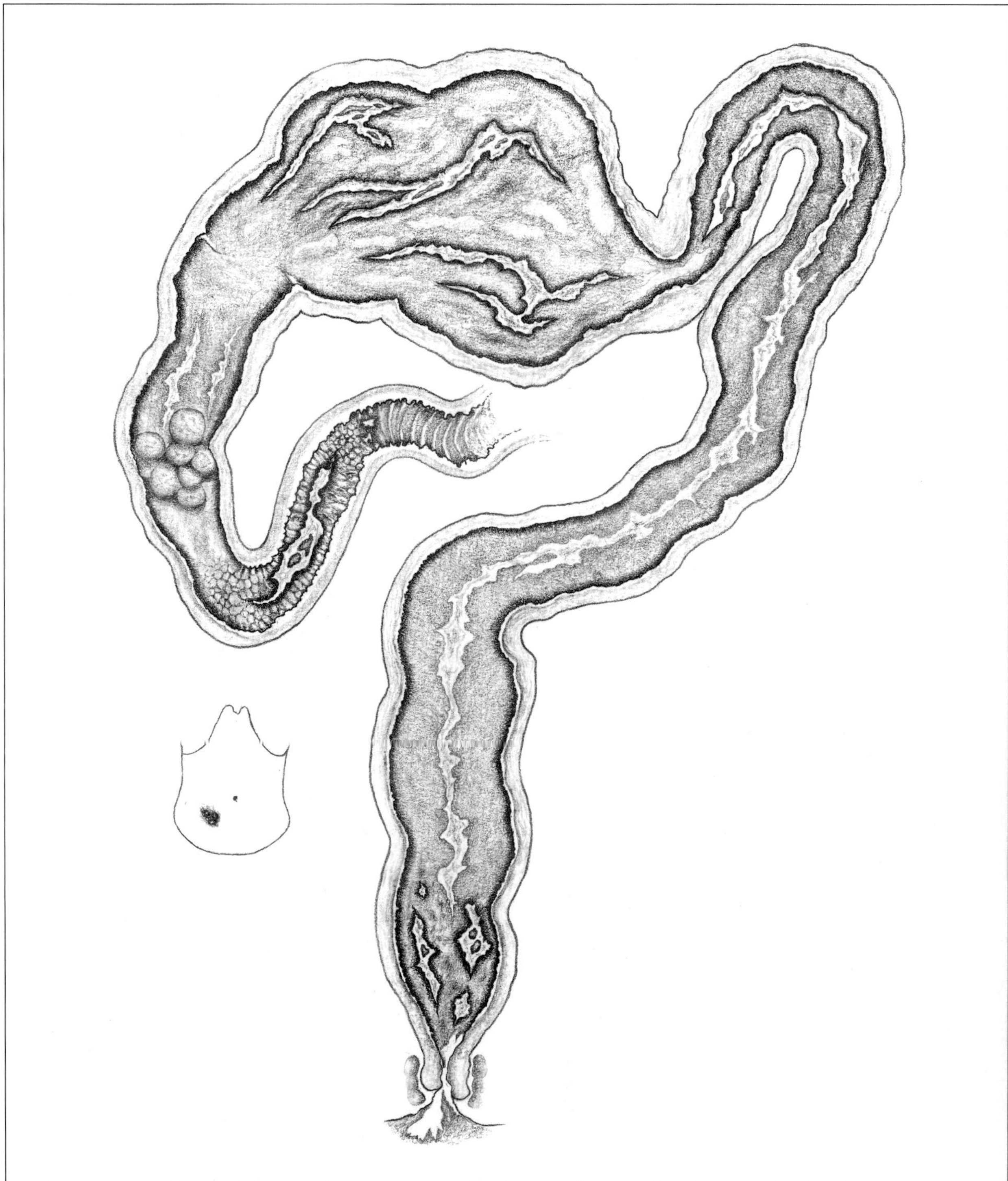

CASE 55 Recurrent Crohn's Disease: Pseudopolyposis

Female, 28 Years (Part 2)

History

One year after the proctocolectomy for chronic Crohn's disease of the terminal ileum and colon (see Case 54), the patient was experiencing episodic abdominal pain, fever, and lethargy. A small bowel x-ray showed nodularity of the mucosa throughout its length. A blood count revealed iron deficiency anemia and a raised erythrocyte sedimentation rate (ESR) (85). Steroid therapy was recommenced and continued for 4 months. A remission for 3 years was obtained with this therapy, albeit with occasional abdominal pain and fever. In May 1993, the patient was admitted to hospital with severe abdominal pain, diarrhea, and fever with a palpable mass in the left iliac fossa (LIF). Radiological investigation demonstrated an intraabdominal abscess.

Operation (5.31.93)

Laparotomy revealed extensive adhesions which were most dense in association with a length of mid small bowel affected by an acute, bordering on chronic, inflammation. There was an interloop abscess present which fixed the inflammatory mass to the left retroperitoneal area. Enlarged lymph nodes were present in the related small bowel mesentery. Proximal to the pathology, the bowel was thickened and dilated due to chronic intestinal obstruction. The abscess was evacuated and 70 cm of small intestine was resected with an end-to-end anastomosis performed with a single layer of interrupted sutures. Long-term suction drains were placed in the region of the abscess.

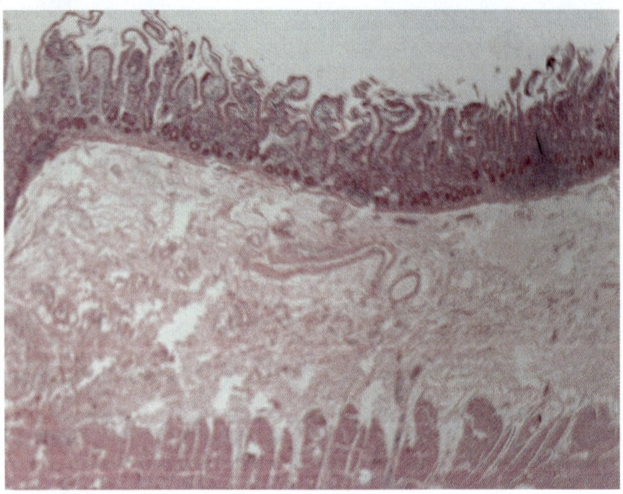

Figure 55.1: Edema has significantly increased the depth of the submucosa, which is responsible for the small pseudopolyps.

Pathology

Examination of the bowel lumen revealed 3 strictures and an obvious "polyposis" of the inflamed mucosa. There were multiple linear ulcers typical of Crohn's disease. The strictures involved all layers of the bowel wall and were due to chronic inflammation, edema, and fibrosis. The inflammatory changes were transmural, and, although no granulomas were identified, the histological appearances were consistent with Crohn's disease. The histological examination of the polyps identified them as "evolving inflammatory polyps" with marked submucosal edema (Figure 55.1).

Follow-Up

Irrigation and drainage of the abscess cavity was necessary for 4 weeks. By 8 weeks, the patient had resumed her favorite sport of horse riding. Since then the patient has remained stabilized on azothiaprine therapy and is without clinical evidence of recurrent disease. She continues to accumulate prizes for her horse jumping in major competitions.

Comment

Recurrence involving the small bowel rapidly supervened within 1 year. The surgical treatment in this patient was resection rather than stricturoplasty, in view of the "clustering" of the 3 strictures. The polypoid mucosa was due to foci of submucosal edema beneath an intact lamina propria and probably represents some of the earliest morphological changes of Crohn's disease. Pseudopolyps in Crohn's disease can be due to a combination of submucosal edema and fissure ulcers producing the "cobblestone" appearance, or caused by severe ulceration leaving islands of polypoid granulation or intact mucosa.[1,2]

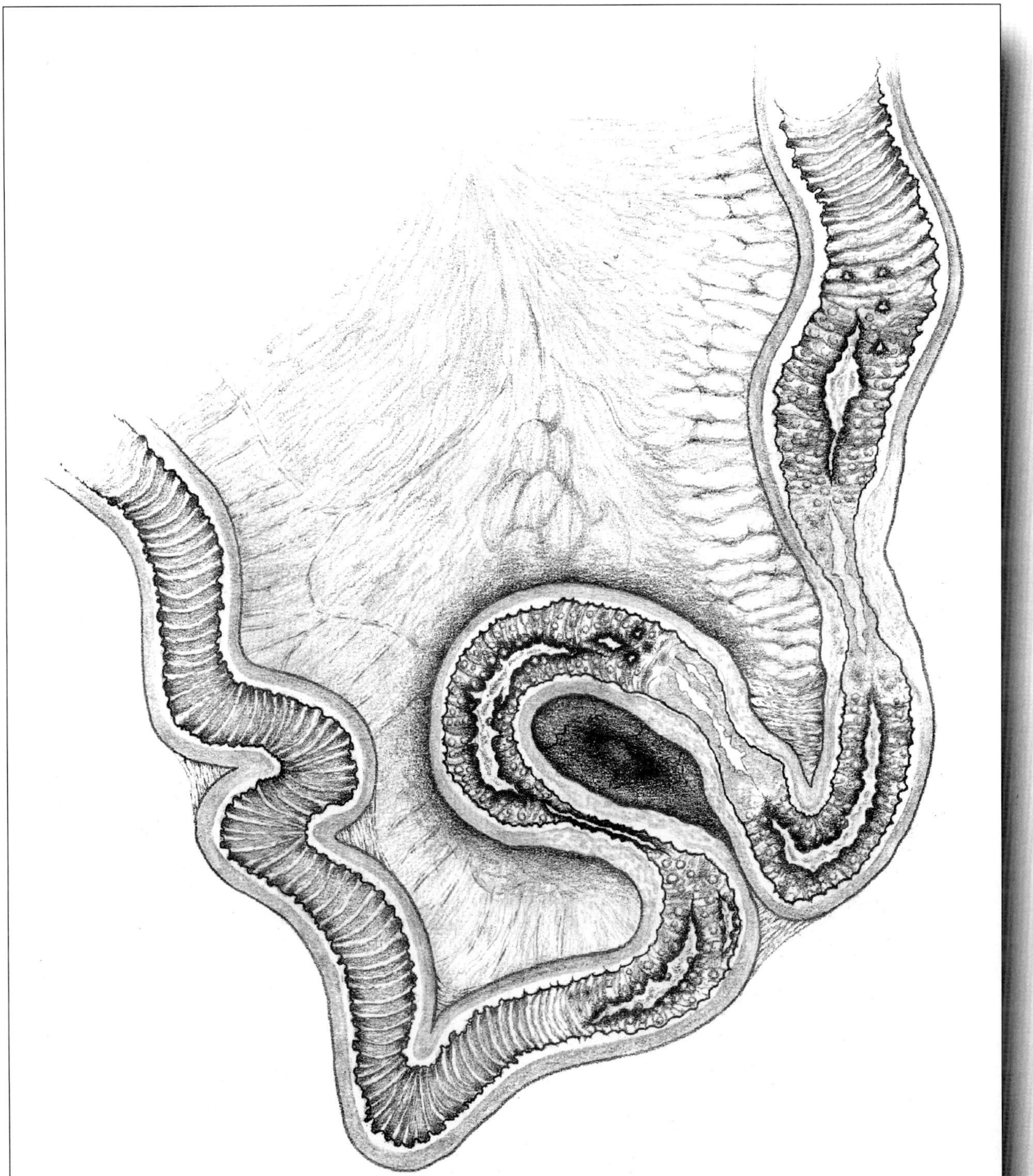

CASE

56 Presentation of Crohn's Ileitis as an Abdominal Malignancy

Male, 54 Years (Part 1)

History

The patient presented with an 18-month history of epigastric and back pain, anorexia, and loss of weight. This was associated with postprandial abdominal distention. His bowel habit was normal. Physical examination revealed a tense palpable cecum. A barium enema showed an unusual extrinsic deformity in the mid transverse colon associated with angulation and narrowing of the colon (Figure 56.1). Carcinoma of the pancreas was considered as a possible diagnosis.

Operation (3.17.78)

Laparotomy revealed a large complex area of Crohn's disease involving the distal ileum, which was attached to the mid transverse colon. At this site, there was an ileocolic fistula. Distal to this were 2 further sites of ileal Crohn's disease, the more distal of which was associated with an ileo-ileal fistula. There was marked dilatation of the ileum (the circumference was 15 cm) immediately proximal to the ileocolic fistula, and proximal to this there were further short skip segments of Crohn's ileitis. Ten centimeters of transverse colon was resected en bloc with 120 cm of ileum. Resection of the small bowel mesentery was difficult, due to the marked lymphadenopathy, and this resulted in extension of the length of small bowel removed due to impaired circulation. The small bowel resected was affected by 4 segments of Crohn's disease. Two minimally affected areas in the proximal ileum were not resected. The two anastomoses were completed with a single layer of interrupted sutures.

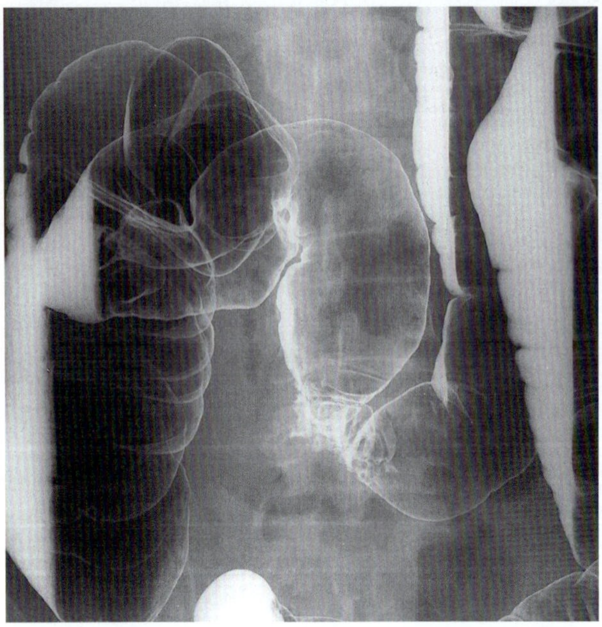

Figure 56.1: The deformity in the mid transverse colon (barium enema 3.3.78).

Pathology

The lumen aspects of the affected ileum showed typical morphology of Crohn's disease. There was linear ulceration, "cobblestone" mucosa, thickened bowel wall, and marked stricture formation. At the site of the ileocolic fistula, the lumen of the ileum permitted only the passage of a probe along the stricture. The fistula opening in the transverse colon was 6–8 mm in diameter, and immediately adjacent to it there were polypoid changes in the mucosa. The rest of the colon mucosa was normal. At this level, there was stenosis of the transverse colon, which was attached to the adjacent ileum by dense, tough adhesions. Histological examination confirmed the diagnosis of Crohn's disease.

Follow-Up

Recovery from operation was uneventful and bowel frequency was × 1 per 24 hours until 2 years after the bowel resection, when diarrhea and loss of weight occurred. He was found to be thyrotoxic. These symptoms partially abated with radioactive iodine therapy. For further follow-up, see Case 57.

Comment

This patient's presentation with epigastric and back pain associated with a very unusual deformity of the transverse colon led to a preoperative diagnosis of carcinoma of the body of the pancreas. Computerized tomography (CT) examination was not available, but colonoscopy would have been an appropriate investigation. It is surprising that, in the presence of an ileocolic fistula, the patient had no disturbance of bowel function. His pain must have been due to the marked degree of bowel obstruction. At the present time, such pathology would be treated with a combination of resection and strictureplasty. The role of strictureplasty and its results have been well defined from the experience at the Cleveland Clinic.[1,2]

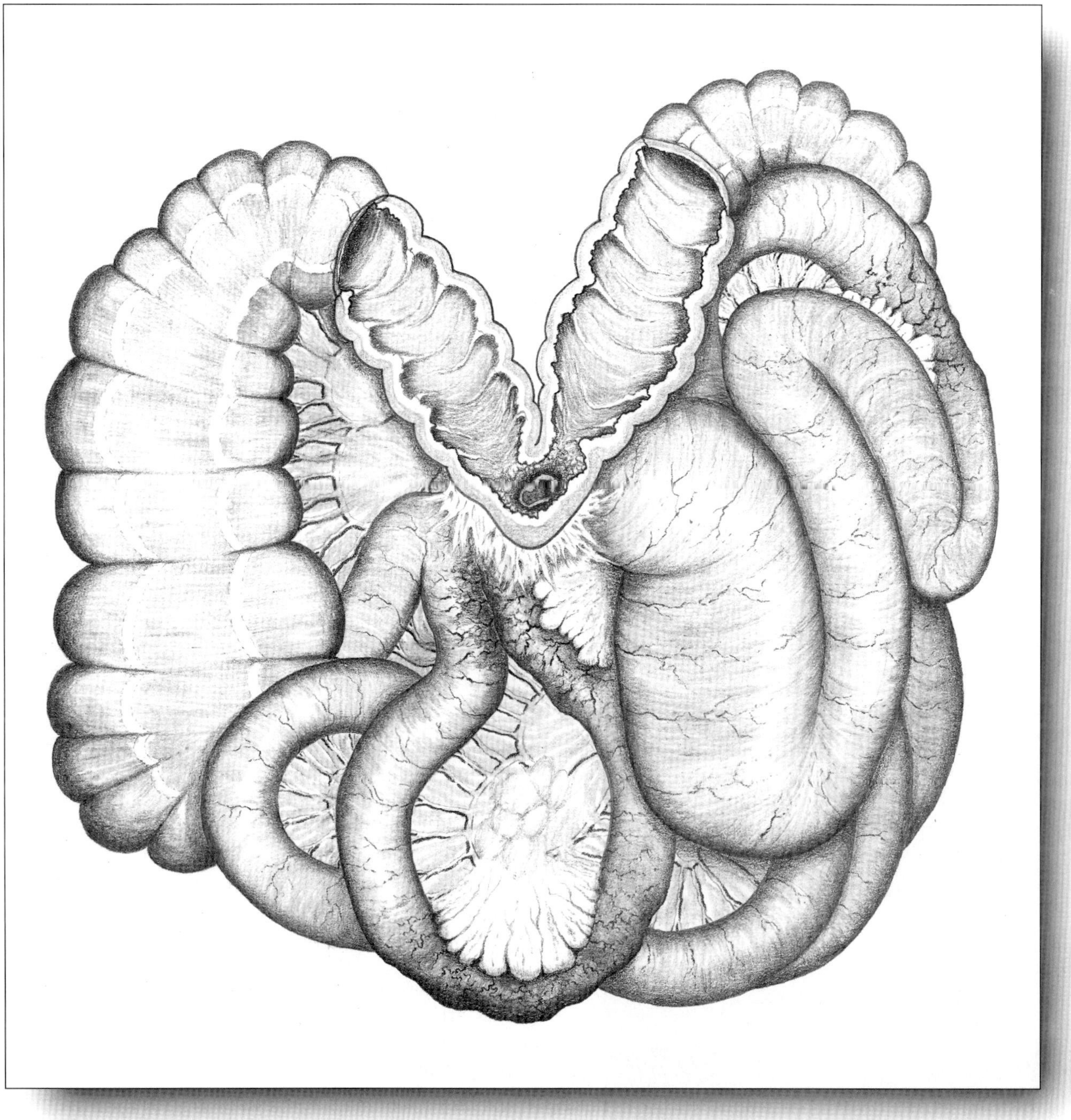

CASE

57 Crohn's Disease 19 Years After Initial Resection

Male, 73 years (Part 2)

History

Four years after a bowel resection for Crohn's disease (Case 56), this patient was admitted to hospital with a 2 week history of lower abdominal pain and alternating diarrhea and constipation. A tender mass was present in the right iliac fossa. A small bowel contrast series showed fixed loops of dilated small bowel indicative of "mild obstruction" (Figure 57.1). Recurrent Crohn's of the small bowel was diagnosed and treatment with prednisolone initiated. The patient's reasonable progress over the next 15 years was interrupted by 3 significant episodes of small bowel obstruction. Radiological investigations demonstrated 2 or 3 small bowel strictures with evidence of chronic obstruction (Figure 57.1). Colonoscopy was normal up to and including the ileocecal valve. The patient now agreed to surgical treatment.

Operation (9.5.97)

There were 2 short strictures a short distance proximal to the previous anastomosis in the ileum. Large "saccular" dilatations had formed in relation to these strictures and this area was affected by adhesions. Proximally, there was an area of induration in the ileum, indicating minimal stricture formation. Excluding this focus of disease, 29 cm of ileum was excised, removing 2 strictures. Care was taken to ensure an adequate blood supply to the terminal ileum in view of the previous resection in this area. The anastomosis was completed with a single layer of interrupted sutures. The fragile mesentery was closed. The residual small bowel measured 150 cm.

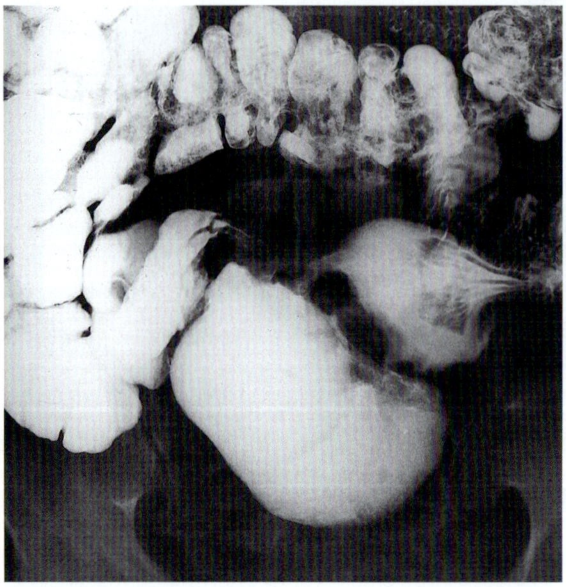

Figure 57.1: Small bowel series (1993) showing evidence of chronic obstruction and at least 2 strictures.

Pathology

The lumen of the resected bowel revealed longitudinal scars of healed ulceration, more marked in the region of the strictures. Two ileo-ileal fistulae were present with adjacent areas of inflammation. Histological examination confirmed the diagnosis of Crohn's disease. In the distal part of the resected small bowel there was a long pedunculated polyp 15 mm, which was inflammatory.

Follow-Up (2004)

There has been no further recurrence of Crohn's disease in 7 years. The patient's bowel frequency is 1–2 per 24 hours. His principal health problem has been the onset of Parkinson's disease.

Comment

Recurrence is a well known feature of Crohn's disease, and it is likely that there is a long period of asymptomatic recurrence before the diagnosis is made. Within 6 months of resection, there is a high incidence of recurrence on endoscopic examination.[1] Reoperation in this patient was performed 19 years after the initial surgery, but the first episode of bowel obstruction due to recurrent stenosis occurred at 4 years postresection. There was no evidence of Crohn's disease at the resection margins in 1978, when the disease-free margins were generous in length. The Cleveland Clinic study has demonstrated that recurrence is not related to the length of normal bowel clearance or disease-positive margins.[1] Borley et al found that there was a significantly higher recurrence rate for ileal disease than for ileocolic or colic Crohn's disease.[3] In a study of 51 patients with intestinal fistulae due to Crohn's disease (including 9 entero-enteric fistulae), Poritz et al. found the fistula was usually at the site of active disease and recommended surgery as the preferred treatment.[4] The pathology found at this patient's reoperation was an inflammatory conglomerate, which did not appear suitable for strictureplasty. Despite the patient's 81 years and shortened small intestine, his bowel function is within normal limits.

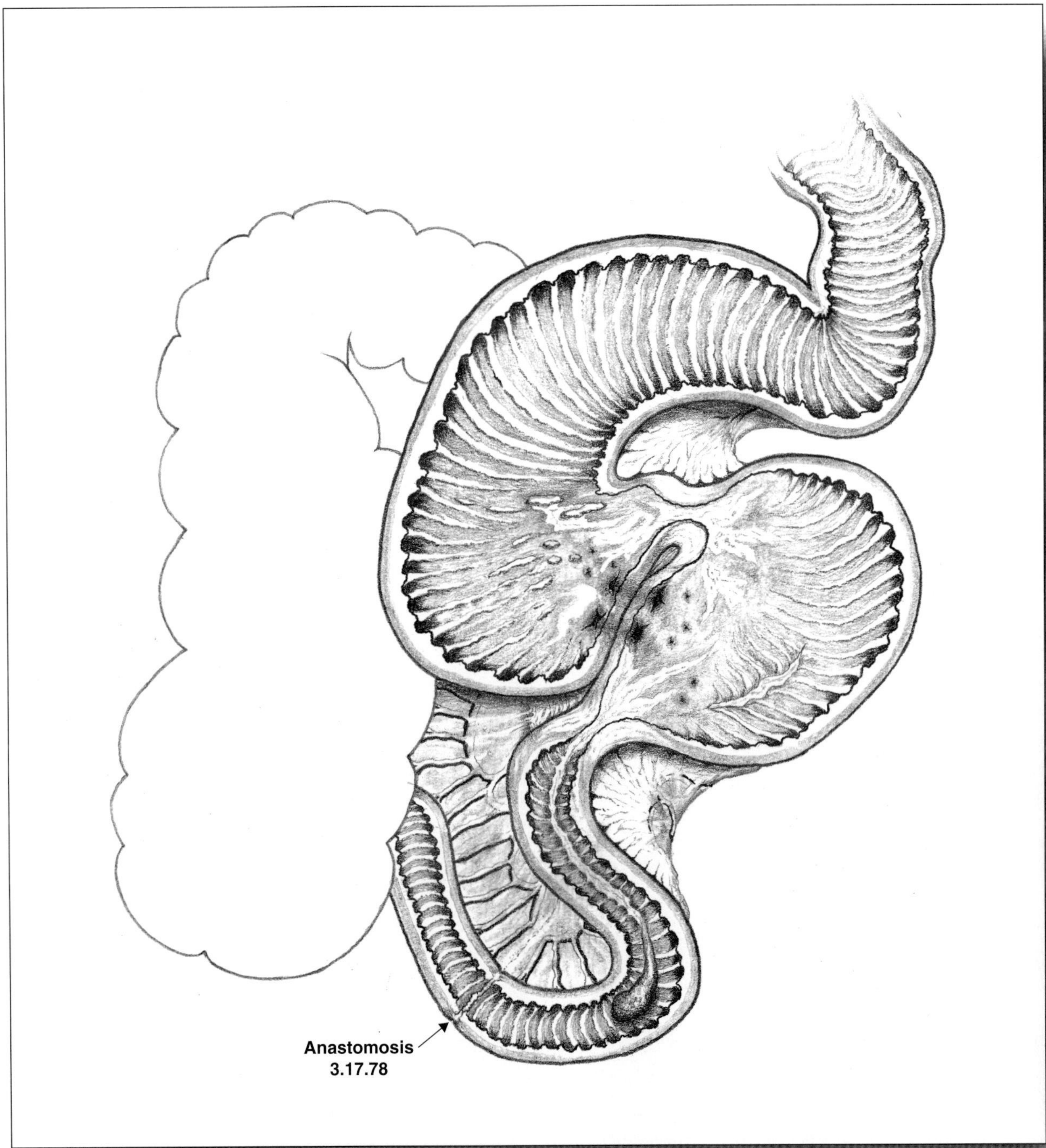

CASE

58 Large Bowel Obstruction: Crohn's Disease

Male, 46 Years

History

In 1976, the patient presented with a 9-month history of diarrhea and anal discharge. Sigmoidoscopy to 20 cm revealed an anterior anal fissure and a mild patchy proctitis. A barium enema demonstrated a long stricture of the descending colon with almost complete obstruction "due to advanced Crohn's disease" (Figure 58.1). Rectal biopsies were consistent with this diagnosis. Over the next 9 months, the patient was treated with oral prednisolone, resulting in intermittent improvement. In April 1977, a cautious barium enema showed persistence of the stricture and gross dilation of the transverse colon (Figure 58.2). Elective operation was arranged but was superceded by urgent admission due to acute bowel obstruction and signs of peritonitis.

Operation (5.24.77)

The colon was markedly distended (12 cm in diameter) proximal to the chronic inflammatory process in the descending and sigmoid colon. This part of the colon was thickened, contracted, deeply congested, and adherent to the left paracolic gutter with dense adhesions. In the anterior wall of the transverse colon, there was a 4-mm perforation with some minimal fecal spill and localized peritonitis. The small bowel was normal in appearance without distention. Colectomy and ileo-rectosigmoid anastomosis were performed, associated with a proximal loop ileostomy.

Pathology

The bowel wall proximal to the stricture was thickened, indicating chronic obstruction. The perforation in the transverse colon showed nonspecific necrotic changes and was not the site of the Crohn's disease. The stricture was due to marked thickening in the wall of the colon due to long standing fibrosis. In addition, prominent polypoidal change in the

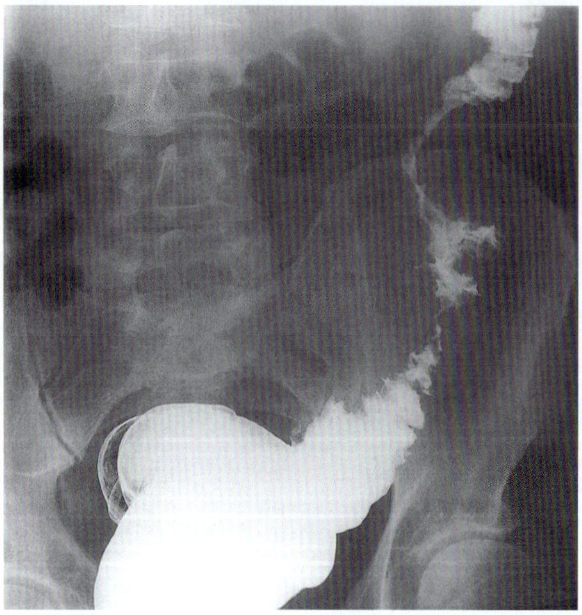

Figure 58.1: The x-ray demonstrates a long, tight stricture of the descending colon (7.6.76).

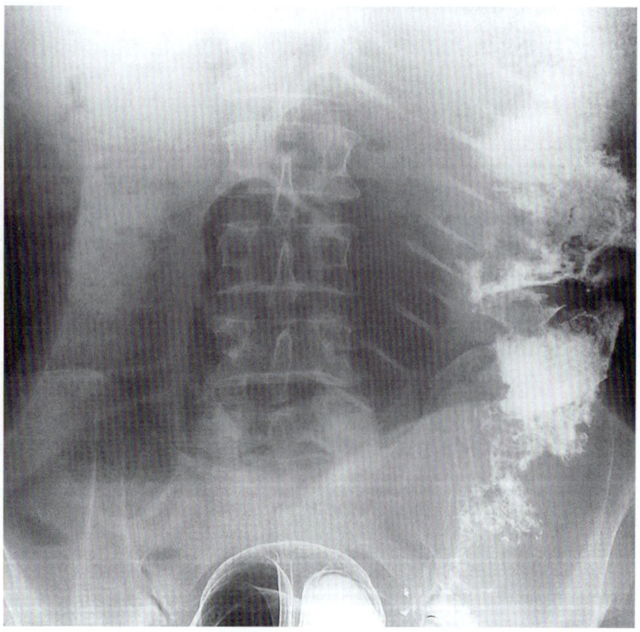

Figure 58.2: Large bowel obstruction is apparent on limited contrast enema 3 weeks prior to emergency operation. The transverse colon diameter measures 13 cm.

mucosal surface had further compromised the lumen of the bowel. There was ulceration present, partly obscured by the polypoid mucosa. Two linear ulcers measured 3 cm and 5 cm in length. Histological examination confirmed the diagnosis of Crohn's disease.

Postoperative Course

This was complicated by a profuse hemorrhage from a gastric ulcer, adrenal hypofunction, and prolonged ileus requiring total parenteral nutrition (TPN). Two months after operation, abdominal surgery was required to drain subphrenic abscesses (right subhepatic and left perisplenic).

Follow-Up

The proctitis in the lower rectum persisted with exacerbation, causing stool frequency of up to 12 × per day during the worst periods. Medical treatment was continued with maintenance azathioprine, sulphasalazine, and local steroids. In 1994, reflux esophagitis and stricture (biopsies: benign) were diagnosed. In 1998, the patient was found to be suffering from carcinoma of the stomach antrum, which was inoperable and caused the patient's death in 1999.

Comment

The management of this patient was less than ideal in that elective surgery should have been performed instead of an emergency procedure precipitated by a life threatening complication. While the short history of 9 months and the patient's obesity (weight: 321 lbs) were relative contraindications, the presence of a tight stricture, obstructive symptoms, and a constant requirement of 30 mgm of prednisolone daily were indications that elective operation was appropriate. The perforation of the transverse colon appeared to be caused by the extreme dilatation of the obstructed colon. Perforation of the colon in Crohn's colitis has been considered to be a rare complication.[1] This is probably due to the fact that the presence of a stricture in the colon is an indication for elective surgical treatment. Strictures of the colon in Crohn's disease should always raise the possibility of supervening carcinoma. Even if examined by colonoscopy biopsy, the diagnosis may not be apparent until a resected specimen is examined histologically. Although it is now recognized that there is an increased risk of colorectal cancer in Crohn's colitis, the number of cases reported are few: St Marks Hospital, UK: 15 in 52 years;[2] Queen Elizabeth Hospital, Birmingham, UK: 8 in 30 years;[3] and Mount Sinai Hospital, New York: 30 in 29 years.[4] These reports indicate the risk of colorectal cancer is increased in long standing disease, particularly when the disease commences at a young age.[3,4] Patients with extensive colitis were found to have an 18-fold increased risk of colorectal cancer.[3]

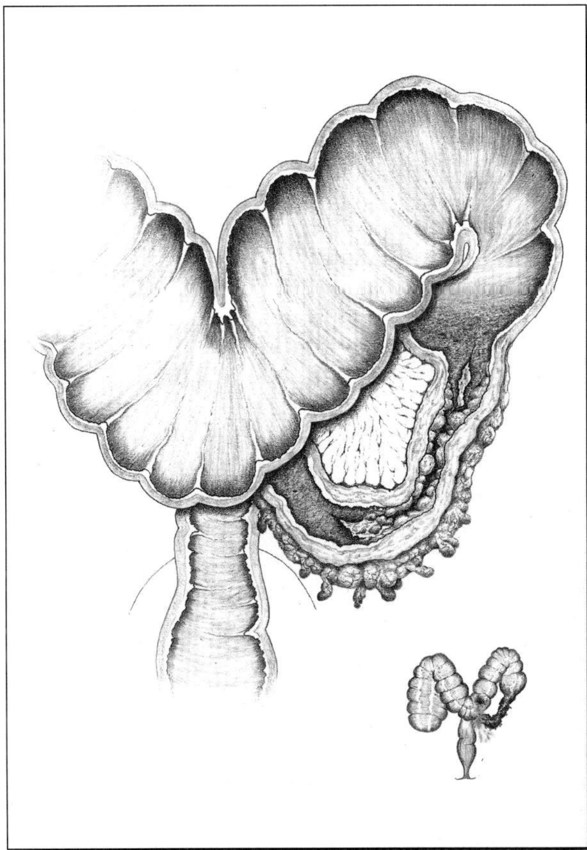

For a full-page image of this figure see the appendix.

CASE

59 Subacute Toxic Megacolon Due to Ulcerative Colitis

Male, 29 Years

History

Ulcerative colitis had been diagnosed more than 2 years previously. A severe attack of colitis supervened in April 1992, necessitating 2 admissions to the hospital with clinical signs of septicemia and dilatation of the colon. With conservative treatment (steroids) he made very slow progress over a period of 3 months, but was readmitted with abdominal pain and constipation. The patient looked unwell, groaning with pain. There was generalized abdominal distention and tenderness most marked in the right iliac fossa. A plain abdominal x-ray showed dilatation of the colon and a large collection of feces in the right colon. On referral, laparotomy was advised.

Operation (7.31.92)

At operation the colon was grossly dilated with inflammatory changes on its serosal surface. The lumen was loaded with soft feces and the wall of the bowel was thickened and friable. The colon was adherent in 3 sites, over a broad attachment to the anterior abdominal wall (1), liver–stomach (2), and a loop of jejunum (3). To minimize fecal spill, the colon was gently irrigated, via an ileotomy, with 22 liters of saline solution (evacuated per rectum) until clear of feces. Separation of the colon from the adhesions revealed 3 massive perforations at least 40 mm in length where the colon wall had disintegrated, forming extensive ulcers, the base of which was the adherent structure. The large bowel was resected to the level of the mid sigmoid. An end ileostomy and sigmoid mucous fistula completed the procedure. Peritoneal contamination was minimal.

Pathology

The lumen aspect of the bowel showed extensive ulceration that had left a few "islands" of inflamed mucosa on the surface of the denuded muscle. Areas in the cecum showed macroscopic and microscopic changes consistent with acute-on-chronic ulcerative colitis.

Further Progress

Recovery from operation was slow but uneventful.

Operation (7.19.93)

The distal sigmoid and rectum were excised and a restorative proctocolectomy and loop ileostomy performed.

Operation (11.1.93)

Closure of the loop ileostomy.

Comment

At the time of this patient's first 2 admissions, he suffered acute toxic megacolon and should have been assessed by a surgeon. The importance of combined physician and surgeon management had been ignored.[1] The patient was fortunate that free perforation of the colon and fecal peritonitis did not occur. Turnbull et al. were the first to emphasize the pathology of large penetrating ulcers in acute toxic megacolon sealed off by the omentum, viscera, or parietes.[2] This patient's incomplete recovery from the acute phase of the illness left the colon chronically dilated and malfunctioning as an adynamic obstruction. At the time of his elective operation, he was fit enough for an abdominal colectomy to be performed. The Turnbull "blowhole" ileostomy–colostomy procedure was not considered. Preliminary colon irrigation via an ileotomy substantially reduced the risk of fecal contamination when the large defects in the bowel wall were exposed by mobilization. The technique of irrigation was similar to that advised by Khoo et al, who propose the method as a technique to facilitate resection for toxic megacolon.[3] The Cleveland Clinic experience of the "blowhole" operation has been significantly reduced. In the 18 year period, 1983–2001, it has been employed in only 6/328 (1.9%) of patients with toxic colitis due to inflammatory bowel disease (IBD).[4]

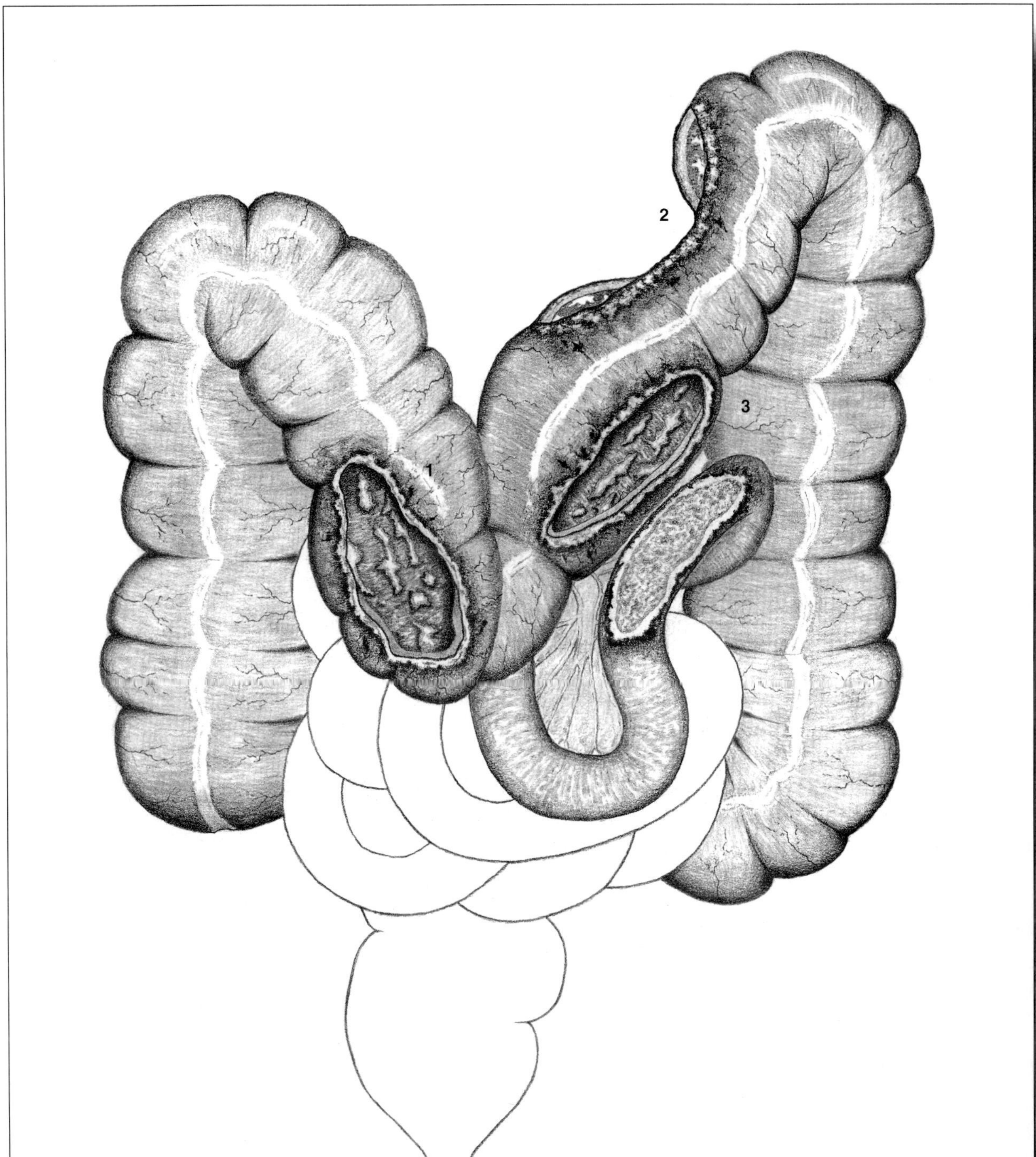
2
3
1

CASE

60 Colitis and Pseudopolyposis

Male, 68 Years

History

This patient underwent urgent laparotomy (February 1989) for toxic megacolon that was initially interpreted as mechanical large bowel obstruction. The surgeon performed a loop colostomy in the transverse colon. The true nature of the disease was revealed with a subsequent colonoscopy, which demonstrated severe colitis from the rectosigmoid to the cecum. The patient made a satisfactory recovery and was referred for further management 6 months after the urgent operation. Colonoscopy revealed an active colitis commencing at the rectosigmoid, with extensive polyposis extending to the transverse colon. The colon proximal to the colostomy was diffusely inflamed without obvious ulceration or polypoid lesions. The mucosa of a large prolapsed transverse colostomy was relatively normal.

Operation (10.16.89)

Adhesions involving an otherwise normal small bowel were dissected. There were vascular changes on the serosal surface of the colon consistent with an underlying inflammatory process. The colon was resected from the cecum to the rectosigmoid junction, and an end-to-end anastomosis between terminal ileum and rectosigmoid was completed with a single-layer interrupted suture of 3/0 polyglactin 910 (vicryl).

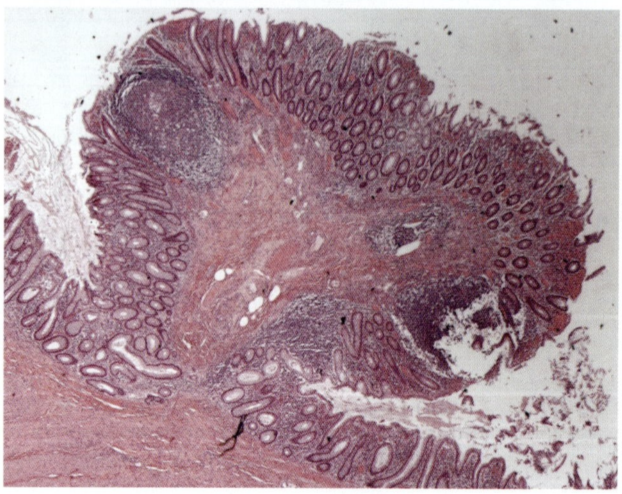

Figure 60.1: Inflamed mucosa forms an inflammatory polyp, which is one variety of pseudopolyp.

Pathology

The mucosa proximal to the colostomy was actively inflamed, showing hyperemia, edema, and small foci of bleeding. The mucosa of the colon between the colostomy and the splenic flexure showed a cobblestone effect with some linear ulceration, indicating an active chronic colitis. The colon distal to this was contracted, with its lumen covered with small sessile pseudopolyps between which the surface of the lumen was scarred without active ulceration. The pathology report stated that the mucosa of the distal 5 cm of the specimen was "almost normal" in appearance. The histological features of the bowel wall confirmed the diagnosis of chronic ulcerative colitis with pseudopolyp formation (Figure 60.1).

Postoperative Course/Follow-Up (2005)

Recovery from operation was satisfactory. Two months after operation, his bowel frequency was Day/Night: 4/1. On flexible sigmoidoscopy, the mucosa of the rectum appeared normal, the anastomosis was at the 18 cm level. These features remained unchanged throughout a follow up period of 5 years which included regular sigmoidoscopy examinations. The patient reports that he is well for his 84 years, more than 15 years since the operation.

Comment

The clinical details preceding the patient's emergency laparotomy are not available, but the surgeon recorded that he undertook the operation for large bowel obstruction. Subsequent findings suggest the event was acute toxic megacolon due to ulcerative colitis (UC). The rectal sparing raised the possibility of Crohn's disease (CD) (excluded by the histological examination) and facilitated the ileo-rectosigmoid anastomosis. Interestingly, the patient's colon exhibited 3 distinct morphological types of ulcerative colitis. The pseudopolyps were principally "mucosal islands" consistent with a previous severe episode of colitis. Goligher reported that 20% of his patients with total or substantial colitis were found to have pseudopolyps.[1] Pseudopolyps are more common in UC than CD, may be localized to a segment of colon, and do not usually involve the lower 10 cm of rectum.[1] They may be sessile, pedunculated, or filiform, usually less than 15 mm in size, but they can form large masses.[2,3] Histologically, they may be islands of normal or inflammatory mucosa, excessively regenerative glands, or epethelialized foci of granulation tissue. The morphology of the colon may persist with little change, and the inflammatory change may even become quiescent. The pseudopolyps have no specific malignant potential.[1,3,4,5] Their presence alone is not an indication for colectomy.[1] Macroscopic Dysplasia Associated Mass Lesion (DALM) may be differentiated by its morphology and histological appearance.

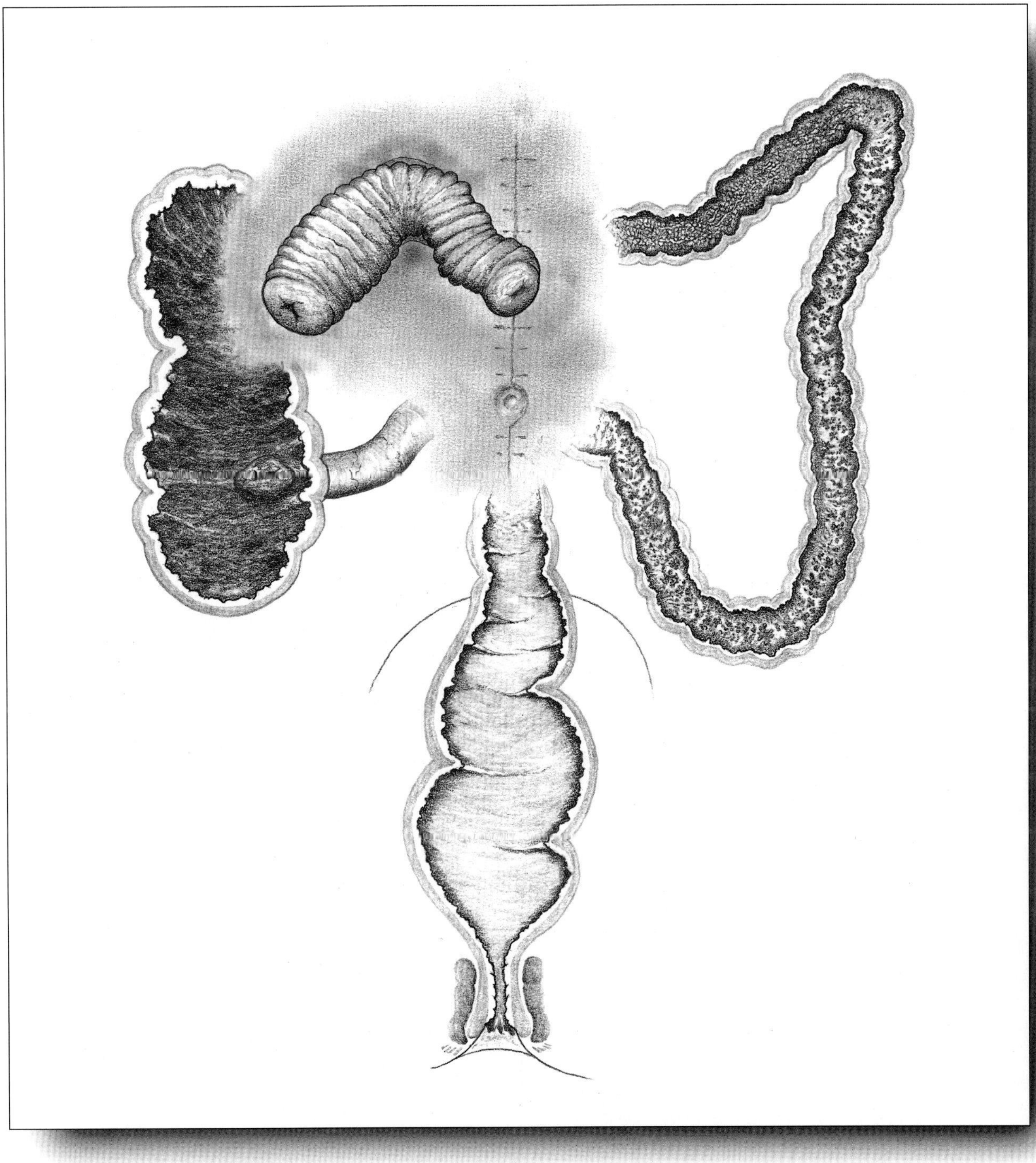

C A S E

61 Ileorectal Anastomosis for Chronic Ulcerative Colitis: Early Diagnosis of Carcinoma: Late Diagnosis of Large Polypoid Lesion

Female, 51 Years

History

The patient's colitis had been diagnosed at 10 years of age, and after 18 years of medical treatment, her diarrhea was still disabling (Day/Night = 8/1). Sigmoidoscopy revealed chronic changes of proctocolitis without obvious ulceration. A biopsy showed histological changes consistent with chronic ulcerative colitis. Colonoscopy was not performed (1974). A barium enema had demonstrated a smooth stricture of the transverse colon.

Operation (4.23.74)

Colectomy and ileorectal examination was performed. The distal level of resection was 2 cm below the sacral promontory.

Pathology

In the distal half of the resected specimen, the muscle wall of the colon was thickened and the mucosa showed multiple small areas of ulceration.

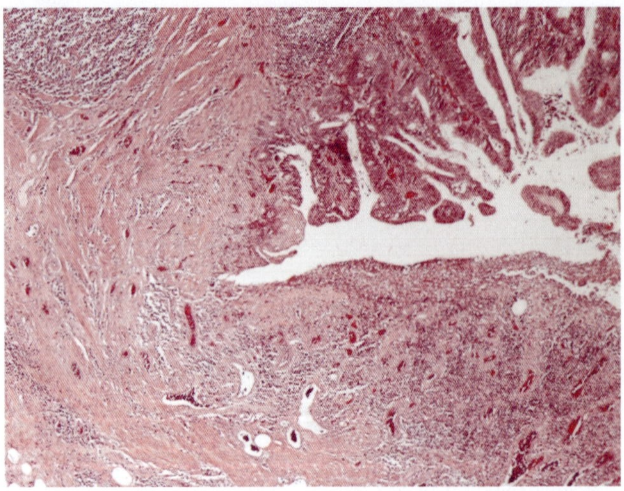

Figure 61.1: Intense inflammation in a macroscopic lesion interpreted as a Dysplasia Associated Mass Lesion (DALM).

The stricture in the transverse colon was less obvious than on x-ray. Histological examination confirmed the diagnosis of chronic ulcerative colitis. There was no evidence of carcinoma or dysplasia.

Follow-Up

In a few months, the patient's bowel frequency became stable (4–5/24). She attended sigmoidoscopy assessment regularly. After 1981, no biopsies were performed for dysplasia (at the patient's request) as rectal bleeding, requiring transfusion, had occurred after 2 of these examinations. The endoscopic appearance of the chronic proctitis did not change until 1990, when 4 small white ulcers were noted below the anastomosis at 14 cm. The ulcers appeared to be inflammatory and biopsy was not performed. Sigmoidoscopy on 12/19/97 revealed a small (5 mm) sessile polyp on the posterior wall of the rectum at 11 cm. On palpation, it felt soft and its appearance was benign. Diathermy snare removal was performed. Histological examination showed well differentiated adenocarcinoma arising in a dysplastic villous adenoma.

Operation (1.5.98)

The small bowel was dissected free of many adhesions. A restorative proctocolectomy and loop ileostomy were performed.

Pathology

Examination of the specimen revealed that the site of the small carcinoma was related to a flat pale polypoid change in the mucosa 50 mm in its largest diameter. Histologically, this was regarded as Dysplasia Associated Mass Lesion (DALM) (Figure 61.1), but the distinction between this and an inflamed villous adenoma can be difficult. There was no evidence of residual carcinoma. The ulcers near the previous anastomosis were consistent with ulcerative colitis. Six mesorectal lymph nodes showed no metastases. Long standing anal fissures showed no specific features.

Operation (5.18.98)

Closure of ileostomy.

Comment

The patient remains free of recurrent cancer 7 years since resection of the rectum. Although regular examination with a rigid sigmoidoscope detected an early carcinoma, it failed to diagnose an extensive flat lesion. Flexible endoscopy with its magnification would probably have been more successful. If the patient had permitted routine random biopsies, it may have detected the dysplastic polyp. The risk of supervening carcinoma after ileorectal anastomosis (IRA) has been well documented, and early diagnosis, even with careful surveillance, is not always possible. Johnston et al reviewed 155 patients with ulcerative colitis treated by resection and IRA.[1] During the follow up period (3 months through 40 years), 11 patients developed carcinoma in the residual rectum. The estimated probability of developing rectal cancer was 17.1% after 27 years. The 11 tumors were advanced stage, high histologic grade, and the median cancer specific survival was 14 months.

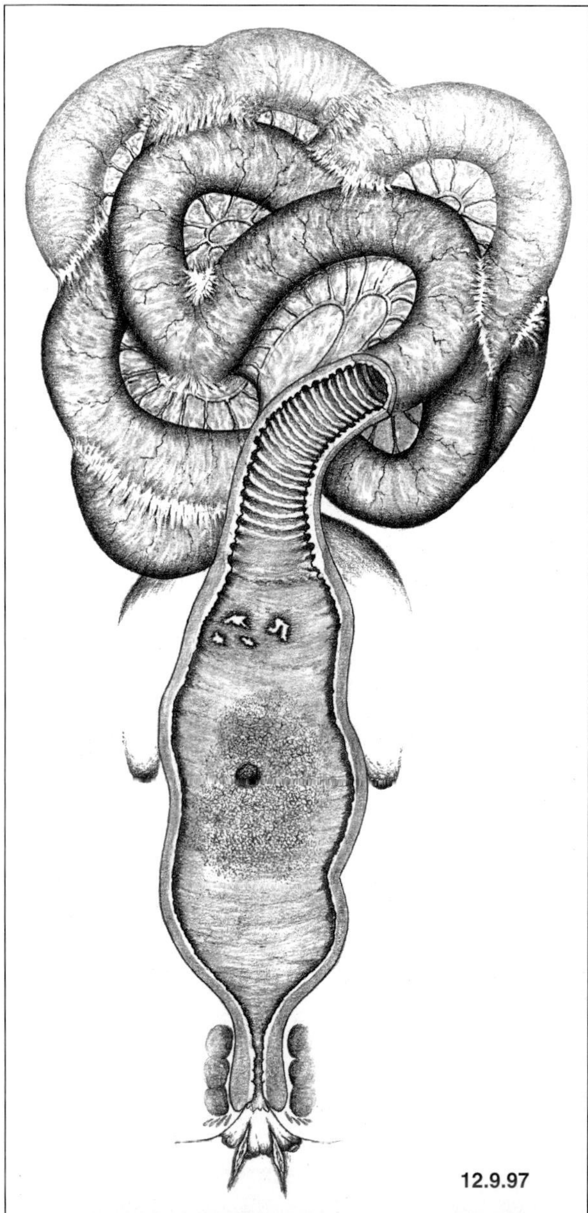

For a full-page image of this figure see the appendix.

CASE

62 Childhood Ulcerative Colitis: Rectal Cancer

Male, 34 Years

History

The patient, aged 9 years, was first seen by the author within a few days of the first episode of diarrhea and rectal bleeding (1972). Within 1 week, a significant proctocolitis to 20 cm was apparent. Treatment with intermittent courses of prednisolone and maintenance with sulphasalazine was supervised by the attending gastroenterologist. In 1982, colonoscopy revealed total chronic colitis with pseudopolyp formation, and biopsies were consistent with ulcerative colitis. The patient's family rejected proctocolectomy at this time. An exacerbation of the colitis resulted in a short hospital stay in 1988. Follow-up colonoscopies revealed slow progressions of the colitis with pseudo polyps, contraction and rigidity of the distal colon. No dysplasia was identified in random biopsies. Colonoscopy (9.23.94) identified chronic active disease in the right colon and more acute inflammation in the left colon and rectum. The patient was advised to undergo restorative proctocolectomy but declined. Thirteen months later, cystoscopy was performed to investigate dysuria and hematuria. Inflammatory changes were present in the bladder. Sigmoidoscopy now revealed an obstructing carcinoma in the upper third of the rectum (Figure 62.1).

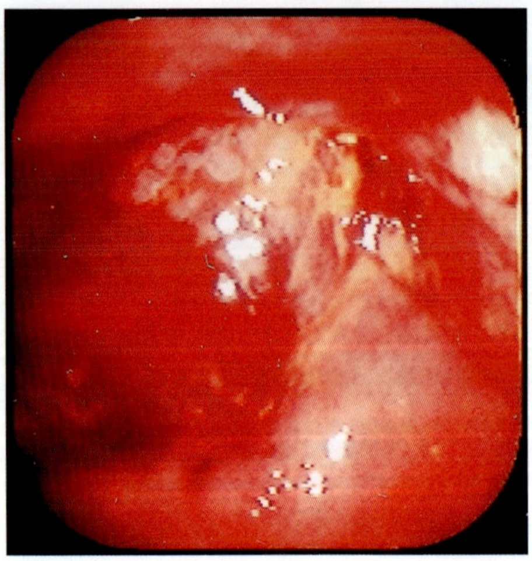

Figure 62.1: Carcinoma at 12–13 cm seen on sigmoidoscopy (11.16.95).

Operation (12.4.95)

A large malignant mass in the rectum was found attached to the upper surface of the bladder. There were no metastases identified beyond this mass. The colon was dilated, indicating obstruction was well established. There was a marked inflammatory reaction in the right anterior aspect of the pelvis. Proctocolectomy–end ileostomy was performed with en bloc partial cystectomy. The omentum was mobilized and used to fill the pelvic space.

Pathology

The carcinoma was annular, causing constriction of the lumen. Its length was 60 mm. A perirectal abscess between the rectum and the bladder was draining pus into the lumen of the bladder, but no fistula from the rectal lumen was identified. A segment of vas deferens was attached to the right aspect of the specimen. Histologically, the tumor was a well differentiated mucinous adenocarcinoma which extended locally beyond the muscularis propria, but did not invade the bladder wall. No metastases were detected in the examination of 12 lymph nodes (Dukes C, T_3 N_0 M_0). Chronic ulcerative colitis without dysplasia was present throughout the large bowel.

Postoperative Course/Follow-Up

Recovery from operation was complicated by a deep venous thrombosis and gastrointestinal bleeding induced by heparin therapy. Sexual function in relation to surgery had been a concern for the patient, but this proved not to be a problem, and his wife's pregnancy commenced 3 months after the proctocolectomy. Unfortunately, abdominal metastases became apparent 18 months after operation. There was no response to chemotherapy and the patient died 25 months after the resection.

Comment

The patient's colitis-cancer was diagnosed after 23 years of active disease. It was an unusual experience for a surgeon to follow the patient's inflammatory bowel disease a few days after its commencement until the patient's death. It was regrettable that at least twice the patient almost underwent elective surgery. In 1982, a permanent ileostomy was rejected, and, in 1994, the discussion on postoperative impotence proved to be a deterrent. Dysplasia was never detected on repeated colonoscopic biopsies. The extensive tumor was diagnosed 13 months after a colorectal surgeon performed a colonoscopy. There had been no alteration in bowel symptomatology. The practice of regular cancer surveillance in these patients unfortunately does not always yield early-stage disease,[1] although Lennard-Jones et al from St Mark's Hospital found that 70% of tumors diagnosed in patients attending a surveillance program for total ulcerative colitis were either Dukes A or B.[2] They also agreed that surveillance for mucosal dysplasia had limitations. The original paper by Morson and Pang described it as "a useful but imperfect marker" in colitis–cancer detection.[3] Currently, the problems are that to be effective, extensive biopsy sampling is necessary, interpretation by an expert pathologist can be difficult, and up to 25% of established colitis–cancers are not associated with dysplasia.[4]

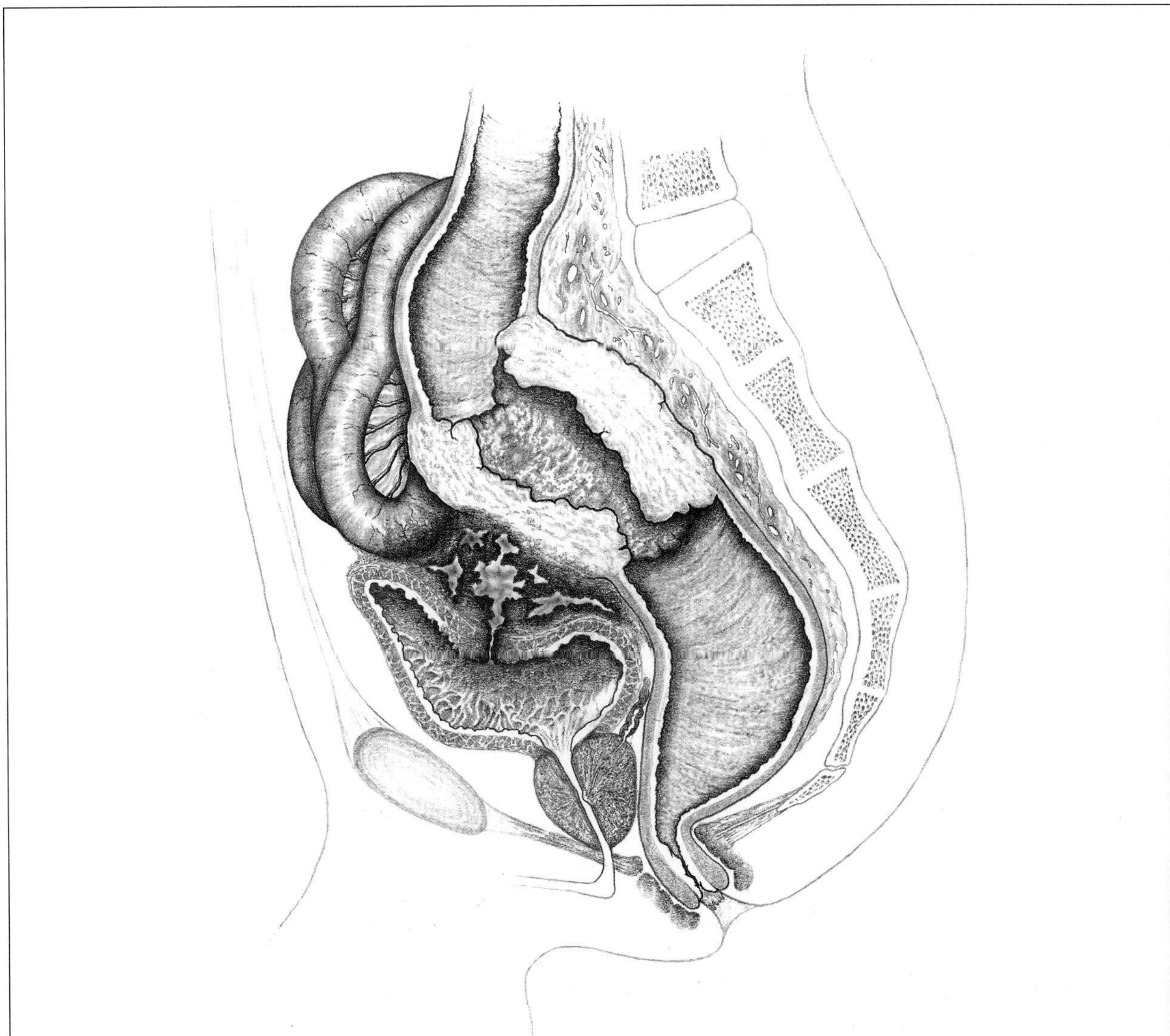

For a full-page image of this figure see the appendix.

CASE

63 Obstructive Colitis

Female, 55 Years

History

The patient had been aware of constipation for a period of 4 months and, for 6 weeks, had noticed a frequent and frustrated desire to defecate. During this latter period, a small amount of bleeding and mucus appeared with the stools. On examination, distention of the left and right colon was palpable. Rectal examination revealed a large firm mass in the pelvis, and flexible sigmoidoscopy revealed edema of the mucosa at 15 cm where the further lumen could not be visualized due to angulation of the rectum. A limited barium enema demonstrated a stenotic lesion in the rectosigmoid (Figure 63.1).

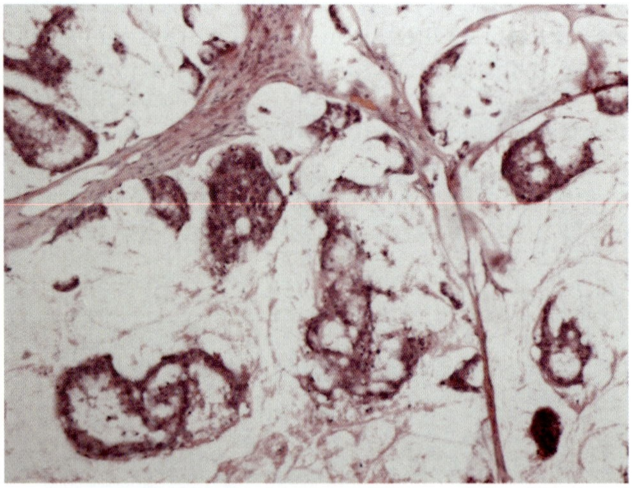

Figure 63.2: Clumps of adenocarcinoma surrounded by pools of mucin. Signet ring cells were identified elsewhere in the tumor.

Operation (1.31.92)

Laparotomy revealed a large malignant tumor of the rectosigmoid with significant serosal involvement over the tumor that was contiguous with the adjacent parietal peritoneum. No metastatic disease was detected on examination of the abdomen. The colon was markedly distended and loaded with feces. The wall of the sigmoid and left colon was thickened and edematous. A low anterior resection was performed, including the abnormal left colon to include the

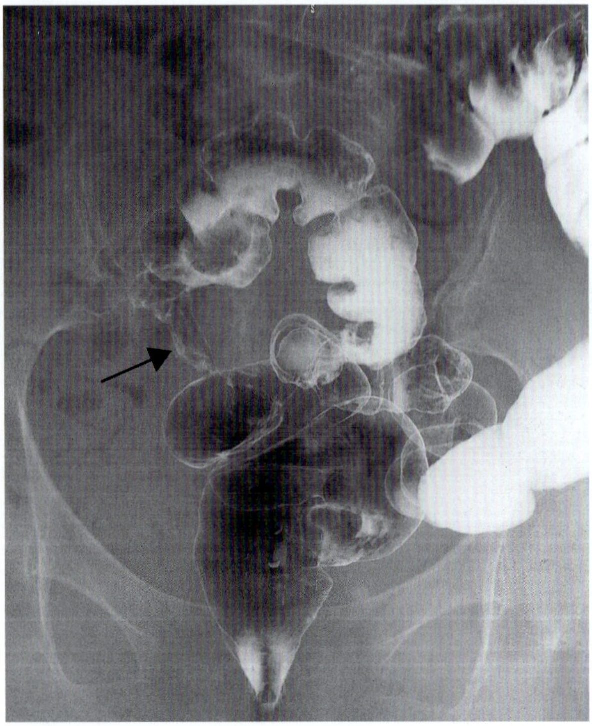

Figure 63.1: Barium enema showing a malignant rectosigmoid stricture (arrow).

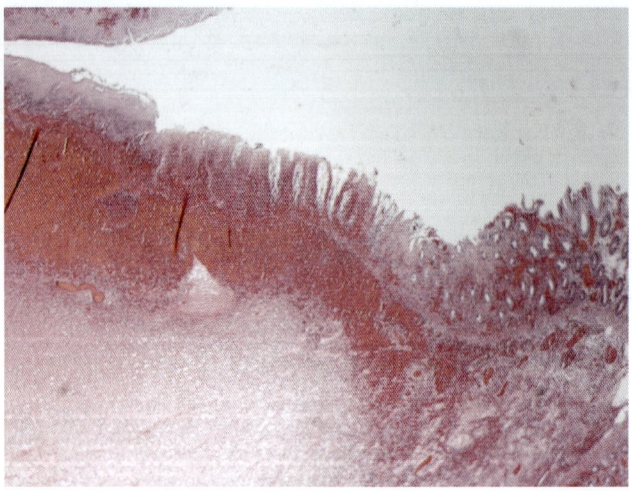

Figure 63.3: Typical changes of ischemia causing hemorrhagic infarction. Necrosis has occurred in the lamina propria.

splenic flexure. This procedure was combined with on-table lavage and a loop ileostomy.

Pathology

Examination of the specimen revealed a stenotic tumour 65 mm in length. Commencing 50 mm proximal to the lesion and reaching the splenic flexure, the mucosa was intensely inflamed with longitudinal and parallel ulceration. The lymph nodes noted in the mesentery were small. Histologically, the tumor was a poorly differentiated mucinous adenocarcinoma (Figure 63.2) with a prominent signet ring cell population extending through the bowel wall into the pericolic tissue. The ulcerated mucosa showed features of acute hemorrhagic infarction extending into the submucosa without evidence of preexisting inflammatory bowel disease (Figure 63.3). Six lymph nodes contained metastatic mucinous adenocarcinoma. There was extensive lymphatic and perineural invasion of the perinodal tissue (Dukes C, T_3 N_2 M_0).

Follow-Up (2005)

The ileostomy was closed 3 months after operation, by which time adjuvant chemotherapy had been commenced with 5-Fluorouracil and Levamisole. This treatment was administered for 12 months. The patient has continued follow-up surveillance for more than 13 years without evidence of recurrent disease.

Comment

Despite the ominous nature of the pathology of the tumor, long-term survival has occured. It would seem appropriate to attribute this success to adjuvant chemotherapy, as the results from surgery alone are very poor for signet ring adenocarcinoma. The ulcerating colitis observed in this patient is distinct from ulcerative and Crohn's colitis and was probably first described in the early 1940s. Further reports have described the characteristic features of the disease.[1,2,3] The colitis may be near total or segmental, and typically there is a zone of normal mucosa immediately proximal to the obstructive pathology which most frequently is a carcinoma. The ulceration may be longitudinal, transverse, or circumferential, and pseudopolyps may be evident.[3] Many of the morphological and microscopic features resemble those of ischemic colitis.[3,4] Boley et al have demonstrated experimentally that as intraluminal pressure rises, blood flow in the mucosal and muscle layers of the bowel wall diminishes.[5] The ischemic effect induced by obstruction is regarded as the mechanism of the colitis. The possible role of intestinal flora is unclear.[3] Teasdale and Mortensen have reported 6 cases with acute features requiring emergency surgery for necrotic changes in the wall of the bowel.[6]

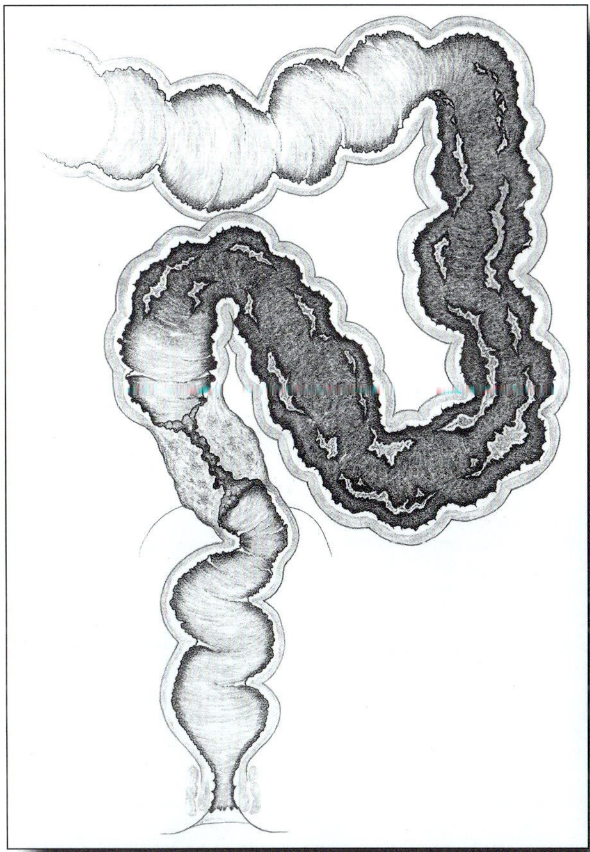

For a full-page image of this figure see the appendix.

CASE

64 Pseudomembranous Colitis and Toxic Megacolon

Female, 67 Years

History

The patient was admitted to hospital with a respiratory infection which had been treated with erythromycin. The patient also suffered from bronchiectasis and asthma. Prednisolone and trimethoprim were administered in view of poor lung function. Ten days after admission, there had been no bowel action for 3 days. At the time of the initial surgical consultation, the abdomen was distended with absent bowel sounds. The patient was afebrile with a pulse rate of 110 and a white cell count of 57,400. During the next 4 days, the patient's bowel function varied from diarrhea to no bowel action or flatus in a 24 hour period. Abdominal distention persisted. Radiological investigation revealed a grossly dilated colon (Figure 64.1) without evidence of mechanical obstruction. The diagnosis remained obscure. On the fifth day of admission, the patient complained of severe abdominal pain in the right upper quadrant. The abdomen was distended with localized tenderness. A computerized tomography (CT) examination revealed a small collection of free gas adjacent to the transverse colon.

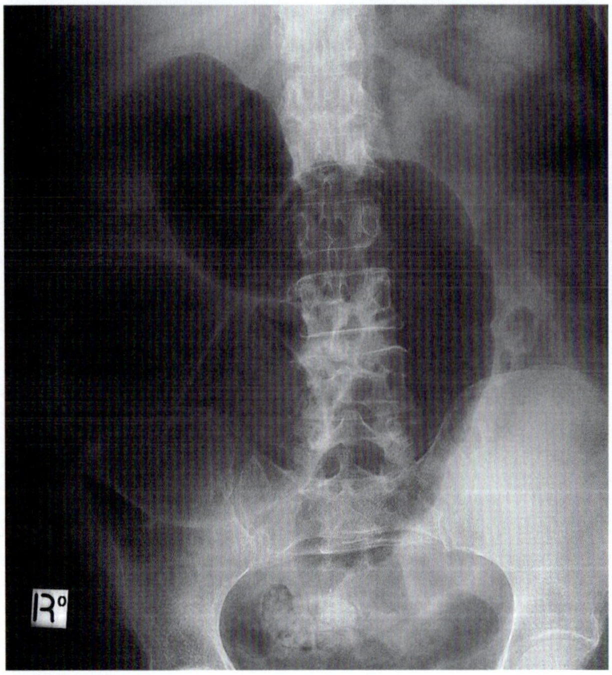

Figure 64.1: A plain x-ray demonstrates the dilatation of the colon.

Operation (8.10.94)

Laparotomy revealed distended colon with areas on the right colon and mid transverse colon showing necrosis and imminent perforation. The precise site of the free gas leak was not identified. The intraoperative diagnosis was ischemic colitis. A subtotal colectomy with anastomosis and proximal ileostomy was performed.

Pathology

The macroscopic appearance of the mucosa was classical of pseudomembranous colitis (PMC). There was extensive loss of mucosa of the left colon leaving "islands" of intensely inflamed mucosa covered with small foci of yellow pseudomembrane (Figure 64.2). Histologically, the suspect areas in the colon revealed full thickness necrosis. The pseudomembrane showed numerous neutrophils and gram positive organisms consistent with a diag-

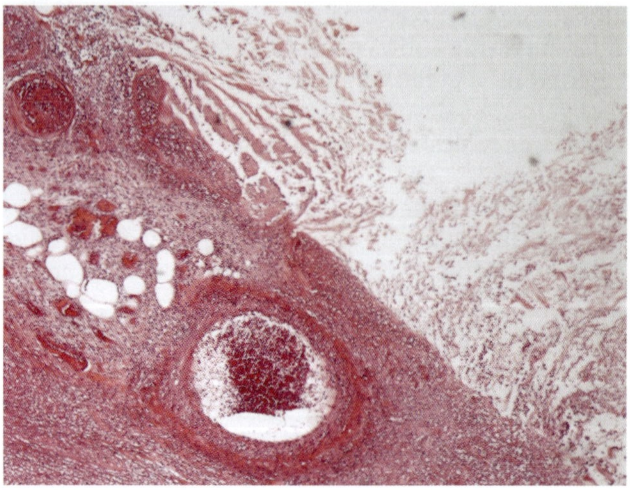

Figure 64.2: The pseudomembrane is superficial to the submucosa. Complete loss of mucosa has occurred.

nosis of PMC. Clostridium difficile was not identified on culture.

Progress

Recovery was complicated but satisfactory after 4 weeks. The ileostomy was closed 7 months after the resection.

Comment

In a review of the surgical aspects of clostridium difficile colitis, Bradbury and Barrett emphasize there has been a dramatic increase in the diagnosis of Clostridium difficile infection amongst surgical patients.[1] This has been due to increased awareness, better methods of diagnosis, more widespread use of antibiotics, and the increasing numbers of elderly and immunocompromised patients.[1] A wide range of antibiotics has been associated with PMC. Erythromycin and trimethoprim used in this patient are less commonly associated than other antibiotics. In the patient described here, the diagnosis was not realized until the resected specimen was examined immediately after operation. The intraoperative diagnosis was ischemic colitis. Stool cultures did not reveal Clostridium difficile, and stool assay for toxin A was not performed. Longo states that this assay is the most reliable test to establish the diagnosis.[2] The very high white cell count is characteristic of PMC, It was not appreciated prior to operation that PMC could cause toxic megacolon (TM). Gan and Beck stress that TM can be caused by a wide variety of inflammatory conditions of the colon, which include various infections and ischemic colitis.[3] Prendergast et al report the incidence of TM in PMC to be 2%.[4] Surgical treatment is required in very few patients and, if necessary, is associated with a reported mortality of 38%.[5] If TM develops, the mortality rate can reach 80%.[4]

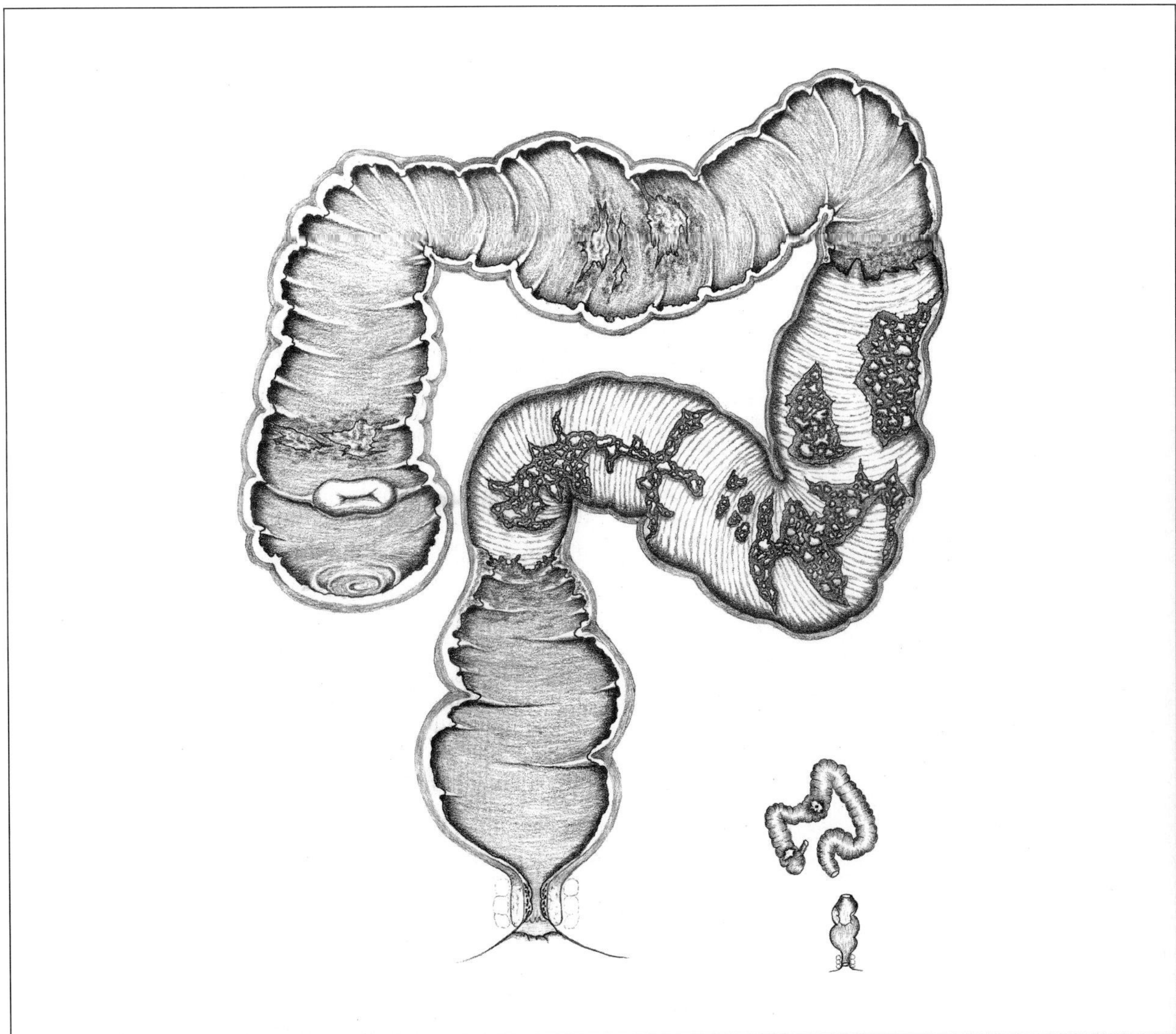

For a full-page image of this figure see the appendix.

CASE

65 Ileocecal Tuberculosis Mimicking Crohn's Disease or Vice Versa?

Female, 62 Years

History

In 1986, the patient was suffering chronic abdominal pain and was investigated in the Department of Surgery at the Aga Khan University Karachi, where a diagnosis of ileocecal Crohn's disease was made. The patient lived in isolation 1000 km from Karachi, and her family in Australia preferred that further treatment occur in Sydney. Investigations indicated the need for operation, which was performed (12.22.86). Right hemicolectomy with 75 cm of ileum was performed for an inflammatory mass of the cecum, cecoileal fistula, and two small bowel strictures. The histology was nonspecific chronic inflammation. Tests for tuberculosis were negative. Recovery was satisfactory and the patient returned to Pakistan until 1990 when she presented with colicky abdominal pain, diarrhea, and marked loss of weight. Endoscopic and x-ray investigations now demonstrated an enteroduodenal fistula and an inflammatory stricture at the ileocolic anastomosis. Extensive tests for tuberculosis (TB), performed in Pakistan, were negative. The patient returned to Australia for further surgical treatment. The Mantoux test was positive and there was a calcified focus in the mid zone of the right lung. A 10-day period of total parenteral nutritional (TPN) therapy was administered prior to operation.

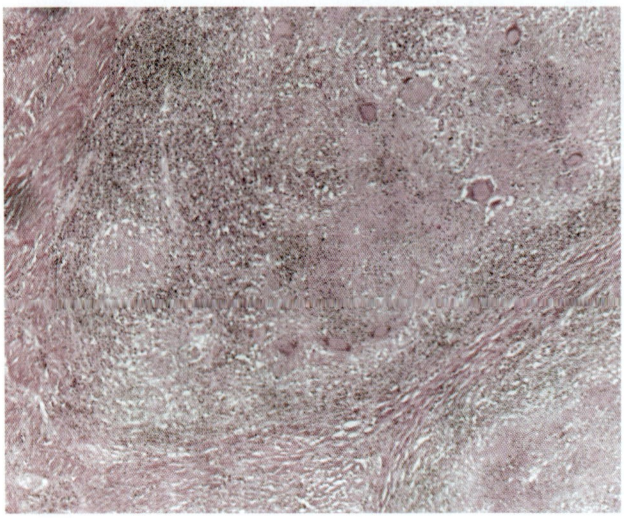

Figure 65.1: Typical tuberculous caseation and fibrosis with Langhans' giant cells. These granulomas were present in the wall of the small bowel and mesenteric lymph nodes.

Operation (5.27.93)

There were extensive adhesions associated with a large inflammatory mass involving the ileocolic anastomosis, adjacent ileum, and duodenum. The terminal ileum was dilated due to chronic obstruction. Firm enlarged lymph nodes were present in the small bowel mesentery and "knobbly" hard nodes were adjacent to the transverse colon. The ileocolic anastomosis and 27 cm of ileum were resected with reanastomosis. The small fistula defect in the duodenum was repaired.

Pathology

The opened specimen revealed a smooth thickened stricture at the site of the previous anastomosis. Proximal to the stricture was a fistula communicating with a loop of ileum. This fistula was also in continuity with the ileoduodenal fistula. Immediately proximal and distal to the stricture, the mucosa was inflamed, atrophic, and featureless with plaques of fibrin exudate obscuring superficial ulceration. These appearances were not typical of Crohn's disease. The histological examination revealed "non specific inflammation" and the diagnosis remained uncertain. Some years later further tissue blocks were examined and the slides reviewed by five pathologists. The bowel wall and mesenteric lymph nodes now showed chronic transmural inflammation, with fibrous ulceration and granulomas with Langhans giant cells (Figure 65.1). Some granulomas were suppurative and others were caseous. Special staining (Zeihl-Neelsen, auramine rhodamine) failed to demonstrate any mycobacteria. Examination of lymph nodes showed granulomas with extensive caseation. Three pathologists regarded tuberculosis as the most likely diagnosis.

Postoperative Course

The patient's general condition remained poor with difficulty in establishing adequate oral intake. Upper gastrointestinal (GIT) bleeding and systemic candidiasis complicated the patient's weakened state. She succumbed 4 weeks after operation. No autopsy was performed.

Comment

The diagnosis of TB was not made until after the patient's death when the slides were examined for a further opinion in an academic department of pathology. No acid fast bacilli (AFB) were seen or obtained by culture from the tissue removed at both resections. Confirmation of intestinal tuberculosis is known to be difficult. Findlay et al report the positivity of tests as follows: Mantoux 31%, chest x-ray 29%, histology 56%, and tissue culture 27%.[1] Where doubt exists, a therapeutic trial of antitubercular treatment has been recommended,[2] and such treatment would have benefited this patient. The original description of regional ileitis (later known as Crohn's disease) was based on the review of pathology specimens at Mount Sinai Hospital, New York. The authors referred to ileocecal tuberculosis in the differential diagnosis and stated, "In all of our first cases of regional ileitis, the diagnosis of ileocecal tuberculosis was the unvarying best possibility."[3]

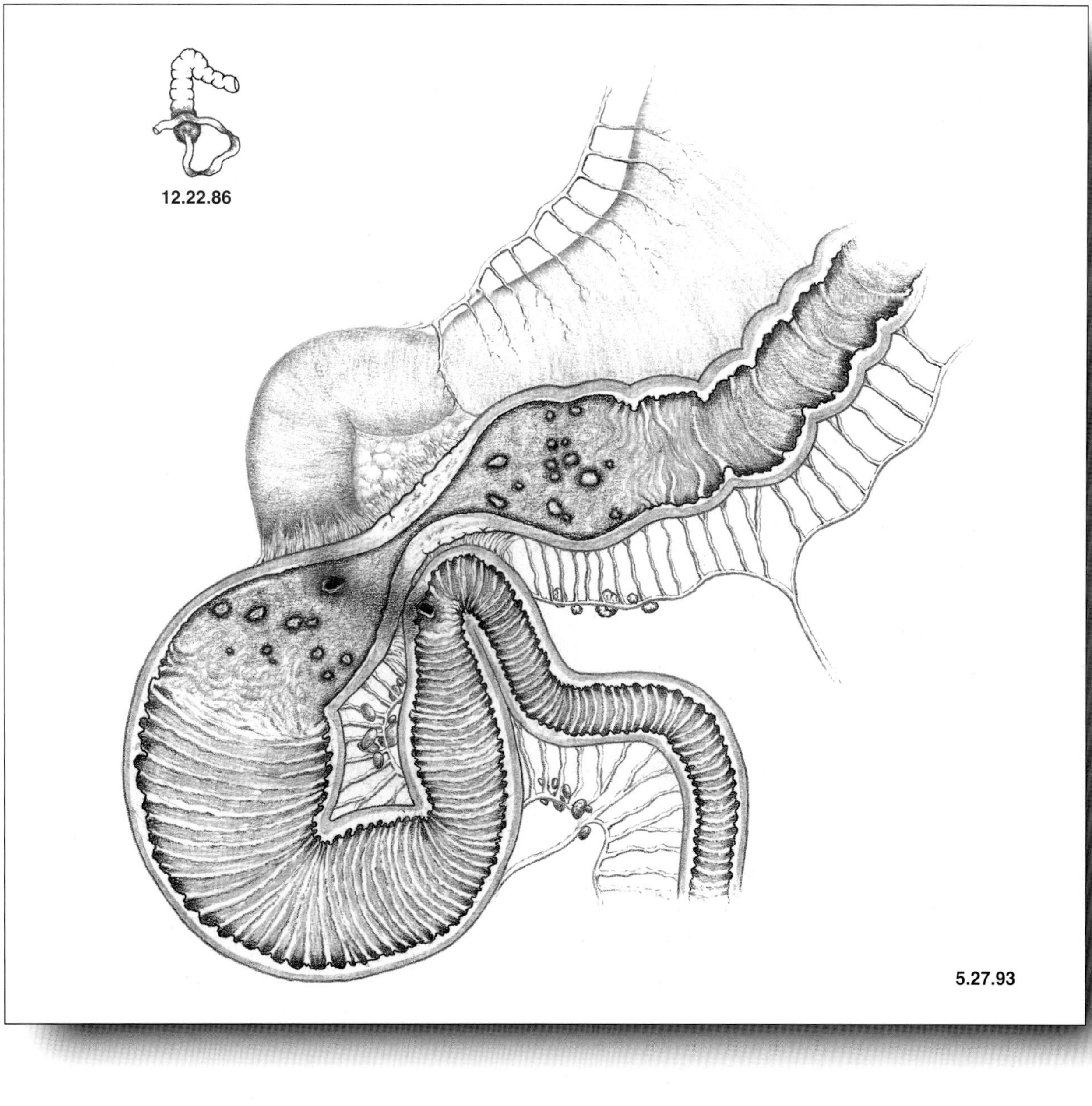

PART VII Lymphoma

CASE

66 Burkitt's Lymphoma (Ileum) with Intussusception

Female, 10 Years

History

The patient had suffered from recurrent abdominal pain for 1 year. The pain, central and in the right iliac fossa, had been worse for 1 week, requiring daily attention from the family doctor. On admission to the hospital, clinical examination revealed a long mass lying transversely in the upper abdomen. A contrast enema confirmed the diagnosis of intussusception (Figure 66.1). The apex reached the splenic flexure.

Operation (1.11.96)

Laparotomy confirmed the extent of the intussusception, which was easily reduced. There were 4 discrete firm lesions palpable in the terminal ileum, the distal one of which was the apex of the intussusception. The related small bowel mesentery contained enlarged lymph nodes. The bowel was obviously viable. There were several hard nodules (2 mm) over the surface of the right colon. A right hemicolectomy, including 70 cm of ileum, was performed.

Pathology

There were a total of nine mucosal lesions of the ileum, 3 of which were polypoidal and firm (15 mm–30 mm). The distal lesion and 1 other were ulcerated. There were 5 soft plaque-like abnormalities along the ileum (10 mm–20 mm). Sections of the polypoid lesions revealed a pale surface, and one of these lesions extended through the full thickness of the intestinal wall. Histologically, the lesions showed atypical lymphocytic infiltration consistent with a diagnosis of Burkitt's Lymphoma (Figure 66.2). The nodules (nodes) on the surface of the right colon and the mesenteric lymph nodes showed no significant abnormalities.

Progress and Investigations

Postoperative recovery was satisfactory. Investigation to stage the patient's disease showed no other foci of lymphoma. The non-Hodgkin's lymphoma (NHL) classification was Stage III (Murphy classification: childhood NHL).

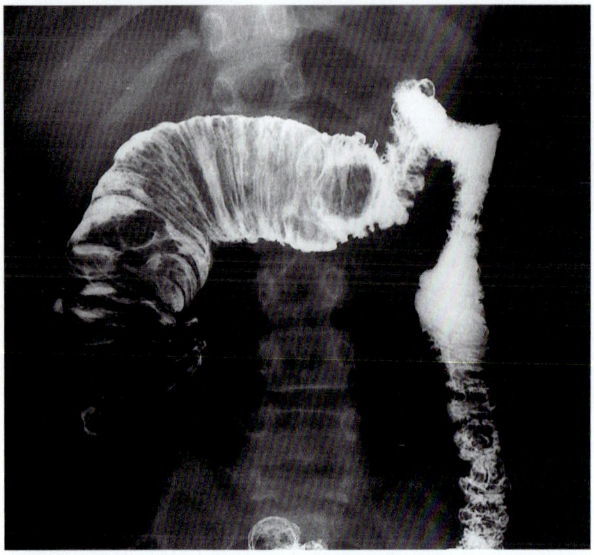

Figure 66.1: The barium enema shows the intussusception has reached the splenic flexure.

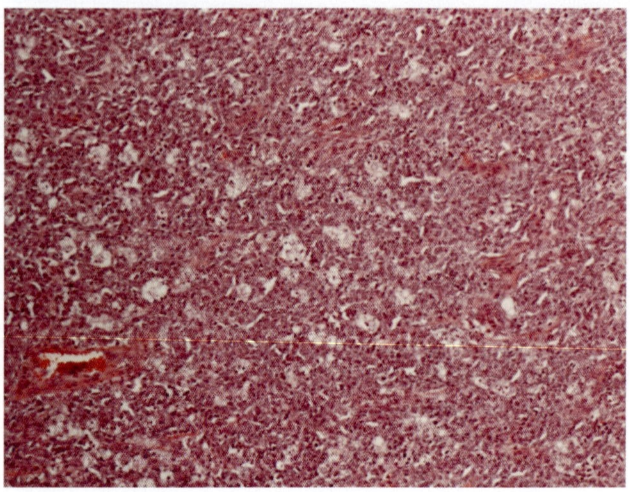

Figure 66.2: The small bowel lesion shows a diffuse infiltrate of lymphoid cells with the "starry sky" appearance.

Chemotherapy

The patient was treated with 6 courses of chemotherapeutic agents, which included cyclophosphamide, vincristine, methotrexate, doxorubicin, and cytarabine.

Follow-Up (2005)

The patient remains well without evidence of recurrence, 9 years since the resection.

Comment

In Western countries, Burkitt's Lymphoma is sporadic and accounts for 2% of all lymphomas. They usually present as abdominal tumors, as in this case, and may affect the jaw and peripheral lymph nodes, particularly in the neck. It is associated with the Epstein-Barr virus (EBV) in 20% of cases (Western disease). The histology shows diffuse changes with sheets of monomorphic neoplastic lymphoid cells evenly interspersed with histiocytes, producing the characteristic "starry sky" pattern.[1] The prognosis without treatment is very poor, howcvcr chemotherapy has been effective in inducing dramatic and complete tumor regression, as in this patient.

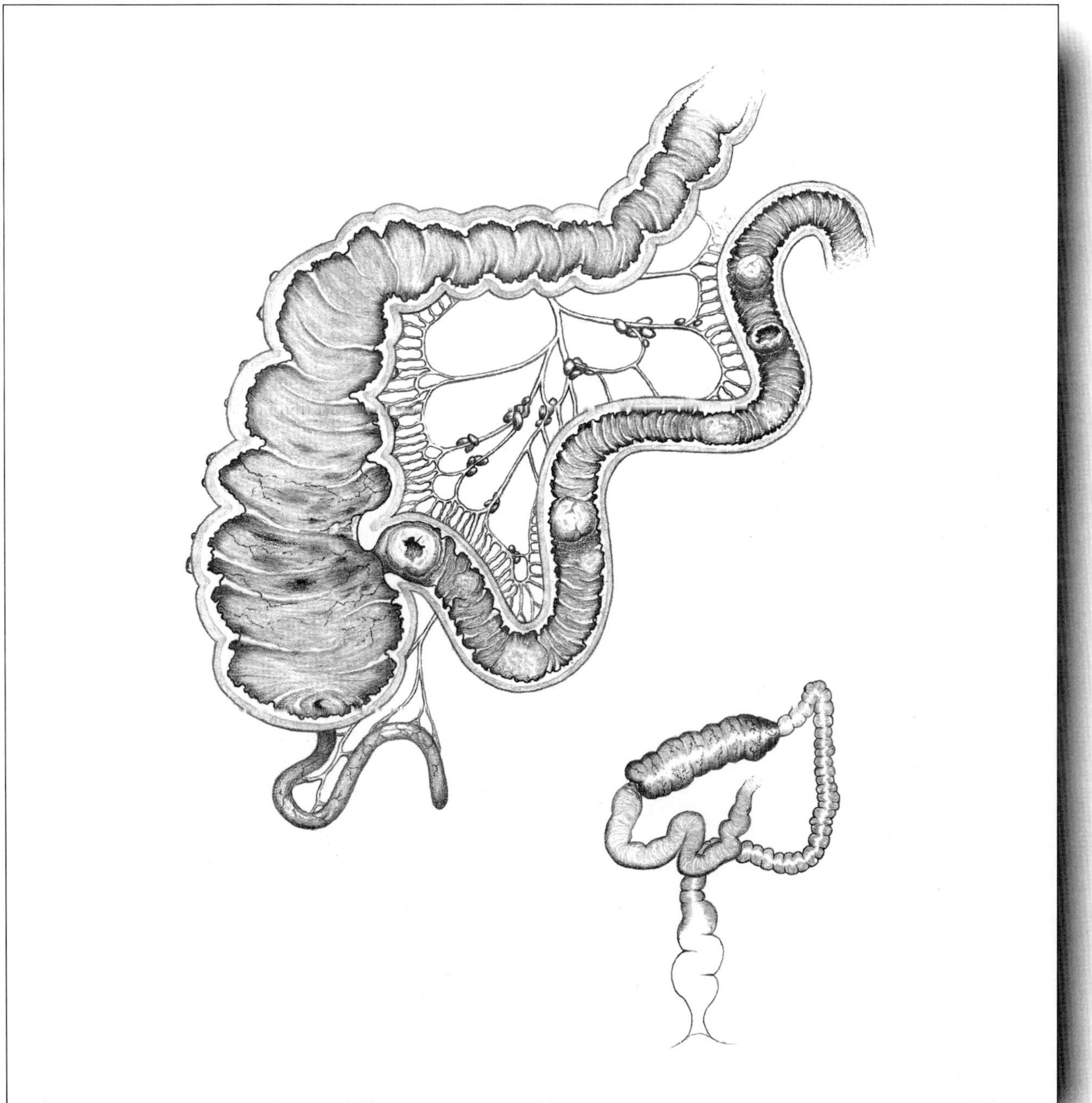

CASE

67 Ileocecal Lymphoma

Male, 82 Years

History

The patient had noted the recent onset of abdominal distention with 2 episodes of acute lower abdominal pain within 2 months. These symptoms were accompanied by a loss of weight. The stools had become black in color over a period of 7 days. Examination revealed a large nontender spherical mass occupying the right lower abdomen. A barium enema demonstrated dilatation of the terminal ileum with distortion of the mucosal pattern. A computerized tomography (CT) examination revealed a mass in the lower abdomen 10 × 10 × 8 cm extending into the cecum and ascending colon. A collection of contrast appeared within the mass, suggesting a bowel perforation was present. Colonoscopy revealed a large polypoid mass in the medial aspect of the proximal ascending colon and cecum, which obscured the ileocecal valve.

Operation (12.4.93)

A large confluent mass was confirmed in the ileocecal region. Its bulky nature suggested the possibility of a lymphoma. The mass appeared to infiltrate the ascending colon, terminal ileum, and mesentery. Enlarged lymph nodes were present along the ileocolic vessels. There was no other pathology detected within the abdomen. A right hemicolectomy was performed, including removal of 50 cm of terminal ileum.

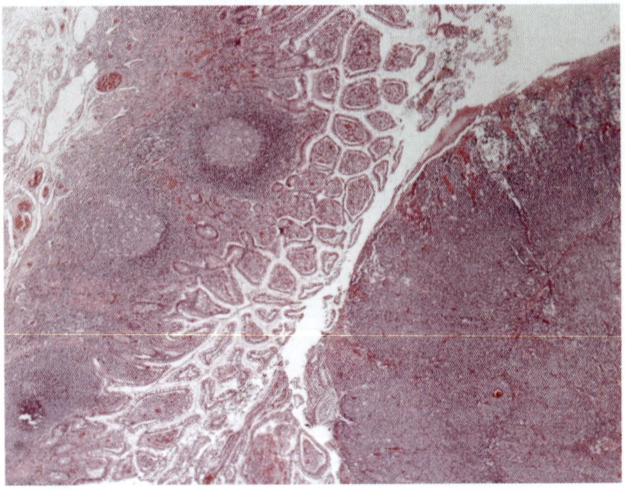

Figure 67.1: The left of the field shows 2 lymphoid follicles with germinal centers. The lymphoma is on the right. Small bowel villi are seen in transverse section.

Pathology

The mass "encased both the terminal ileum and the proximal right colon." On section, it was pale in color with a central cavity that communicated with the terminal ileum in two places. The mucosa of the ileum was otherwise normal. Within the mesentery, seven enlarged, firm lymph nodes were present. Histological examination confirmed the diagnosis of lymphoma (Figure 67.1). The tumor was a non-Hodgkin's large B cell type with a diffuse pattern. It was consistent with the so-called MALT lymphoma (arising from mucosal associated lymphoid tissue). The mesenteric lymph nodes were not involved with lymphoma. In the cecum, a flat pale polyp was present measuring 50 × 50 mm, which on examination was a dysplastic tubulovillous adenoma.

Follow-Up

Six weeks after operation, a right-sided abdominal mass was present and a gallium scan confirmed 4 foci of lymphoma within the abdomen. Over the next 7 months, 5 courses of chemotherapy were administered (cyclophosphamide, mitozantrone, vinblastine). The response to treatment was satisfactory and the patient remained in remission until 1997, when the disease recurred. At the age of 87 years, no further treatment was advised. The recurrent lymphoma was not the cause of death 4 years 9 months after operation, when he died unexpectedly during sleep.

Comment

This patient's clinical presentation and tumor morphology were typical of small bowel lymphoma. Such lesions represent 20% of small bowel tumors[1] and may be associated with Coeliac or Crohn's disease as well as immunodeficiency states. Preoperative diagnosis is unusual, but at operation a pale bulky tumor will suggest the diagnosis is lymphoma. In this patient, the MALT B cell tumor was low grade, which is usually associated with a more favorable prognosis. Adjuvant chemotherapy is frequently associated with resection of the disease, particularly if regional lymph nodes are involved.[2]

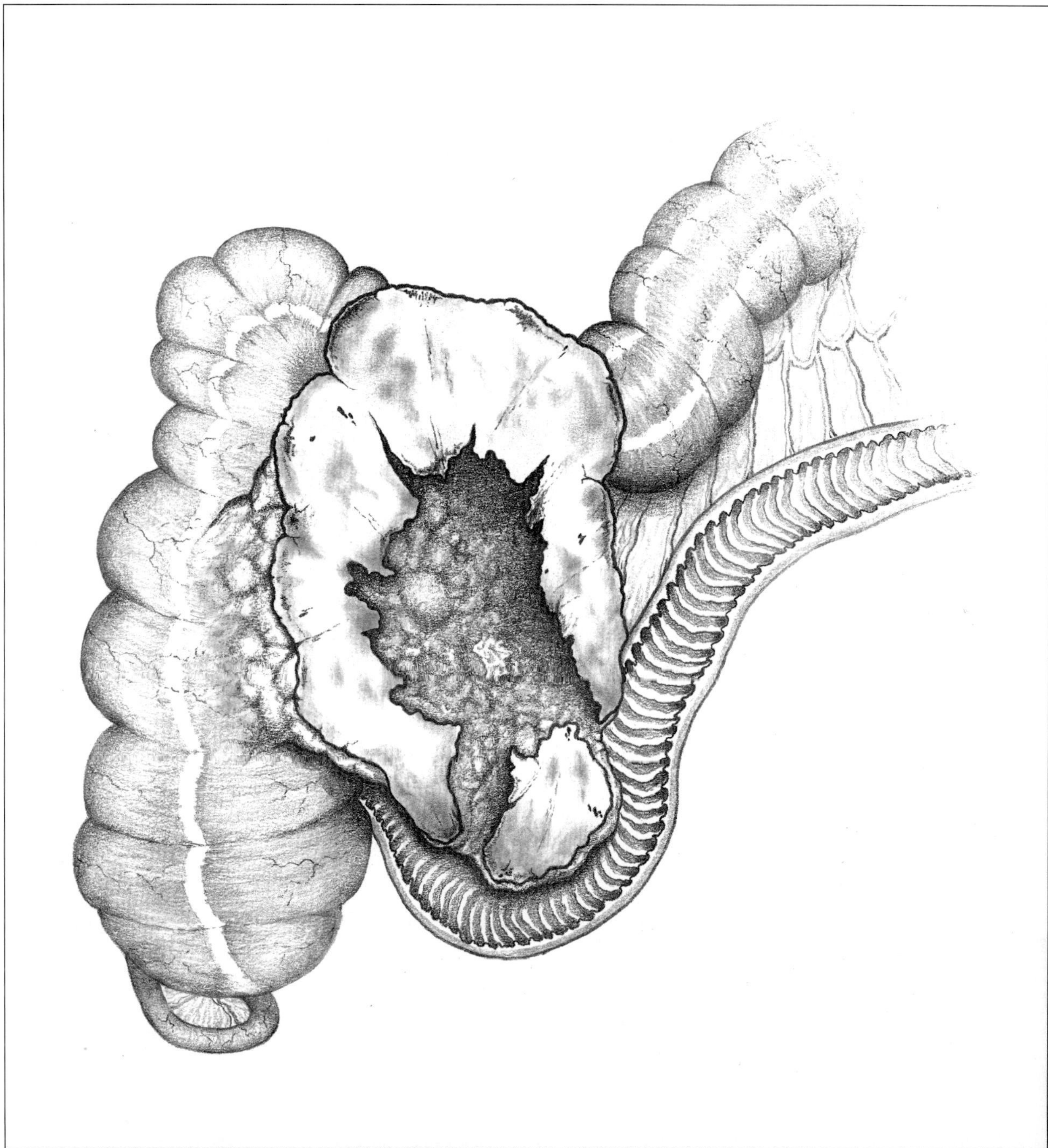

CASE

68 Multiple Lymphoma and Ulcerative Colitis

Female, 49 Years

History

The patient had noticed a few weeks of minimal dark red bleeding from the rectum and was examined by colonoscopy. There was diffuse low grade colitis (Figure 68.1) affecting the colon with a loss of vascular pattern and diminution of the haustral indentation. In the lower third of the sigmoid colon (at 20 cm), there was nodularity of the mucosa with associated hyperemia and small submucosal hemorrhages. Biopsy of this area revealed non-Hodgkin's lymphoma (NHL) of a diffuse type. Immunochemistry was positive for the B cell marker L26. Other biopsies of the mucosa showed nonspecific chronic inflammation. Staging investigation by gallium and computerized tomography (CT) scans revealed no other foci of lymphoma. Surgical treatment was advised in preference to chemotherapy.

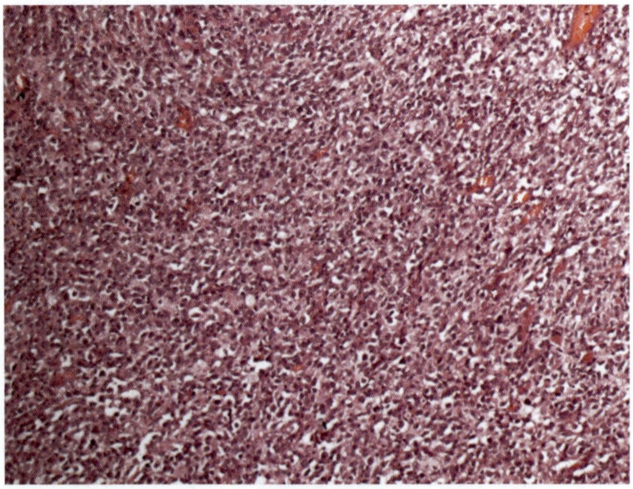

Figure 68.2: Diffuse large B cell lymphoma.

Operation (11.14.94)

The small bowel and colon were normal in appearance, with some thickening apparent in the lower third of the sigmoid colon on palpation. Small firm lymph nodes were palpable in the mesentery of the sigmoid and descending colon. The spleen was enlarged 40–50% of normal size. The extent of the resection was related to distribution of the palpable

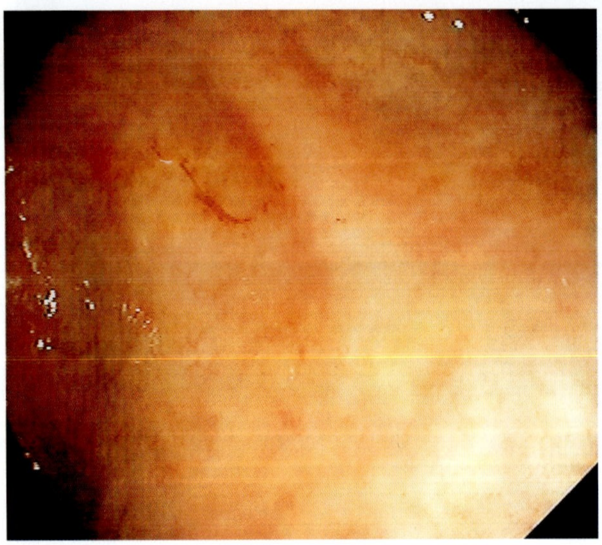

Figure 68.1: Endoscopy shows chronic inflammatory changes in the mucosa of the ascending colon (1998).

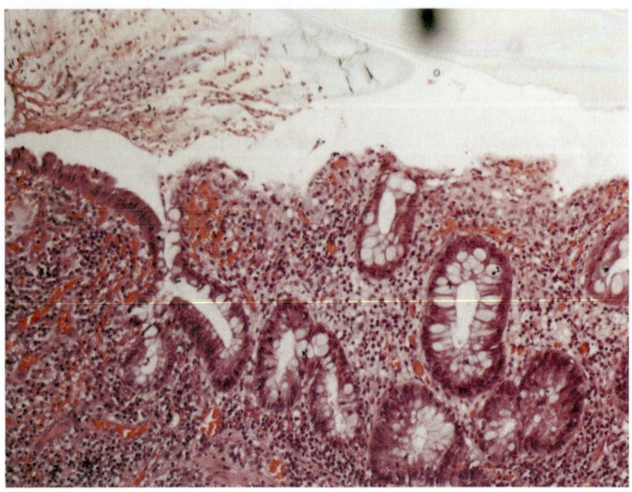

Figure 68.3: Evidence of Colitis: surface ulceration and distorted mucosal glands.

lymph nodes. The proximal level was the upper descending colon, and the distal level was mid rectum. The anastomosis was performed with a circular stapler.

Pathology

In the mucosa of the distal sigmoid, there were 5 pale, firm nodules 3–5 mm in size with surrounding congestion and areas of mucosal hemorrhage. Histologically, the nodules were malignant lymphoma of large cell B type (Figure 68.2). There were diffuse as well as follicular areas of lymphoma in the bowel wall. There was no evidence of lymphoma in any of 11 lymph nodes examined. Macroscopic evidence of colitis was minimal, but microscopic examination confirmed the presence of colitis (Figure 68.3).

Follow-Up (2005)

No chemotherapy was administered, since the localized disease appeared to be adequately removed by operation. Periodic examinations by gallium and CT scans have shown no evidence of recurrent lymphoma. The patient remains well more than 10 years since operation except for occasional episodes of diarrhea, which last for a few days. Surveillance colonoscopies with random biopsies have continued and reveal no change in the endoscopic or macroscopic appearances, which is consistent with a diffuse chronic nonspecific colitis of moderate degree (Figure 68.2).

Comment

Hopefully this patient's prognosis is favorable due to minimal localized lymphoma with no evidence of recurrence in over 10 years. It is unusual for gastrointestinal lymphoma to be a small lesion at the time of diagnosis. The obvious and numerous lymph nodes in the sigmoid and left colon mesentery determined the proximal level of the resection but proved negative for lymphoma. Chronic colitis coexisting with malignant lymphoma is rare and was first reported by Bargen in 1928.[1] Baker reported an incidence of 5 lymphomas in 2500 patients with chronic colitis.[2] It is not yet established whether the association of lymphoma and chronic ulcerative colitis (CUC) is a definite risk factor or coincidence, but some of the literature does support the former.[3] Multifocal involvement is not uncommon in gastrointestinal lymphoma, and the small multiple nodules were of interest in this patient. Wagonfeld et al have described a patient with CUC and 22 lymphomas in the colon.[4] The severity and duration of the colitis is variable in patients with coexistent lymphoma, and the patient described here has been asymptomatic most of the time. Surgery remains the mainstay for colorectal lymphoma. If the lymph nodes are not involved, chemotherapy is usually omitted.

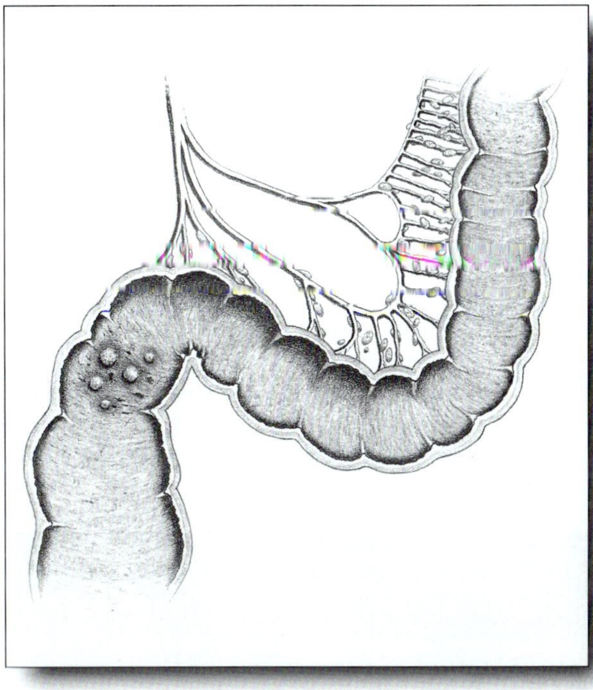

For a full-page image of this figure see the appendix.

CASE

69 Lymphoma of the Rectum

Male 63, Years

History

The patient presented with a history of bright blood on the stool for only a few days. He otherwise felt well. On rectal examination, a large firm polypoid lesion was palpable on the left anterior aspect of the lower third of the rectum 5 cm from the anal verge. It was moveable on palpation. Colonoscopy revealed no other pathology in the colon.

Operation (10.28.99)

The lesion was attached to the wall of the rectum by a broad pedicle, which could be readily constricted by closure of the diathermy snare. The polyp was removed with coagulation current (Figure 69.1) as a total specimen. The underlying rectal muscle remained intact.

Pathology

The polyp measured 25 × 22 × 12 mm. It was pale pink in color, with a lobulated surface. Histologically, the lesion was covered by colonic mucosa with some inflammatory reaction. Beneath the mucosa, there was a nodular mass infiltrating the submucosa composed of a "monotonous population" of intermediate to large sized lymphoid cells. Numerous mitotic figures and apoptotic cells were scattered throughout. Immunoperoxidase stains identified the lesion as a malignant non-Hodgkin's lymphoma of diffuse large B cell type (Figure 69.2).

Further Treatment/Follow-Up (2004)

Investigations revealed no other foci of lymphoma. The patient was treated with 4 cycles of chemotherapy (cyclophosphamide, doxorubacin, vincristine, and prednisolone). The site of the lymphoma healed readily, and regular clinical, endoscopic, and computerized tomography (CT) examinations have shown no evidence of recurrent disease 4 years 6 months after removal of the rectal lesion.

Comment

Gastrointestinal lymphoma accounts for 2%–5% of gastrointestinal tract (GIT) malignancy[1] and is the most common extranodal site.[2] Au et al report the incidence in the GIT as: stomach, 57%: small bowel, 22%; large bowel, 7%; gallbladder, 2%; and multiple sites, 11%.[1] The prognosis for control of this patient's disease is estimated to be in the vicinity of 70%. The technique of diathermy snare with strong coagulation current was used in this patient only because the lesion was in the extraperitoneal rectum.

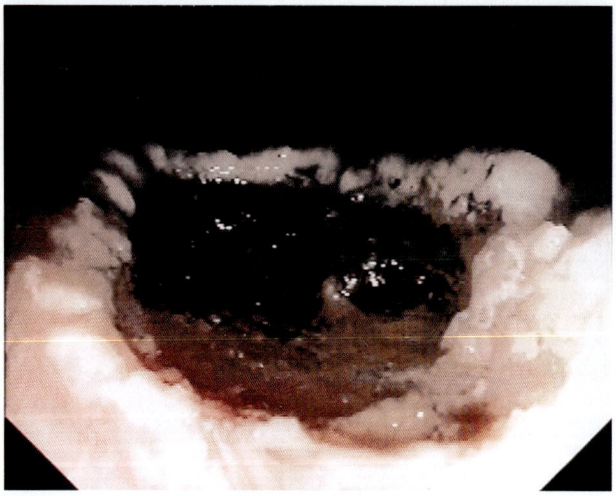

Figure 69.1: Endoscopic view of the defect after diathermy snare removal. Blood clot in the proximal part of the defect.

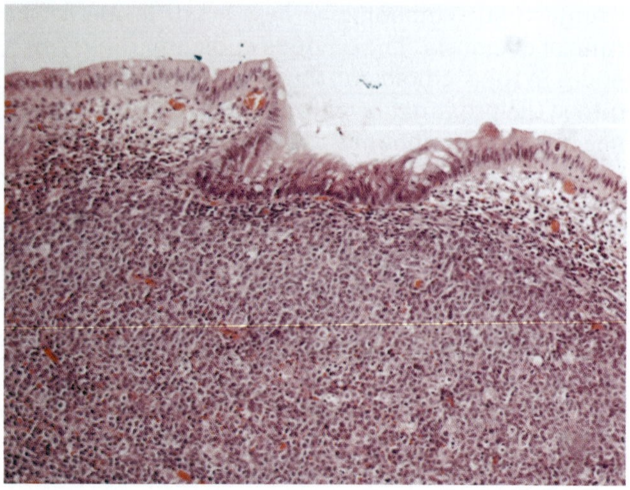

Figure 69.2: The lymphoma is apparent beneath the mucosa.

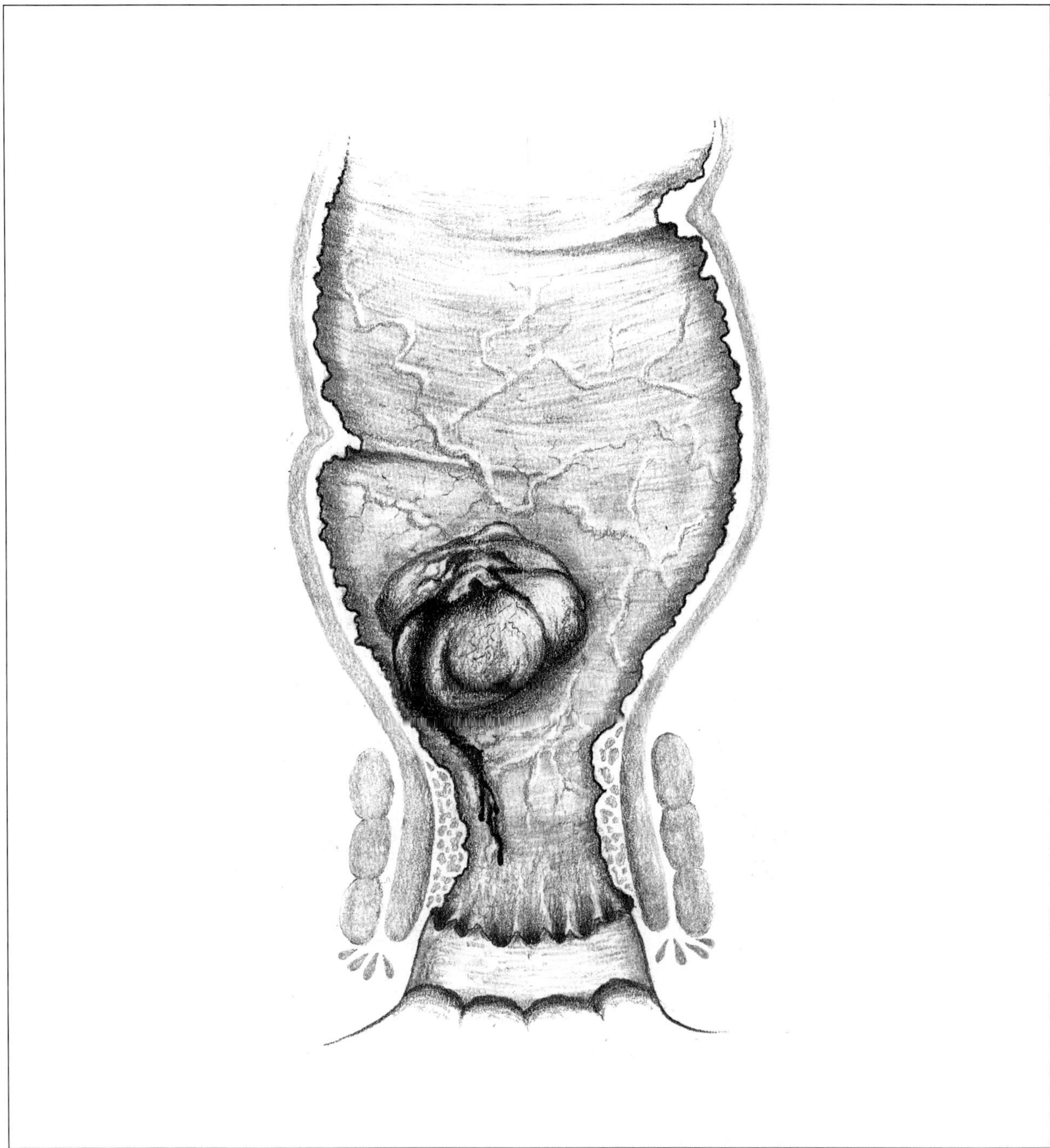

PART VIII Anorectal Disease

CASE

70 An Intrasphincteric Anal Tumor

Female, 59 Years

History

The patient had, for some years, been diagnosed as suffering from an irritable bowel. For a "few months," she had noticed rectal pain on defecation which had become severe and was aggravated by her bowel frequency. She was not aware of any swelling, but there was a sense of blockage during a bowel action. On examination, there was a smooth, rounded, nontender mass on the left side of the anal canal, extending just above the anorectal junction and bulging into the lumen beneath intact mucosa. It extended into the ischiorectal fossa and was readily palpable in the perianal region. Flexible sigmoidoscopy was normal to 30 cm. Transrectal ultrasound (TRUS) revealed a poorly echogenic mass deep to the mucosa within the sphincter muscle. At this examination, fine needle aspiration biopsy was performed. Histologically, this revealed a "smooth muscle tumor" with no evidence of malignancy.

Operation (9.2.91)

Under spinal anaesthetic and with the patient in the prone jack-knife position, a hemicircumferential incision was made over the palpable mass on the left side of the anal verge. Dissection lateral to the external sphincter, "stretched" over the mass, identified the inferior hemorrhoidal nerve. Incision of a thin rim of sphincter muscle revealed the surface of the tumor that was then dissected free from its location entirely within the external sphincter muscle without loss of muscle tissue. The space within the muscle was closed over a small soft rubber drain.

Pathology

The egg shaped tumor, with a well defined capsule (Figure 70.1), measured 50 × 38 × 35 mm, and the surface was smooth with some shallow lobulation. On section, it was pale yellow in color and homogeneous in texture without hemorrhage or necrosis. Histologically, it was uniformly cellular, being composed of spindle cells exhibiting mild atypia with 4 mitoses per 50 high-power fields (Figure 70.2). The tumor was regarded as being "most likely benign." Since the original pathology examination, immunohistochemical staining with C117 has been performed, confirming that the lesion is a gastrointestinal stromal tumor (GIST).

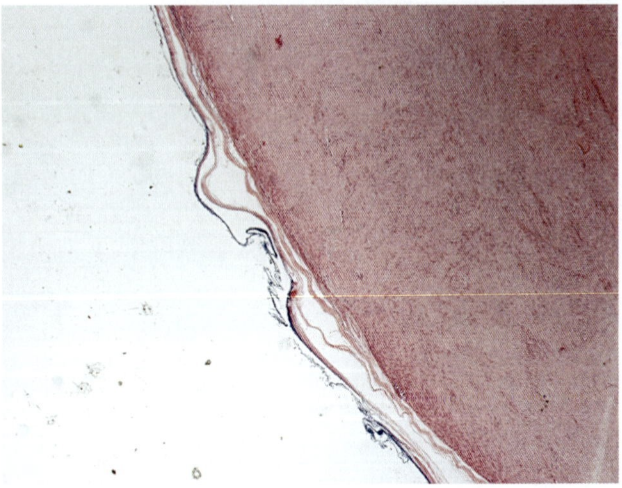

Figure 70.1: Section shows a circumscribed tumor with a well defined capsule.

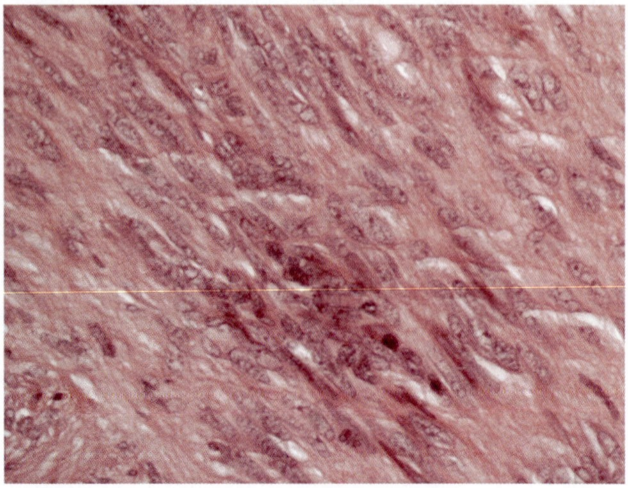

Figure 70.2: Higher power magnification shows a dense field of plump spindle cells, typical of a GIST.

Follow-Up (2005)

There has been no recurrence of the tumor since operation more than 13 years ago. Anal sphincter function is normal without any degree of incontinence. The patient is examined by panendoscopy and colonoscopy on a regular basis for a hiatus hernia, gastric polyps, and symptomatic diverticular disease.

Comment

Tumors of the anal sphincter are rare and stromal tumors the more so.[1] Topographical tumors, more common in other sites, have been reported involving the anal canal: spindle cell lipoma;[2] neurofibrous;[3] and granular cell tumor.[4] Other lesions that may clinically suggest a tumor in this region are chronic intersphincteric abscess, oleogranuloma, and endometrioma.[5] The cloacogenic carcinoma may present as a subepithelial mass in the anal canal. Tan et al have managed a similar tumor to the one described here. Their tumor was initially locally excised and found to have a mitotic count of 4 per 50 high-power fields.[1] Subsequently, abdominoperineal excision of the rectum was performed, which revealed residual stromal tumor with a mitotic count of 2 per 10 high-power fields. This emphasizes the difficulty of assessing the malignant potential of these tumors. Precise preoperative imaging is essential in planning the surgical approach to a tumor involving the anal sphincter, and currently either endoanal ultrasound or magnetic resonance imaging (MRI) with endorectal coil appear to be equally accurate.[6] Local excision to provide a "total biopsy" would appear to be the first step in management. If there is then doubt concerning malignancy, the area can be readily monitored by the available imaging techniques.

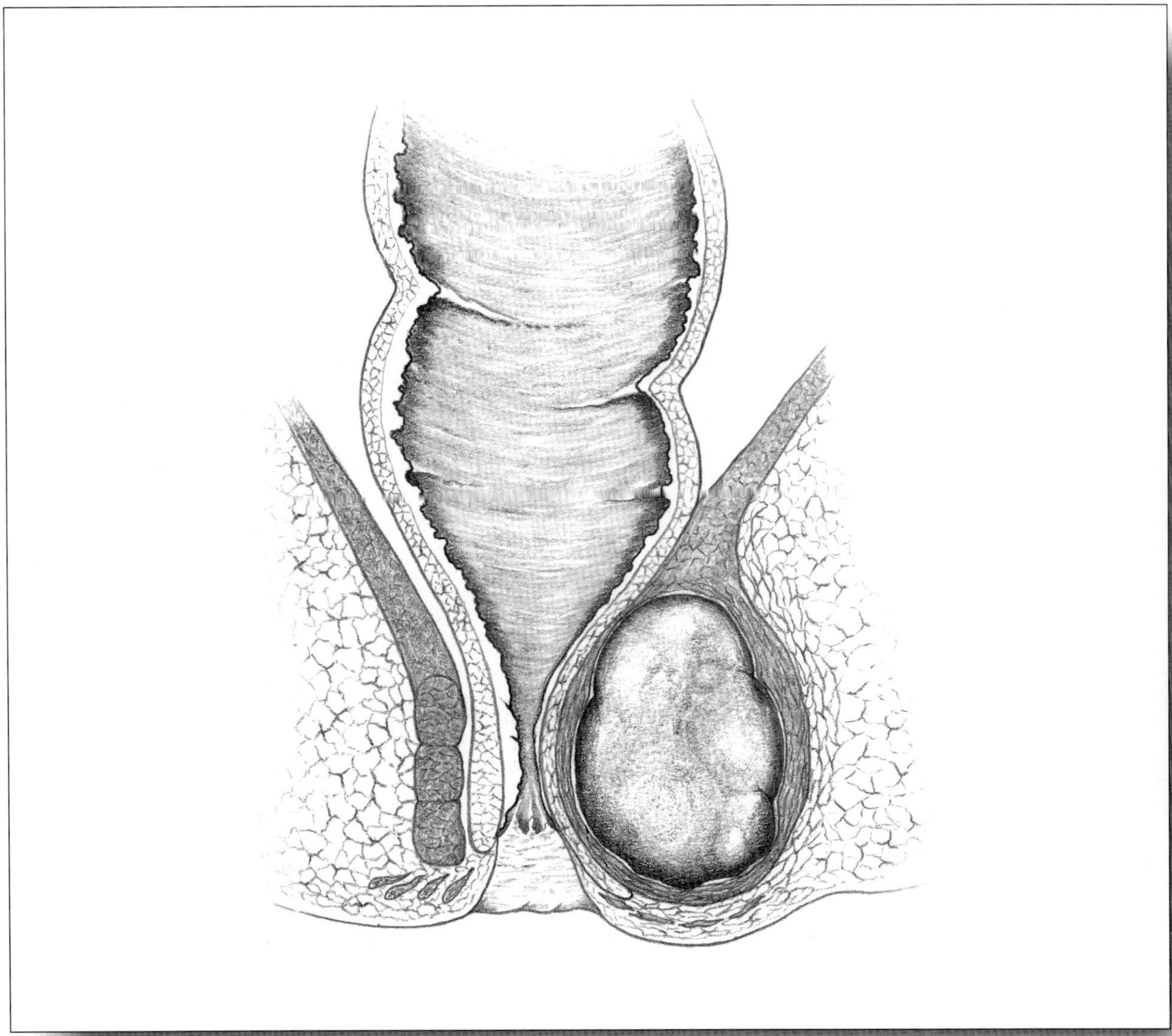

CASE

71 Aggressive Pelvic Angiomyxoma of the Pelvis

Male, 64 Years

History

The patient had been aware of a swelling in the (left) ischiorectal region for 2 years, which altered in prominence with posture, i.e., it appeared to be less obvious when laying on his right side. On examination, a soft cystic swelling was apparent, filling the left ischiorectal fossa. Computerized tomography (CT) examination revealed the ischiorectal lesion was in continuity with a large pelvic mass, mainly left-sided with clearly defined margins. There was displacement of pelvic structures. The maximum diameter was 75 mm. It did not appear to be connected with the small or large bowel. Needle biopsy was nondiagnostic.

Operation (6.4.90)

The surgical approach was abdomino-ischiorectal. The tumor was closely associated with the rectum, which it displaced from the left side. The areolar tissue around the tumor was dense and fibrous. The tumor was dumbbell shaped with an isthmus where it passed through the levator ani. Large vessels were present over its surface. The margins of the levator ani defect were rigid and difficult to dilate in order to extract the tumor via the pelvis. The tumor was removed intact. Profuse venous bleeding was controlled with packs.

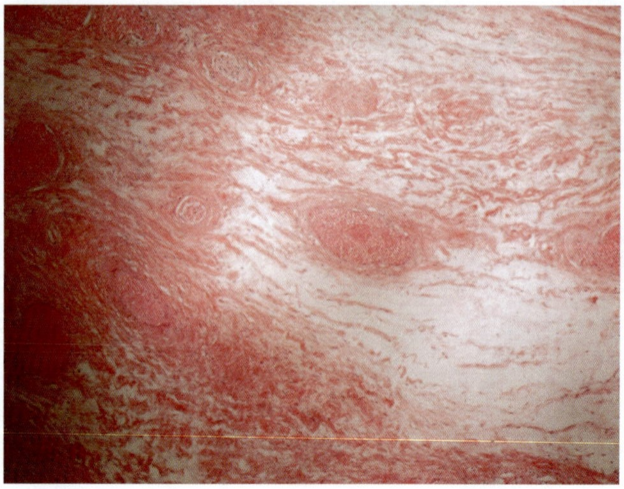

Figure 71.1: Histological appearance shows a myxoid stroma and thin-walled vascular spaces.

Pathology

The tumor size was 17 × 11 cm. There was a thin capsule of fibrous tissue. The consistency was "doughy." The cut surface was pale gray and soft with evidence of some fibrous tissue. Histological examination revealed spindle cells in a loose myxoid stroma (Figure 71.1) with scattered mast cells. Moderate numbers of blood vessels were present. There was no evidence of malignancy. Diagnosis: aggressive angiomyxoma.

Follow-Up (2004)

The patient has been free of recurrence for 14 years. For some years prior to operation, he had been troubled by intractable nausea, which was immediately relieved by removal of the tumor.

Comment

This rare mesenchymal tumor, more common in females, can be troublesome with local recurrence, but there is no tendency to metastasize.[1] The tumor usually involves the pelvic soft tissues and often attains a large size,[1] as occurred in this patient. Wilson reported an identical case, although it was larger, measuring 45 cm in length.[2] The need for radical operation does not appear to be mandatory but will depend on the operative findings. Nyam and Pemberton report an angiomyxoma in a similar anatomical location but with invasion of the rectum.[3] The patient was treated with preoperative embolization, external radiotherapy, intraoperative radiotherapy, and abdominoperineal excision of the rectum.

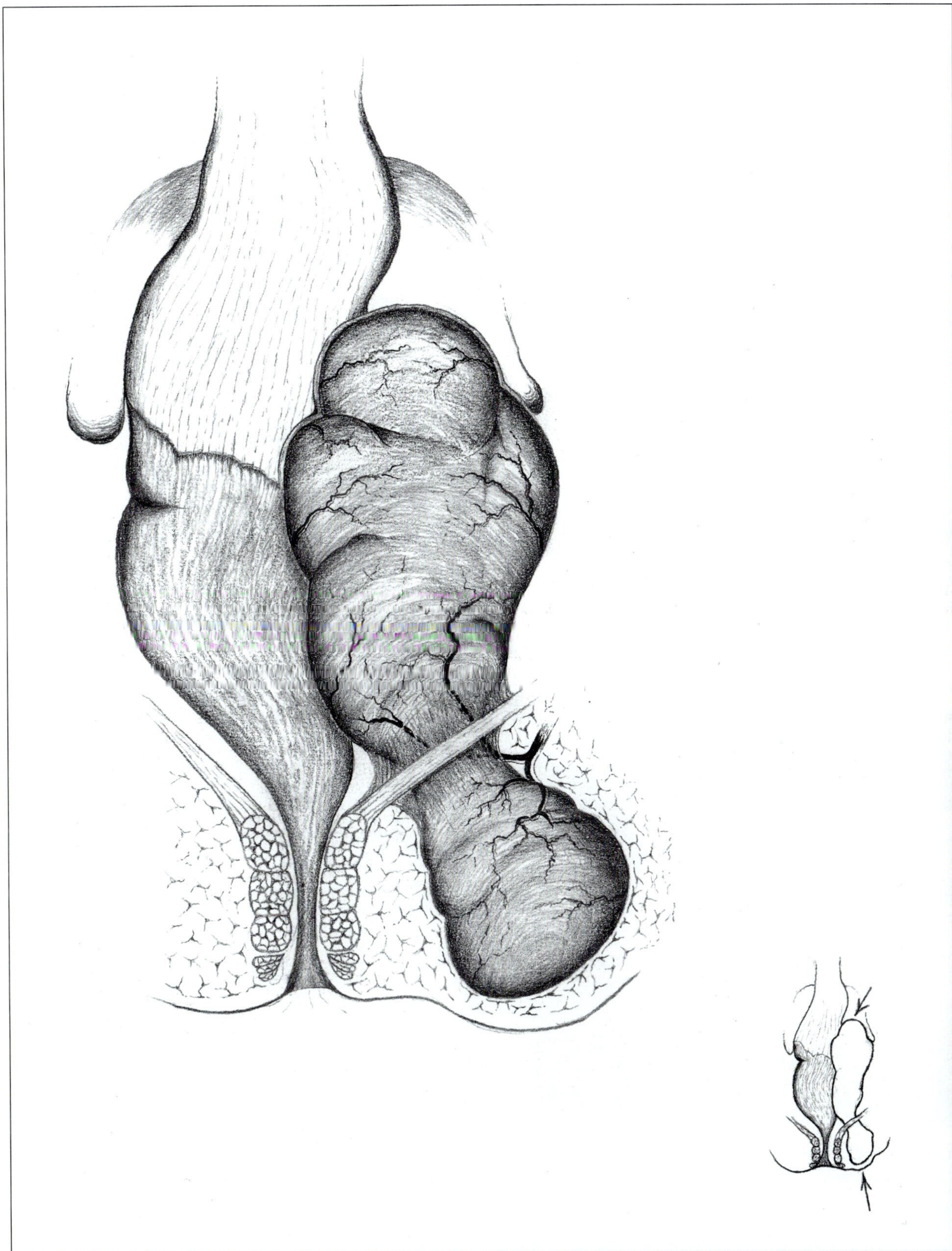

CASE

72 Implantation Metastasis into an Anal Fistula

Male, 63 Years

History

The patient had been diagnosed with an anal fistula 8 years previously. During this period, intermittent discharge occurred in the left perianal region. He complained of a further swelling in the area, increasing in size over a period of 3 weeks. There were no bowel symptoms. There were 2 firm nodules in the left ischiorectal fossa surrounded by inflammation. Adenocarcinoma was confirmed, "erupting" through the perianal skin. There were enlarged hard lymph nodes in the left inguinal region. Sigmoidoscopy and biopsy identified an ulcerating carcinoma of the sigmoid colon at 20 cm.

Operation (8.7.63)

An abdominoperineal resection of the primary tumor with en bloc resection of the lesion in the ischiorectal fossa was performed. The large defect in the buttock was left open to heal by secondary intention.

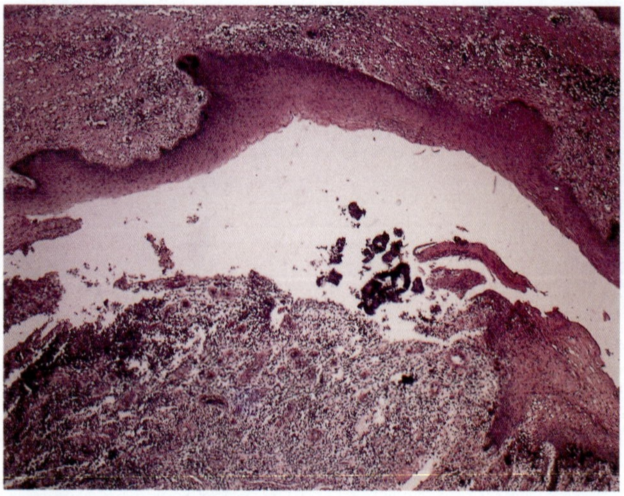

Figure 72.1: Free cancer cells are present in the proximal part of the fistula track.

Pathology

The primary tumor was a well differentiated adenocarcinoma confined to the muscular wall of the colon. There was an adjacent polyp containing a focus of adenocarcinoma. The internal opening of the anal fistula was identified on the dentate line with a track leading to the 2 nodules of adenocarcinoma. Free cancer cells were identified in the fistula track (Figure 72.1). Both sites of cancer were histologically similar. There were no metastases in the mesenteric lymph nodes or in multiple sections of the bowel between the primary tumor and the anal canal.

Follow-Up (1976)

The perineal wound healed in 10 weeks. The inguinal lymphadenopathy subsided completely and no biopsy was performed. The patient remained free of recurrence for a known follow up period of 13 years and 3 months.

Comment

Distal implantation by a proximal adenocarcinoma into an anal fistula may have been first described by Guiss.[1] Implantation into other anal lesions, including hemorrhoidectomy wounds, has also been reported.[2,3] From a pathological viewpoint, a high anterior resection and radical excision of the ischiorectal anal canal lesions would have been feasible in the patient reported here, as there was no intervening focus of malignancy. Using immunohistochemical stains, Hyman and Kida identified a sigmoid carcinoma and a metastasis in an anal fistula as the same malignancy.[4] Although this investigation was not performed in the patient described here, the perianal lesion is regarded as an implantation metastasis, rather than a synchronous primary tumor. Adenocarcinoma arising in a long-standing fistula is most frequently a colloid carcinoma.[5]

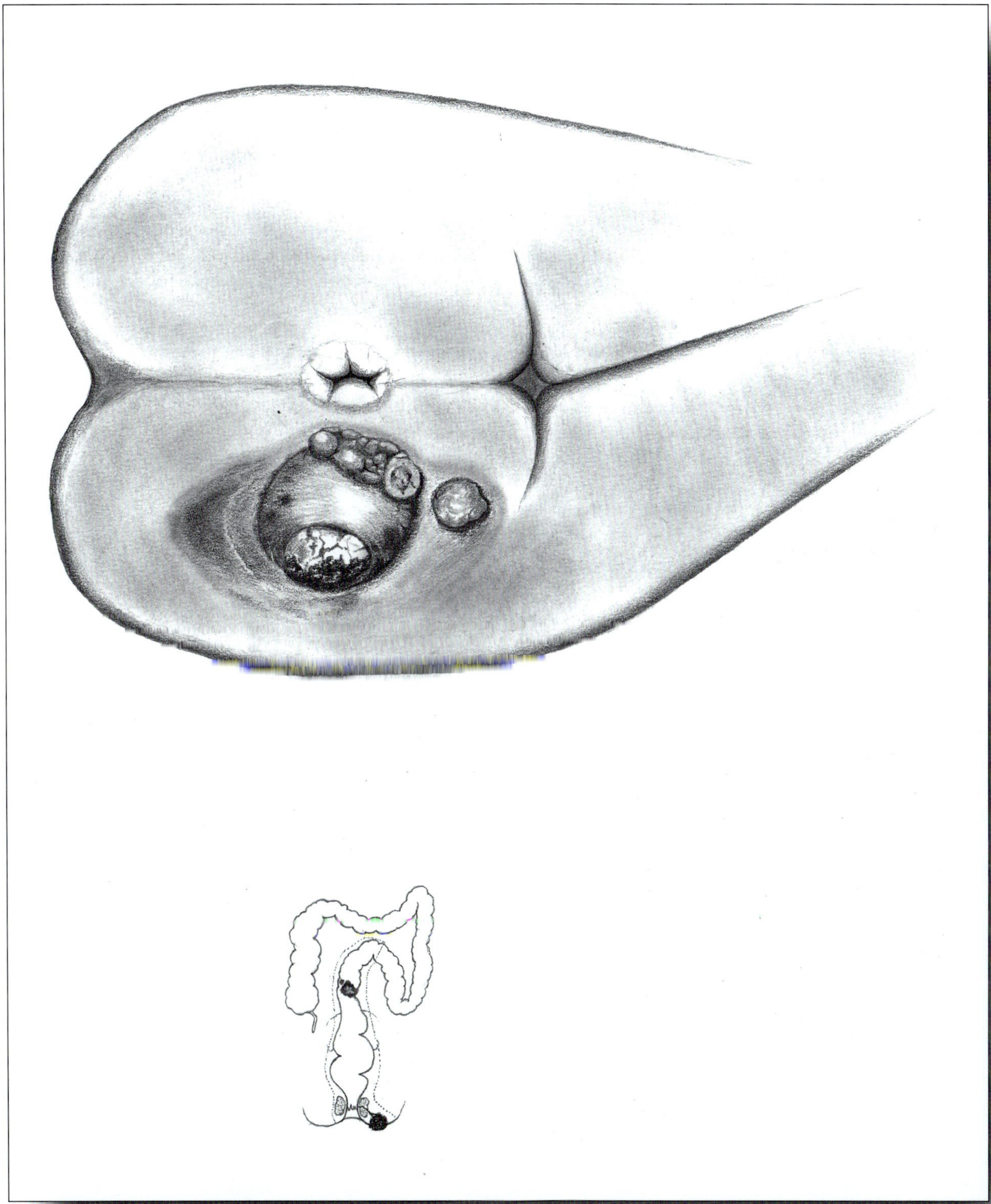

CASE

73 Local Excision of a Rectal Carcinoma Can Be an Easy Operation

Female, 86 Years

History

The patient, who suffered from severe cerebral dementia, was under supervision in a nursing home for the aged. The nursing staff noted rectal prolapse of at least 8 cm in length. An "ulcerated area" on the apex of the prolapse was biopsied and the diagnosis of adenocarcinoma confirmed. The attending gastroenterologist referred the patient. Sigmoidoscopy after reduction of the prolapse located the tumor on the posterior wall of the rectum at 10 cm from the anal verge (there is no available record of a colonoscopy). Abdominal computerized tomography (CT) showed no evidence of major perirectal spread or metastatic disease.

Operation (5.20.83)

With the rectum prolapsed, a "disc" local excision was performed (coagulation diathermy), including a >5 mm margin of normal tissue. The excision exposed the mesorectal fat, but the peritoneal cavity was not exposed. The defect in the wall of the rectum was closed with interrupted sutures.

Pathology

The tumor was a flat plaque 4.5 cm in diameter, deeply penetrating the muscle wall but not extending beyond it. Mesorectal fat, 15 mm in thickness, was attached to the deep surface. Histological examination revealed a well differentiated adenocarcinoma. The excision margins were negative for carcinoma.

Follow-Up (1987)

Postoperative healing of the rectal wall was satisfactory. No surgery was performed for the rectal prolapse, which did not reappear with any significant frequency. The patient was last examined 4 years, 5 months after the local excision, at the age of 91 years, when sigmoidoscopy was normal to 25 cm and there was no evidence of recurrent carcinoma.

Comment

The rectal prolapse greatly facilitated the local excision by presenting the tumor at the apex of the prolapse. Rectosigmoidectomy (Altemeier operation) at the same time as the local excision was deferred in the presence of the exposed malignancy. Subsequently, the prolapse was not causing sufficient problems to justify any surgery in a demented patient. It is quite likely that the rectal carcinoma was initiating the more frequent prolapse prior to local excision.

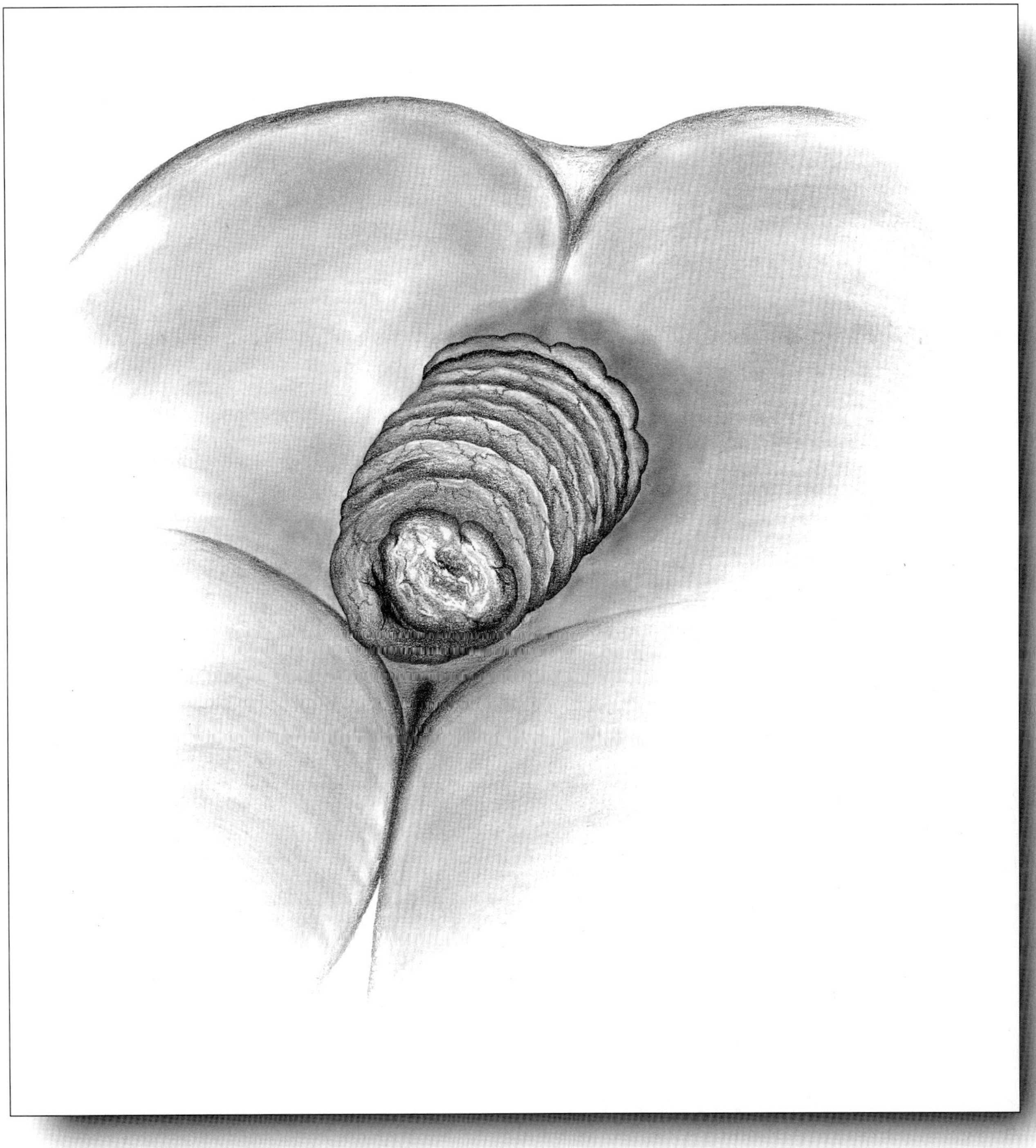

CASE

74 Proctitis Cystica Profunda

Female, 26 Years

History

The patient complained of symptoms for 8 years, which were: rectal discomfort ("a lump"), frequent bowel actions, diarrhea (mucus), intermittent bleeding, and rectal pain. There was evidence of a chronic anxiety state and addiction to analgesics. Sigmoidoscopy and examination under anaesthesia revealed 2 hard areas of leukoplakia, a fibrous stricture of the mid anal canal, and squamous metaplasia immediately above the dentate line. The mucosa above this area was hyperemic, redundant, and polypoid to a level of 8 cm, above which the mucosa was normal. Straining revealed marked internal rectal prolapse. Biopsy of the hyperemic mucosa showed histological changes "consistent with Morson's solitary rectal ulcer" (Figure 74.1).

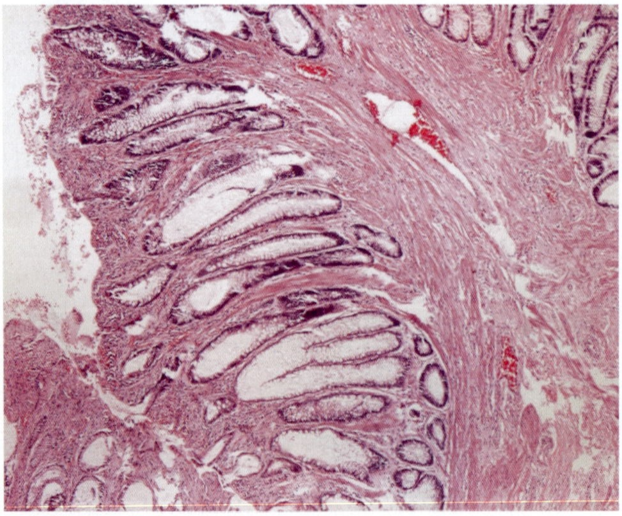

Figure 74.1: Thick extensions of the muscularis mucosa are seen radiating between the mucosal glands towards the ulcerated surface.

Operation (1.30.79)

Ripstein rectopexy was performed.

Follow-Up (1995)

The rectal symptoms were relieved and most of the macroscopic features of the rectal mucosa resolved permantly. The leukoplakia was unchanged. Two months after operation, bowel function was satisfactory, but 6 years later, the patient was complaining of prolonged periods of constipation, abdominal pain, and distention. Investigations revealed a markedly redundant colon. Colon transit studies were not performed. On 8/26/85, abdominal colectomy was performed for intractable constipation. During the period 1989–1991, several operations were required to cure a complicated anal fistula. The patient continued to complain of chronic abdominal pain and remained addicted to analgesics.

Comment

The morphology and histology were consistent with the diagnosis of proctitis cystica profunda. An association with rectal prolapse of 54% has been reported by Stuart.[1] In this patient, complete rectal prolapse may have been "held back" by the anal canal stricture. There was a satisfactory response of the patient's ongoing symptoms to rectopexy, which unfortunately was later complicated by severe constipation requiring further operation. The morphological and histological appearances may cause confusion with carcinoma of the rectum, particularly the presence of displaced, distorted mucous secreting glands within the submucosa. Nagasako et al. report such a case treated by abdominoperineal excision of the rectum.[2] Valenzuela et al. report 2 patients in whom computerized tomography (CT) and magnetic resonance imaging (MRI) demonstrated the disease limited in depth to the submucosal layer. Both patients were treated with a high fiber diet, bulk laxatives, and reeducation to avoid straining. Resolution of the pathology occurred in both patients with this conservative treatment.[3]

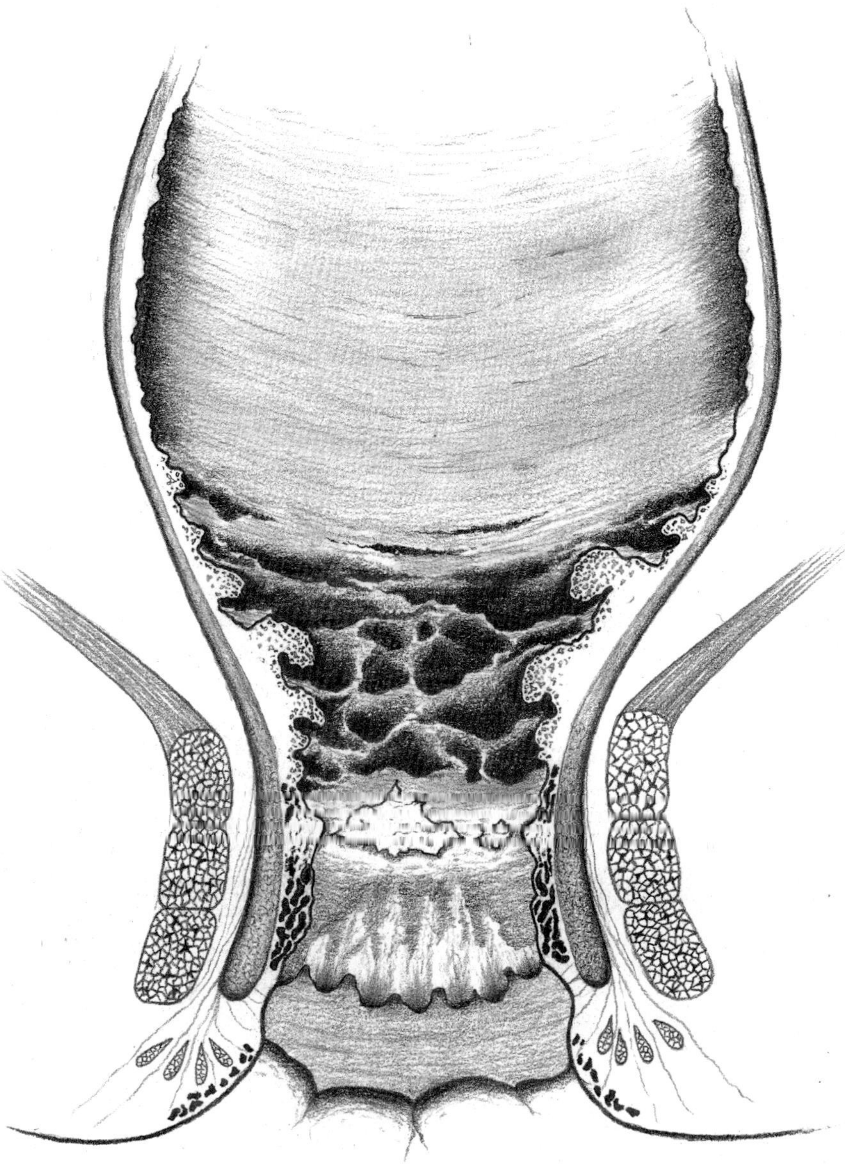

Examination under anaesthesia

11.28.78

CASE

75 Rectopexy for a Rectal Stricture-Ulcer

Male, 38 Years

History

The patient presented in 1985 with a long history of a sense of blockage in the rectum that resulted in prolonged defecation. There had been minor rectal bleeding and mucous discharge for 1 year. There was no awareness of any prolapse. Rectal examination revealed a firm stricture in the mid rectum, confirmed at 8 cm by sigmoidoscopy. The lumen at this point was approximately 13 mm in diameter. There were leukoplakia-like projections on the "rim" of the stenosis and 5 areas of shallow ulceration at this level. The base of the ulcers was yellow-white, firm, and surrounded by erythematous mucosa. Above this level to 15 cm, the mucosa appeared normal. A barium enema demonstrated the abnormality (Figure 75.1). The radiologist stated the appearances were not exclusive of a neoplasm.

Biopsy

Biopsy of the lesion showed distortion of the mucosal glands, chronic inflammation, submucosal fibrosis, and squamous epithelium. These findings along with the sigmoidoscopic appearances were consistent with the diagnosis of solitary rectal ulcer syndrome (SRUS).

Operation (7.29.85)

At laparotomy, there was no apparent abnormality of the rectum or colon. There was no palpable thickening of the rectum at the level of the stenosis. There was a deep rectoprostatic "pouch of Douglas" and virtual absence of normal pararectal fascia ("lateral ligaments"). The rectum was mobilized to the pelvic floor and anterior rectopexy performed using a 4 cm wide band of monofilament polypropylene (Ripstein operation).

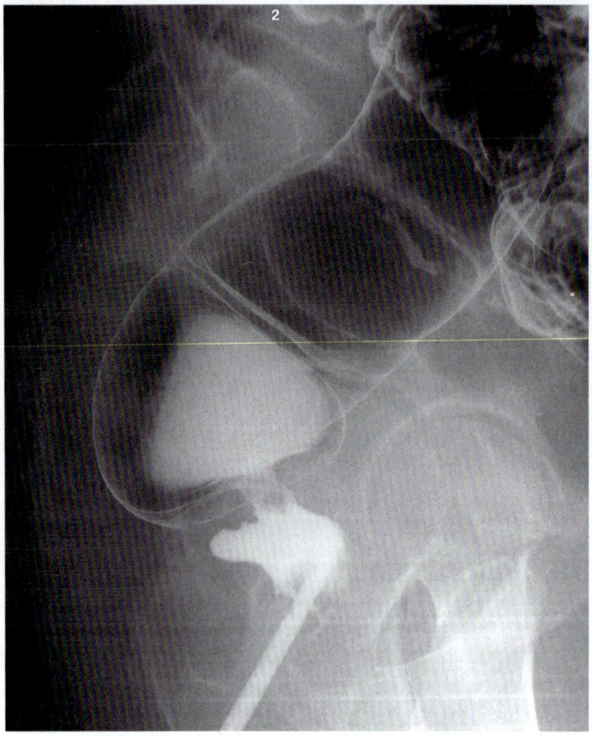

Figure 75.1: The barium enema on 5/14/85 (preoperative) shows an annular irregular stenosis of the rectum with "shouldering." Below this level, the rectum was in spasm.

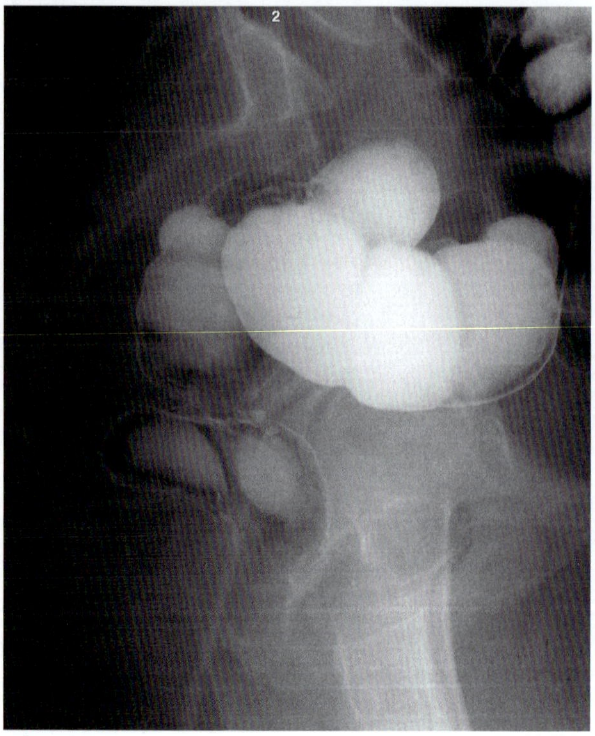

Figure 75.2: Barium enema on 8/19/86 (15 months after operation) shows a persistent area of narrowing. The rectum below this appears normal.

Follow-Up (1990)

Four weeks after operation, the patient reported a significant improvement in bowel function. The sense of obstruction was greatly diminished. Frequency of defecation was reduced, and the stools were now of normal diameter. Rectal examination revealed the stenosis had improved and was now soft and supple. The clinical improvement was maintained and, 13 months after operation, the stenosis was almost impalpable and not apparent on sigmoidoscopy. The ulceration had healed, leaving some erythema and persistent leukoplakia. A barium enema 15 months after operation showed persistent narrowing, which was surprising in view of the clinical and sigmoidoscopic findings (Figure 75.2). When the patient was last examined 5 years after the operation he was asymptomatic and without recurrence of the rectal ulceration.

Comment

The clinical, endoscopic, and pathological features of this condition were defined by the seminal publication of Madigan and Morson in 1969.[1] The ulceration is more common in the incomplete (internal intussusception) variety of rectal prolapse.[2] This patient's rectal ulcers were classical SRUS in appearance, although circumferential ulceration and associated stricture are unusual. The stricture is related to the marked submucosal fibrosis that occurs in association with the ulceration. There was no rectal intussusception detected endoscopically (proctography was not performed). Rectopexy for SRUS has been shown to have a low success rate when not accompanied by complete rectal prolapse,[1] although Nicholls and Simson have reported symptomatic success in 12 out of 14 patients.[3] In the presence of disabling symptoms and no alternative operation, rectopexy in this patient was undertaken as a speculative procedure. It was considered that rectal intussusception may have been an etiological factor but obscured by the development of stenosis. The response to rectopexy was successful and lasting. The persistence of the narrowing radiologically is interesting in view of the near-normal appearance on sigmoidoscopic examination. In the author's series of 216 Ripstein rectopexies (complete prolapse, 180; incomplete prolapse, 36), there was only one other patient with SRUS and stenosis. This patient also responded well to rectopexy. The terminology and classification of the rectal prolapse syndrome, rectal intussusception, solitary rectal ulcer syndrome, and proctitis cystica profunda needs an international consensus.

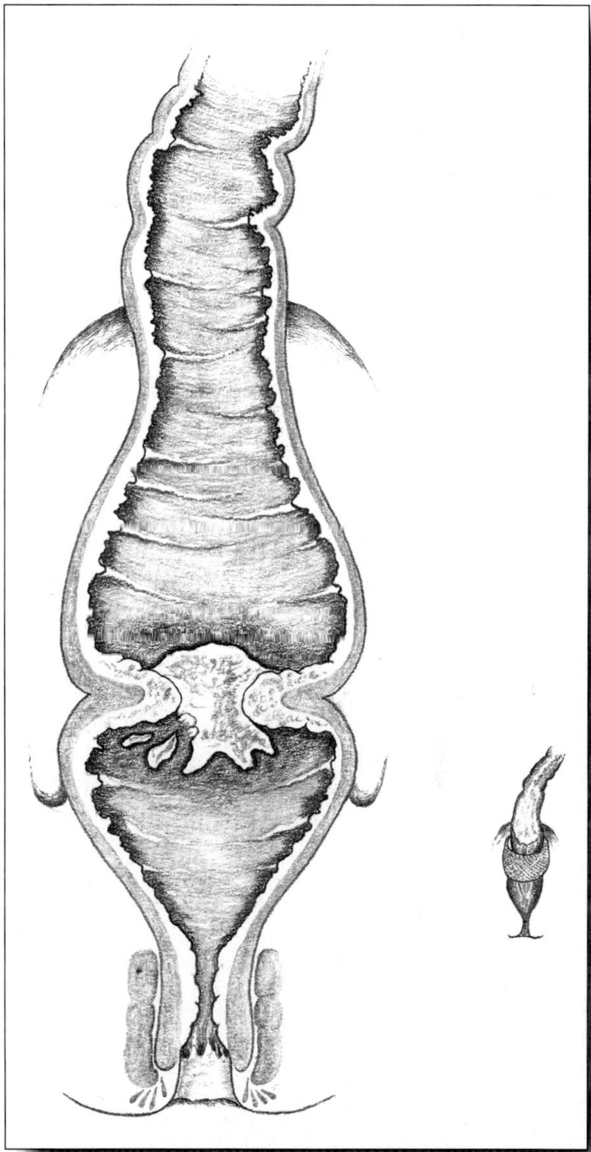

CASE

76 Intersphincteric Anal Fistula with Proximal Perirectal Extension

Male, 34 Years

History

In June 1977, an anal fistula was treated by operation, and, although healing occurred, the rectum was "abnormal". The radiological demonstration of a rectal stricture suggested the possibility of Crohn's disease (Figure 76.1). The patient was referred for further management. Examination under anaesthesia revealed marked rigidity of the anorectal junction and the rectum with a long stricture of the rectum, most marked between 10 cm and 13 cm. An internal opening was identified on the left lateral aspect of the dentate line with an ascending track passing anteriorly. A focus of granulation tissue at 10 cm in the midline anteriorly was identified as a probable secondary internal opening. The rectal mucosa was pale and edematous. Biopsies at various levels showed nonspecific inflammation.

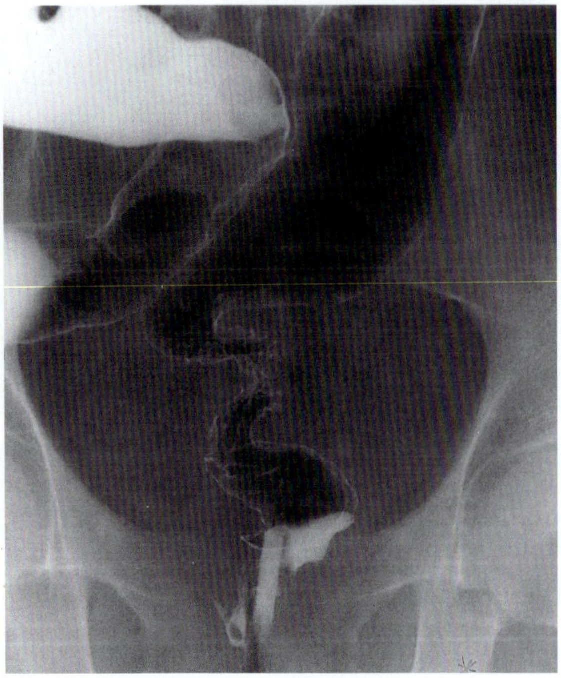

Figure 76.1: The barium enema examination shows a stricture of the lower rectum. Crohn's disease was considered as the likely diagnosis until the fistula openings were identified.

Operation (12.6.77)

Peranal exploration enabled only part of the fistula track to be laid open into the lumen. Access to the upper limit of the track was prevented by the rectal stricture.

Operation (2.21.78)

Laparotomy revealed an extraperitoneal mass on the left side of the rectum but no other intra-abdominal abnormality. A loop ileostomy was performed.

Operation (6.8.78)

A posterior transsphincteric approach was used with incision of the posterior wall of the rectum to the 12 cm level. Access was still difficult due to intense fibrosis of the rectum, and strong retraction was required to facilitate laying open the track into the lumen. Sutures approximated each edge of the track to the divided wall of the rectum to ensure hemostasis and prevent premature healing ("marsupialization").

Operation (9.12.78)

The ileostomy was closed after examination revealed healing of the fistula was complete.

Follow-Up (1980)

Bowel function was satisfactory after 4 months. Examination under anaesthesia (28 months after the fistulotomy) revealed sound healing of the rectum with resolution of the stricture.

Comment

This "upside down" fistula caused significant difficulty in diagnosis until both internal openings were identified. The Parks classification of anal fistulae includes the upward extension of the intersphincteric fistula,[1] but the high level of the track and secondary internal opening in this case was unusual. The transsphincteric operation provided the only access possible for complete fistulotomy. The resolution of the stricture and most of the perirectal induration had occurred within 2 months of the fistulotomy.

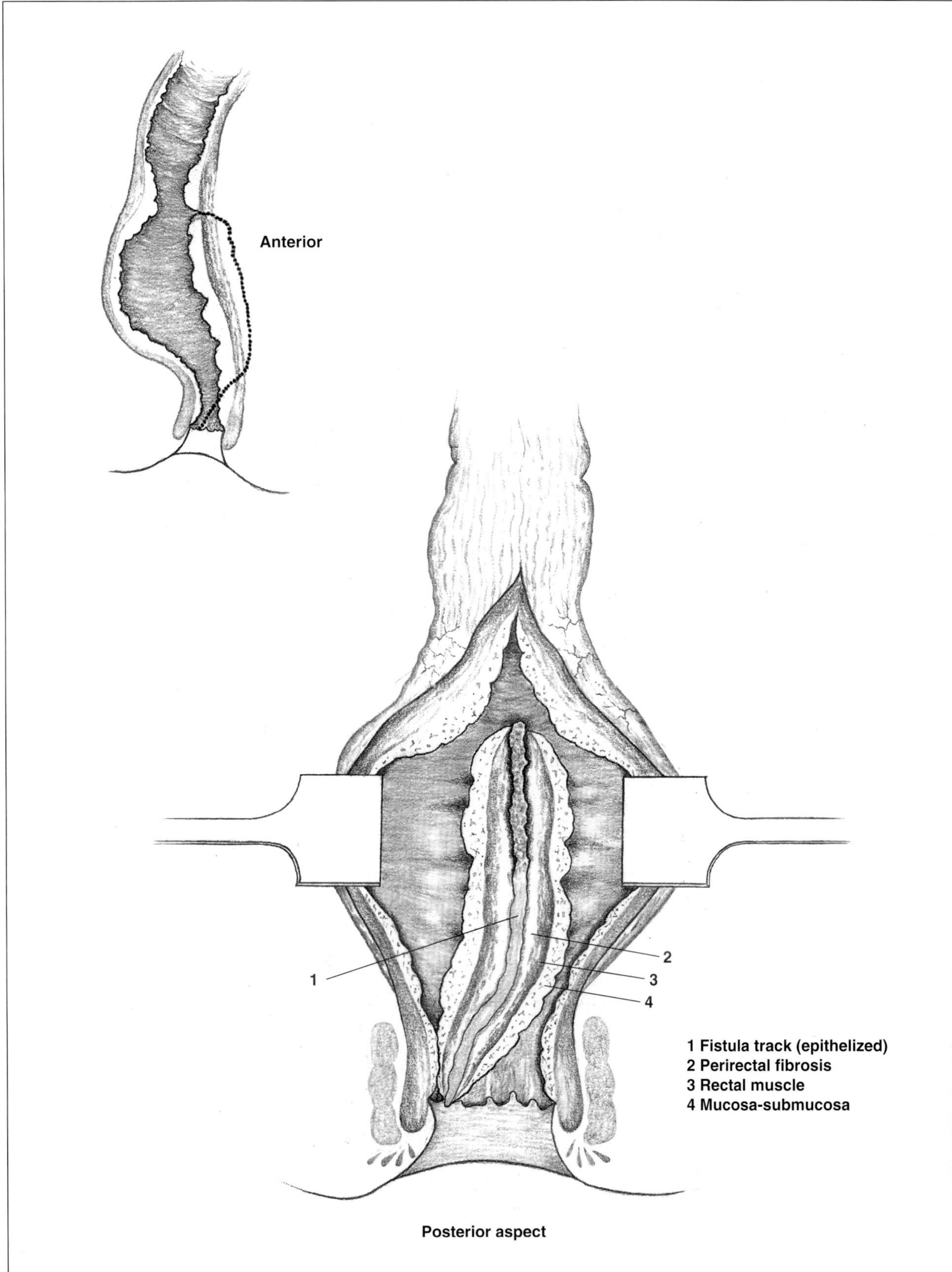
Anterior
1
2
3
4
1 Fistula track (epithelized)
2 Perirectal fibrosis
3 Rectal muscle
4 Mucosa-submucosa
Posterior aspect

CASE

77 Necrotizing Infection After Removal of "Benign" Rectal Polyp

Female, 64 Years

History

On 5.1.90, endoscopic removal of a sessile rectal polyp ($15 \times 15 \times 3$ mm) was performed. It was situated posteriorly in the lower third of the rectum. The histology report noted severe dysplasia ("at least carcinoma in situ") with no evidence of invasive carcinoma. Within a few days, an abscess appeared in the left ischiorectal fossa, which was drained. A fecal fistula was apparent subsequently. The patient was referred.

Operation (5.31.90)

Examination revealed a large area of necrosis in the left posterior wall of the rectum with undermining of the mucosa. This was in continuity with a large supralevator fistula. The internal opening easily admitted an examining digit. Laparotomy, antero-grade colon irrigation, and loop ileostomy were performed.

Progress

The fistula healed and the ileostomy was closed (11.12.90). Follow up examinations revealed satisfactory healing until 2 years after the polyp excision. Examination now revealed a small, firm polypoid lesion at the site of the previous internal opening of the fistula. Biopsy confirmed the diagnosis of moderately differentiated adenocarcinoma. Computerized tomography (CT) examination revealed no evidence of metastatic disease. The anal canal wall was thickened.

Operation (7.13.92)

Abdominoperineal excision of the rectum was performed. There were no intraabdominal metastases.

Pathology

There was a raised ulcer at the site of the excised polyp that was in continuity with a small mass (8×8 mm) in the left parasphincteric area. Histological examination revealed the mass was adenocarcinoma extending into fatty tissue. The mesenteric lymph nodes showed no evidence of carcinoma.

Follow-Up (2004)

The patient remained well until August 1996, when a 2 cm lung metastasis in the right upper lobe (RUL) was detected upon routine chest x-ray. A right upper lobectomy was performed. No further recurrent disease has been detected 11 years and 7 months since rectal excision was performed.

Comment

Histological review of the initial polyp removed in 1990 did not reveal evidence of invasive carcinoma, and yet this relatively small "benign" polyp was ultimately responsible for a rectal excision and a right lobectomy. Necrotizing infection after polyp excision is rare. The healing of the supralevator fistula after a defunctioning ileostomy was encouraging, but direct spread or implantation of carcinoma cells supervened. Local re-excision was considered to be inappropriate.

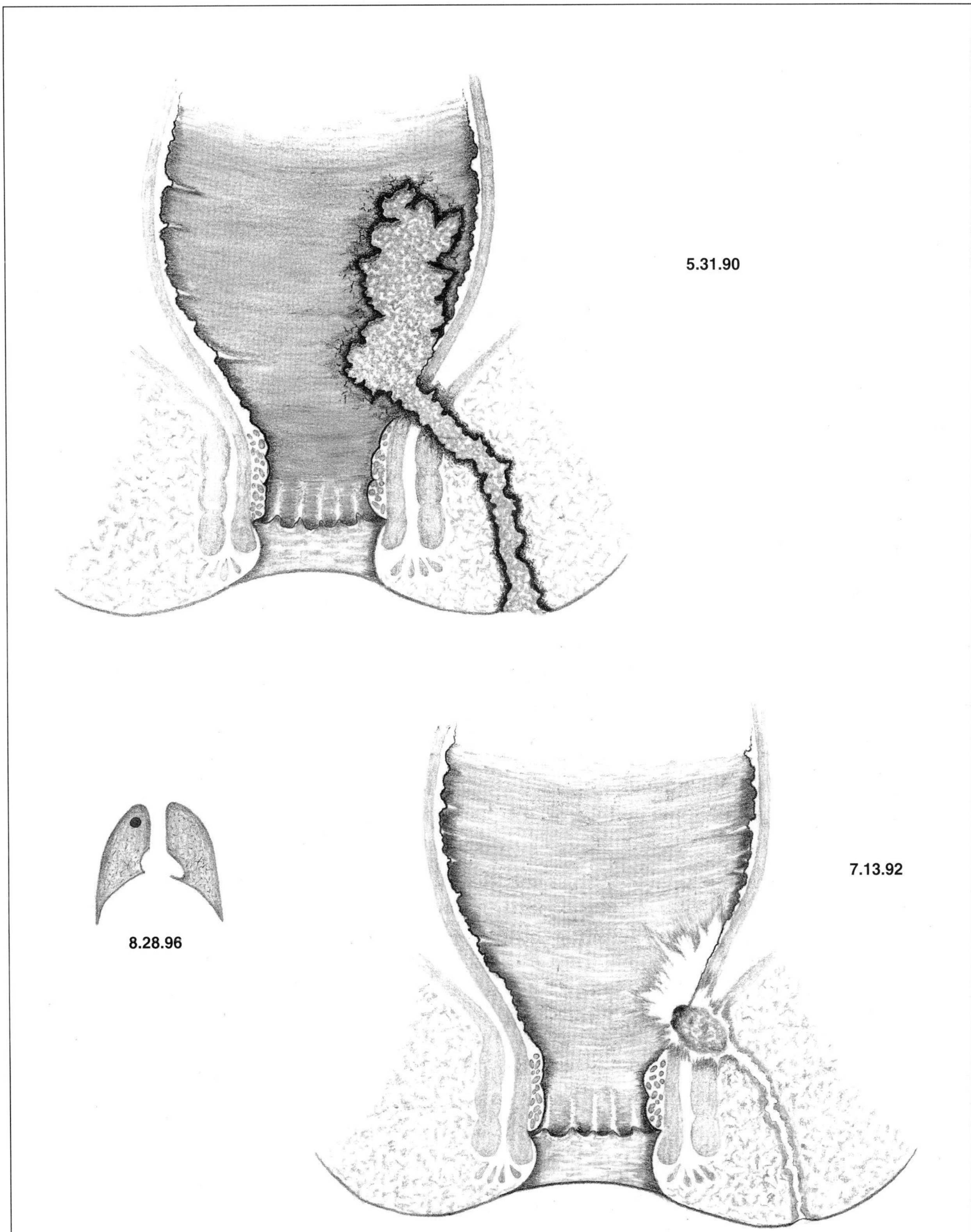
5.31.90
7.13.92
8.28.96

PART IX Various Pathology

CASE

78 Intra-Abdominal Desmoid Tumor Unassociated with Familial Adenomatous Polyposis

Female, 74 Years

History

During the first year of her life, this patient was treated for bilateral congenital dislocation of the hips. At 26 years (1956), a caesarian section was performed, as there was "a pelvic lump present the size of a tennis ball." In 1975, x-rays revealed a large soft-tissue mass in the pelvis, causing a lytic lesion in the sacrum. This was thought to be a chondroma. In 1977, a trans-abdominal biopsy was performed and the diagnosis of desmoid tumour confirmed. On clinical examination, a firm lobulated mass filled the lower half of the abdomen to the level of the umbilicus. Rectal and vaginal examination revealed a hard pelvic mass causing marked compression of the vagina and rectum. A computerized tomography (CT) scan demonstrated considerable destruction of the sacrum. The tumor size was "12 × 12 × 15 cm." Sigmoidoscopy was not possible. A barium enema revealed sigmoid diverticulosis. At a colorectal conference (1981), the unanimous opinion was that the lesion was inoperable.

Treatment

Oral delta testolactone was commenced in 1978 and continued for 32 months. Oral sulindac was administered for 19 months (1984–1985). Intra-aterial perfusion chemotherapy with doxorubicin, vincristine, 5 Fluorouracil, and carmustine was performed in 1986. None of these treatments appeared objectively to reduce the size of the tumor (Figures 78-1 and 78-2).

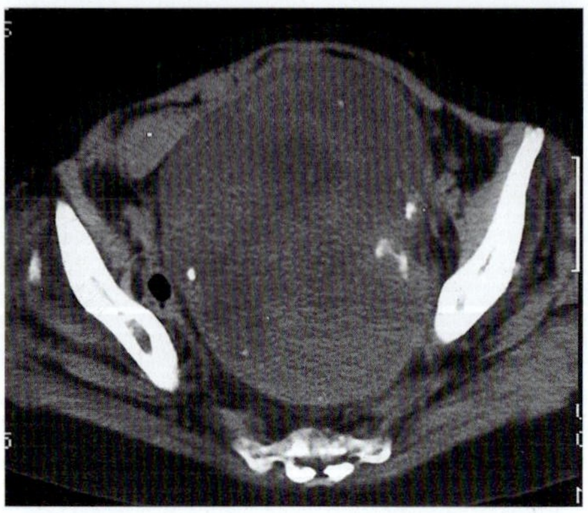

Figure 78.1: CT scan shows the maximum transverse and antero-posterior dimension. (4.24.84).

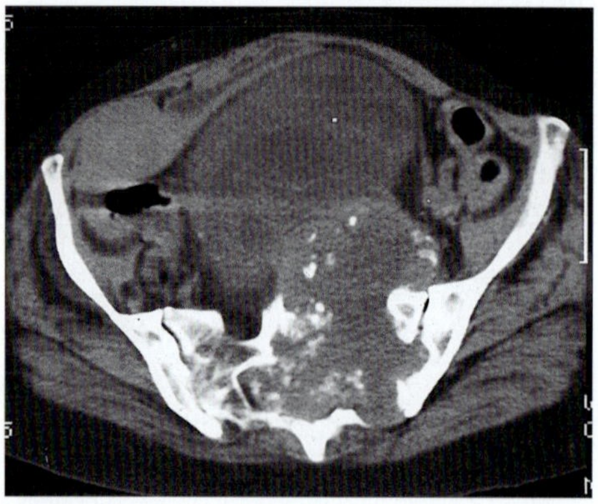

Figure 78.2: CT scan demonstrates the erosion of sacrum and sacral canal. (4.24.84).

Follow-Up (2004)

Clinical and CT examination have not demonstrated any further progression of the tumor since 1981 (Figure 78-3). On CT examination, the tumor dimensions are 12 × 13 × 15.5 cm. Small areas of

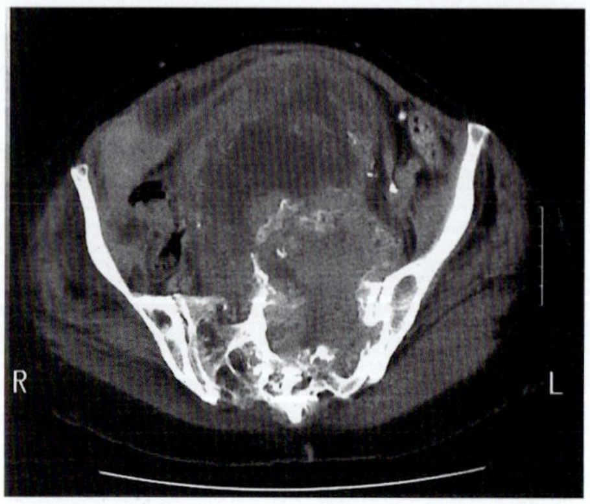

Figure 78.3: CT scan reveals no increase in size in 18 years. Calcification and areas of hypodensity are apparent. (9.30.99).

calcification have appeared, as have stable areas of hypodensity interpreted as cystic or necrotic changes. The colon and bladder are markedly displaced cranially and to the right. The stretched dome of the bladder is at the L4/5 disc level just above the upper surface of the tumor. A left hip replacement was performed in 2004. The patient's general health is good for her 74 years.

Comment

This tumor, present for 55 years is not an example of a familial adenomatous polyposis (FAP) related desmoid. It is better classified as pelvic fibromatosis which occurs in young females (20–35 years) unrelated to pregnancy. Such slow growing, locally aggressive tumors appear to arise from muscle or aponeurosis in the pelvis. The absence of small bowel obstruction suggests it has not primarily involved the bowel mesentery, so common in desmoids complicating FAP. The tumor growth has not progressed since 1981. This could be spontaneous regression known to occur in 7% of desmoids[2] or due to 1 of the 3 nonsurgical therapies administered. The adaptation of pelvic viscera to this massive pelvic tumor is surprising, as there are no significant bladder or large bowel symptoms. In addition, the involvement of the sacral canal has not become symptomatic. Considering the risks of attempted resection, [St Mark's Hospital, London, reports an operative mortality of 8 out of 22 (36.4%)[3]] the nonoperative treatment of this patient appears to have been validated.

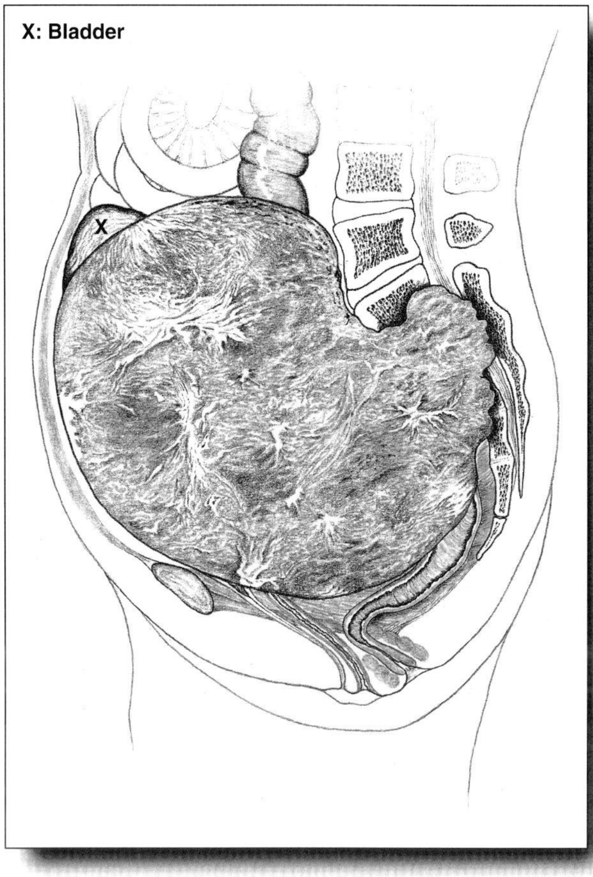

For a full-page image of this figure see the appendix.

CASE

79 Pneumatosis Coli

Male, 53 Years

History

For several years, the patient had been troubled with diarrhea (6 bowel movements in 24 hours). The stools often contained small flecks of red blood and mucus. Initially on sigmoidoscopy, the patient was thought to have a polypoid carcinoma at the 20 cm level. A further opinion confirmed the diagnosis of pneumatosis coli. Sigmoidoscopy revealed tense submucosal cysts between 20 cm and 25 cm, mostly 5 mm in diameter, but also clusters of smaller lesions throughout the mucosa. Many of the cysts were "capped" with hyperemia. There were also small patches of similar hyperemia without mucosal projections. Biopsy was difficult, because the smooth surface and firm consistency of the cysts hindered closure of the forceps. The histology was consistent with the diagnosis. Colonoscopy was not performed. A barium enema revealed typical appearances of pneumatosis in the descending and sigmoid colon (Figure 79.1).

Treatment (9.19.75)

Over a period of 4 days, the patient was given oxygen therapy via a mask at the rate of 14 L per minute.

Follow-Up (1987)

A barium enema examination 6 days after cessation of oxygen therapy showed no evidence of the previous radiological abnormalities (Figure 79.2). Sigmoidoscopy subsequently was normal to 25 cm. The patient's symptoms were improved within days of completing the oxygen treatment, and his bowel habit was no longer a social disability. The patient was last examined 12 years after treatment. His general health was good, bowel actions occurred twice per day, varying in consistency. Flexible sigmoidoscopy to 70 cm showed small pale areas corresponding to the previously involved colon. There was no recurrence of the pneumatosis.

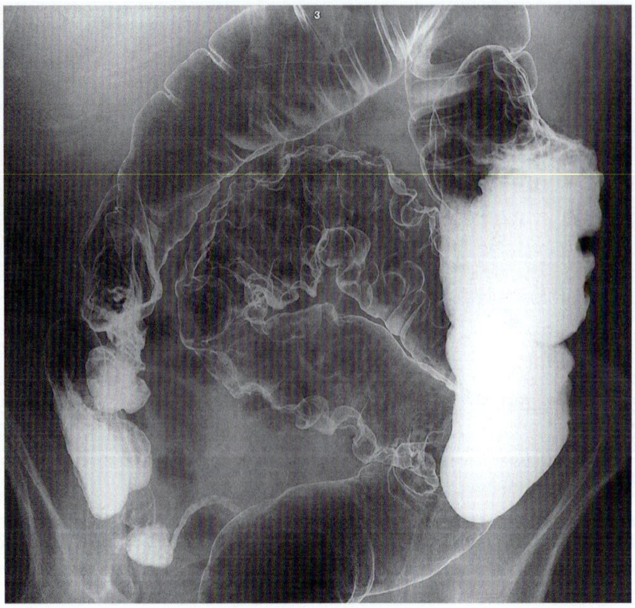

Figure 79.1: Barium enema shows typical appearance of pneumatosis coli in the sigmoid colon.

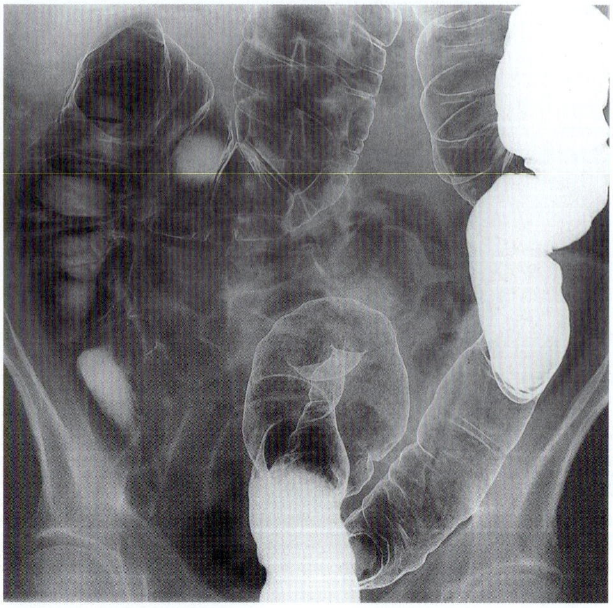

Figure 79.2: Barium enema 6 days after completion of oxygen therapy demonstrates resolution of the pneumatosis.

Comment

The etiology of pneumatosis is unknown, but in some cases it is associated with respiratory, gastrointestinal or psychiatric comorbidity.[1] In the patient described, the disease appeared to be idiopathic, which is usually associated with involvement of the left colon.[2] Oxygen therapy, first advocated by Forgacs et al,[3] was successful long-term in this patient after 1 treatment. It is not unusual for oxygen therapy to be required for more than a single treatment. Complications of pneumatosis occur in 3% of patients (volvulus, necrotizing enterocolitis, rupture of cysts) and may require surgical treatment.[2]

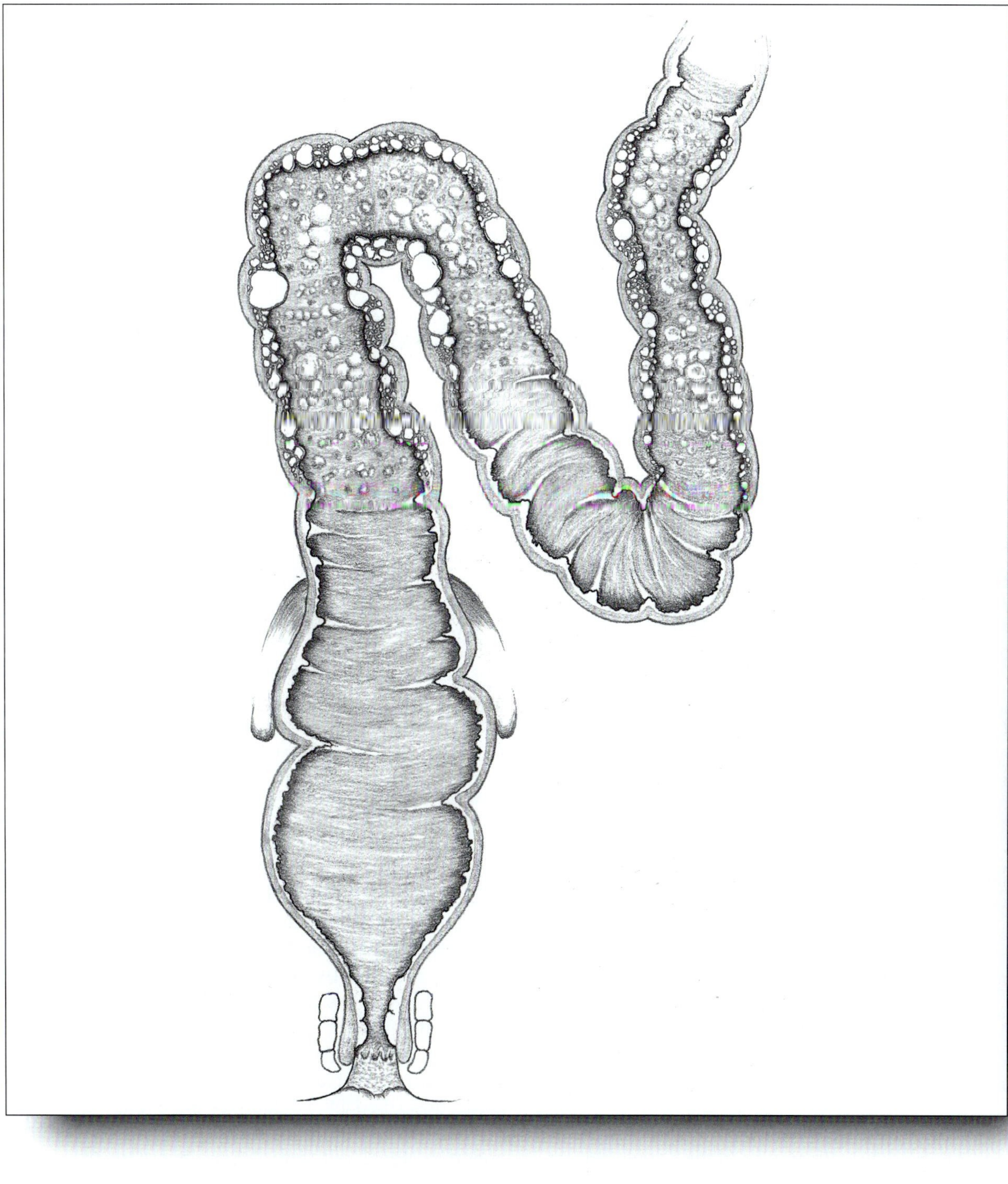

CASE

80 Stercoral Ulceration: Sigmoid Pcrforation

Female, 62 Years

History

In 1987, the patient, aged 52 years, was initially investigated for rectal bleeding and a family history of colorectal cancer. Her general health status was frail, with chronic respiratory disease, severe kyphosis, osteoporosis, recurring vertebral fractures, obesity, and a Cushinoid state induced by years of steroid therapy administered for severe generalized eczema. There was a long history of constipation. Due to respiratory insufficiency and muscle weakness, the patient's ambulatory capacity was limited to a few steps. On January 24, 1997, the patient was admitted to the hospital with severe abdominal pain and clinical signs of peritonitis.

Operation (1.24.97)

Laparotomy revealed a colon grossly loaded with feces that were "lumped" in firm-to-soft masses, rather than scybala, which was oozing into the peritoneal cavity through a 4 mm perforation of the anterior wall of the colon at the sigmoid descending colon junction. This area of the colon showed prominent inflammatory changes of increased vascularity and fibrinous exudate. Fecal peritonitis was present in the lower abdomen. Immediately mobilization of the left colon was commenced, the colon ruptured, and significant fecal contamination occurred. When this difficult situation was controlled, a Hartmann resection was performed. The distal sigmoid was oversewn.

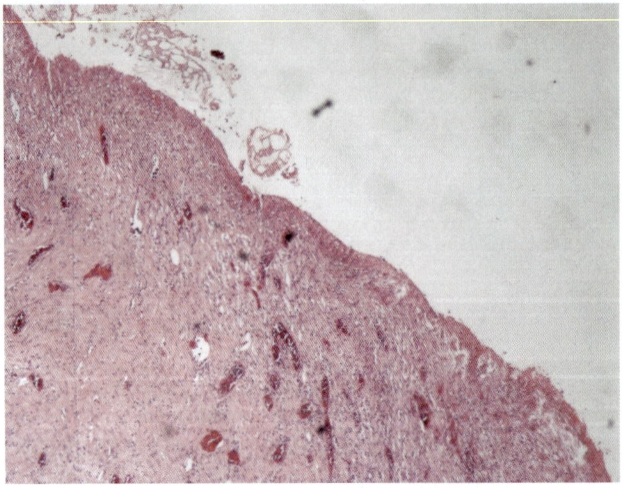

Figure 80.1: The stercoral ulcer shows complete loss of mucosa and nonspecific inflammation in the submucosa.

Pathology

There was a large ulcer involving the mucosal surface of the resected colon, revealing the inflamed and partly necrotic muscle layer. The perforation was in the distal area of the ulceration. The histological changes were nonspecific, consistent with ulceration and necrosis (Figure 80.1).

Postoperative Course

The patient remained in the intensive care unit until she died of respiratory failure 21 days after operation. She remained dependent on respiratory ventilation during this time, until the patient and family requested that this therapy (managed via a tracheotomy) be withdrawn.

Comment

Stercoral perforation is rare, and, adopting strict criteria, Maurer et al have found 81 cases in the literature.[1] These criteria are:

1. sharply demarcated round or ovoid perforation;
2. larger than 1 cm (85%);
3. antimesenteric in position;
4. associated fecalomas; and
5. necrosis and/or ulceration associated with the perforation (74%).

This patient's morphology exhibited 3 of these features. The long history of constipation and the fecal loading found at operation is also consistent with the diagnosis. Immune suppressed patients are vulnerable to this complication.[2] The tissues of this patient, affected by high, long-term doses of prednisolone, were extremely fragile, and this undoubtedly contributed to the complication. There was no evidence that the pathology was primarily ischemic. The histological features (Figure 80.1) are similar to those described by Haddah et al.[3] Colon irrigation prior to bowel mobilization may have prevented the operative fecal contamination, but this maneuver would have been difficult (long-dilated and fragile colon, obesity, high flexures, and the patient not postured in the lithotomy Trendelenberg position). Two senior anesthetists administered the anesthetic because of the anticipated problem of respiratory function. The choice of operation in this condition is significantly influenced by the patient's comorbidities, which are often multiple. They are frequently frail, nursing home residents or institutionalized patients.[3] This patient's anesthetic status for any future elective surgery was regarded as prohibitive, and the Hartmann stoma would have been permanent if the patient had survived. Stercoral perforation is association with a high postoperative mortality. Serpell and Nicholls, in reviewing 64 cases, recommended resection without anastomosis; even so, there was still a high postoperative mortality of 32%.[2]

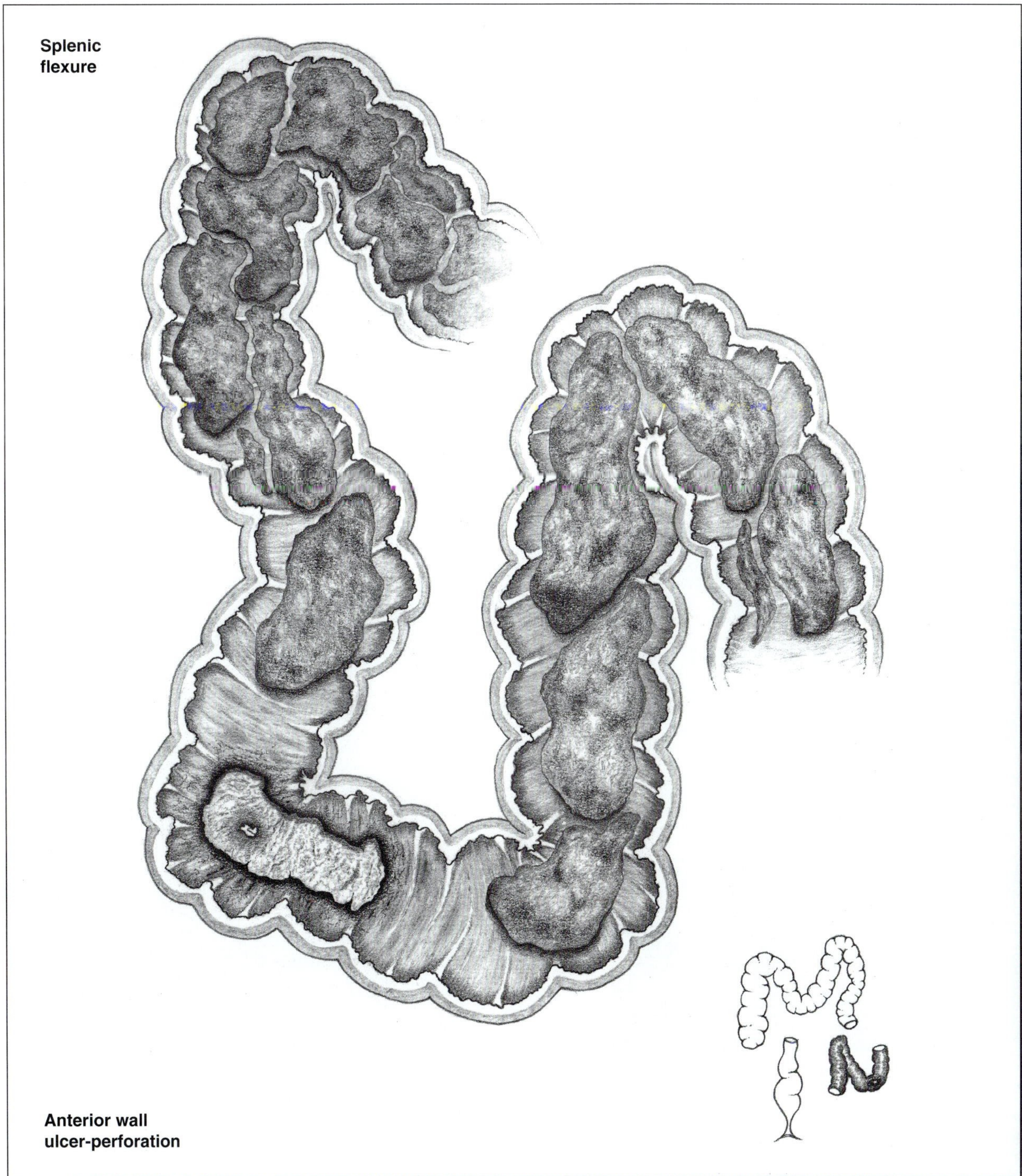

CASE

81 Nongangrenous Ischemic Colitis

Female, 71 Years

History

Two weeks prior to referral, the patient suffered a sudden episode of colicky abdominal pain accompanied by diarrhea that lasted 3 days. On the third day, the patient passed a small amount of dark red blood. A barium enema 1 week after the onset of symptoms showed an area of narrowing at the splenic flexure (Figure 81.1). The mucosal pattern was distorted, and small areas of "thumb printing" were just visible. A colonoscopy subsequently revealed sigmoid diverticular disease and a marked stenosis at the splenic flexure associated with ulceration. Biopsy showed nonspecific inflammatory changes. A limited contrast enema was performed 5 weeks after the onset of symptoms (Figure 81.2). The stenosis measured 10 cm in length, which the radiologist regarded as consistent with a constricting carcinoma. This diagnosis was not accepted. The patient remained asymptomatic, however a third contrast enema, now 6 months after the acute episode,

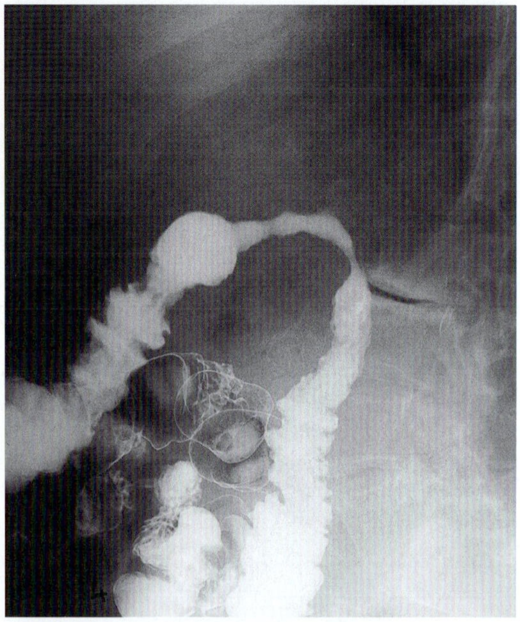

Figure 81.2: Contrast enema at 5 weeks reveals a long stricture with no mucosal pattern.

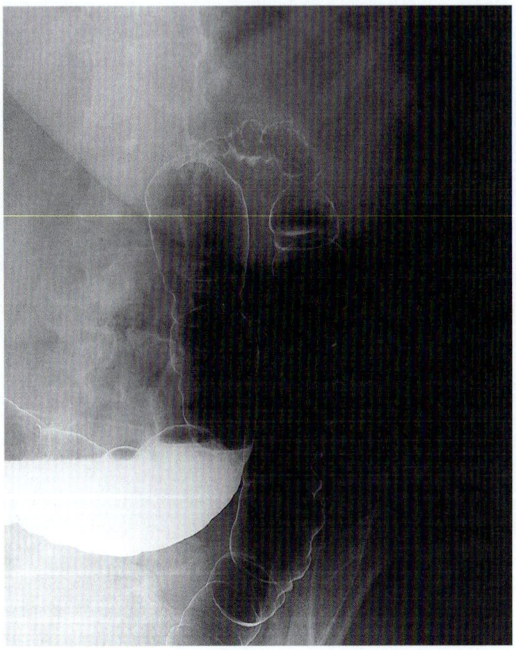

Figure 81.1: Barium enema at 1 week shows early mucosal changes and narrowed lumen at the splenic flexure.

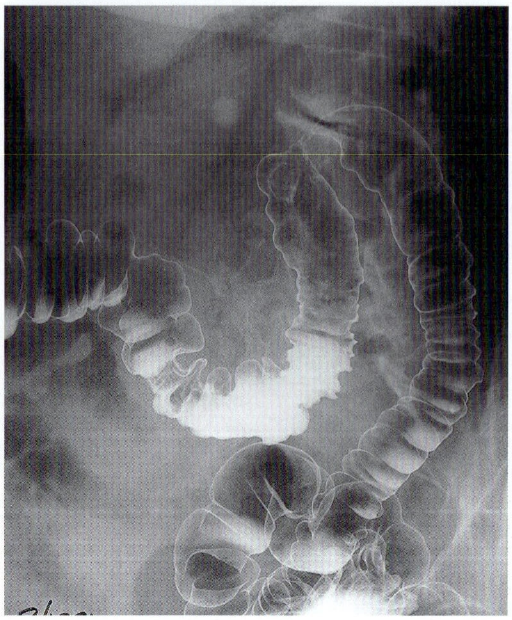

Figure 81.3: Contrast enema at 6 months demonstrates a short persistent stricture.

showed further narrowing of the lumen, which radiologically measured 2 mm in diameter (Figure 81.3).

Operation (9.15.94)

At laparotomy, the short stricture of the splenic flexure was confirmed. The mesenteric vessels appeared normal. Sigmoid diverticular disease, without inflammatory changes, was present. Resection with anastomosis was performed.

Pathology

Inflammatory changes were present on the serosal aspect of the stricture. The muscle wall was thickened (8mm) and white due to fibrosis. The stricture was associated with mucosal ulceration, which was shallow and well defined. The adjacent mucosa was smooth, slightly congested, and featureless. Histologically, nonspecific inflammatory changes were present in the floor of the ulcer and bowel wall. There was no evidence of vascular occlusion or vascular disease. The findings were consistent with ischemic ulceration.

Follow-Up (1996)

The patient's progress was satisfactory with no further gastrointestinal symptoms. Colonoscopy 15 months after operation showed no abnormality other than sigmoid diverticulosis.

Comment

Nongangrenous ischemic colitis is the more common form of this vascular disease of the colon.[1,2] Post ischemic stricturing frequently occurs and in this patient was developing 1 week after the onset of symptoms. At 5 weeks, the radiological opinion suggested the diagnosis was carcinoma. This was excluded by colonoscopy and biopsy. The stricturing had persisted at 6 months, and operation was therefore advised despite the patient's lack of symptoms. Brown, in a review of 17 patients, found that the stricture was often well tolerated and that there was significant resolution in patients, thus avoiding operation.[2] No histological evidence of vascular occlusion was found, which is not unusual in specimens resected some time after the acute event. Nonocclusive ischemia due to inadequate perfusion of the bowel wall was unlikely in this patient, as there were no acute comorbid conditions present usually associated with this form of ischemic disease.[3]

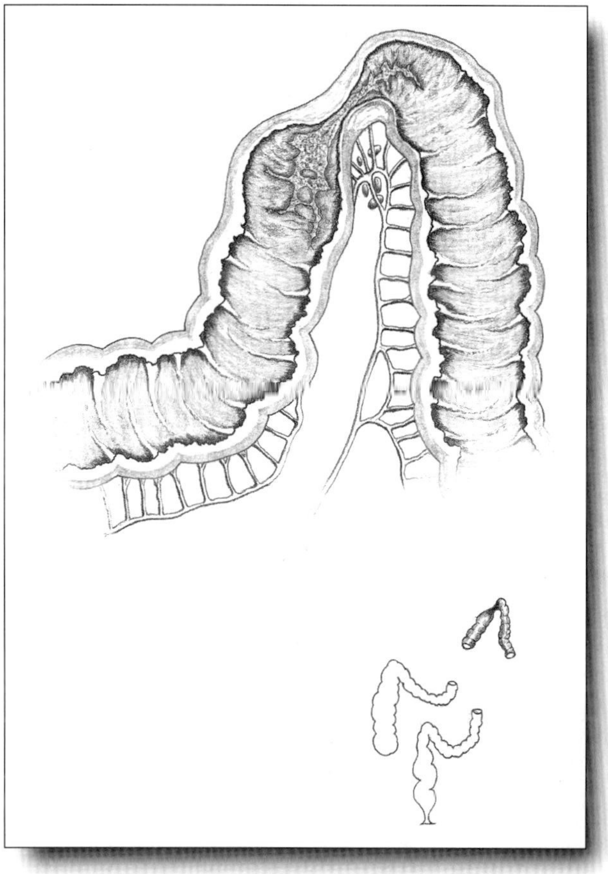

For a full-page image of this figure see the appendix.

CASE
82 Infarction of the Omentum

Female, 63 Years

History

In 1984, the patient underwent a high anterior resection for symptomatic diverticular disease. On July 4, 1996, laparotomy was performed to exclude a sigmoid carcinoma in view of an abnormality on colonoscopy and computerized tomography (CT) examinations. No lesion was identified in the sigmoid colon, but extensive adhesions were found involving the small bowel, omentum, and the anterior abdominal wall. Due to the trauma of a difficult dissection, a small length of ileum was resected. Three weeks after the operation, a severe bout of abdominal pain occurred followed by persistent pain in the left iliac fossa (LIF). A firm mass was palpable in the LIF. A CT examination confirmed the presence of the mass anteriorly with a "fatty central component" (Figure 82.1). The pain continued and became worse in January 1997, when it was associated with a fever. The patient was treated in the hospital with intravenous antibiotics. When this acute episode subsided, the patient continued to suffer significant pain. On referral, laparotomy was advised.

Operation (3.3.97)

An inflammatory, omental mass was found in the LIF, intimately fused with the small bowel, making dissection hazardous. (The adhesions are minimized in the diagram on page 181 for clarity). Incision into the mass revealed inflamed adipose tissue with a central necrotic area, which was curetted and drained. Excision of the mass was not undertaken.

Pathology

The necrotic material was identified as fat necrosis (Figure 82.2).

Follow-Up

Respite from the abdominal pain was only temporary, and within 3 months the patient required narcotics for pain relief. The abdominal mass persisted clinically and radiologically (CT).

Operation (7.14.97)

Extensive dense adhesions were again encountered between the fibrofatty mass, small bowel, and the left lateral and anterior parietes. The mass, measuring 10.5 × 45 × 40 cm, was excised. Anatomically, it was isolated from the stomach and colon by loops of small bowel. There were no significant blood vessels attached to it.

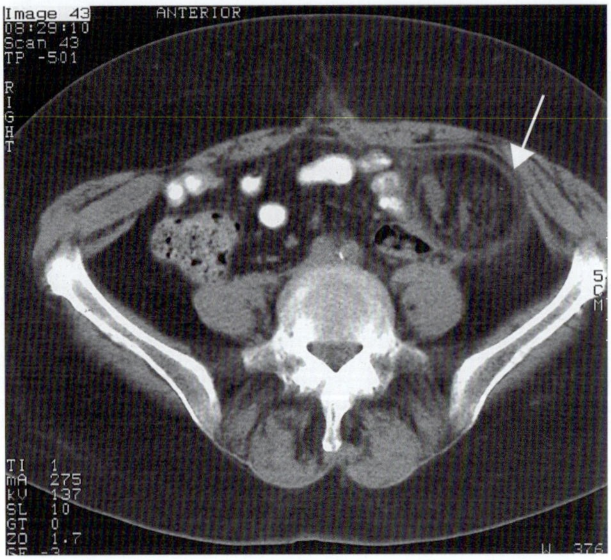

Figure 82.1: CT examination (10.10.96) shows the left-sided abdominal mass (arrow) prior to laparotomy on 3.3.97.

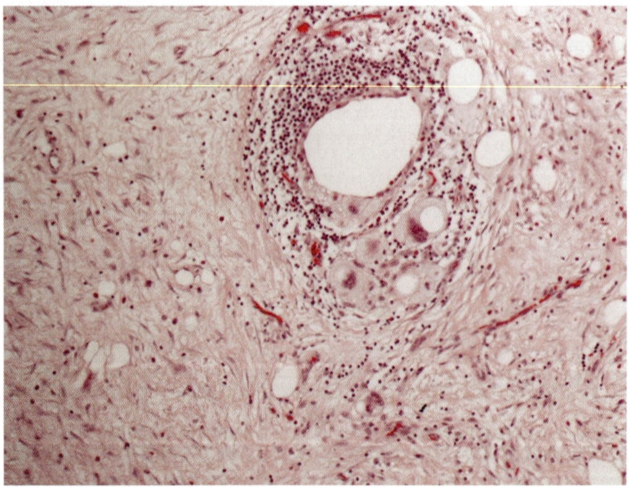

Figure 82.2: Tissue from the abdominal mass (3.3.97) showing fat necrosis. Fat vacuoles are surrounded by inflammation containing histiocytes and foreign body giant cells.

Pathology

Incision into the resected mass revealed yellow adipose tissue with no residual abscess. Microscopic examination revealed areas of foreign body reaction with numerous foamy macrophages and intracellular and extracellular fat vacuoles. The appearances were consistent with organizing fat necrosis.

Follow-Up (2004)

The operation relieved the severe pain, but subsequently, bouts of abdominal pain have recurred without a clear diagnosis. In 2004, relief is obtained with nonnarcotic analgesics and short courses of antibiotics prescribed by her family physician.

Comment

As a result of a difficult abdominal dissection (7.4.96) it seems most likely that acute omental infarction occurred 3 weeks later. This resulted in separation and sequestration of omental tissue, which was sustained by the vascular inflammatory tissue surrounding it, forming a virtual "parasitic" fibrofatty mass within the abdomen. The excision (7.14.97) did resolve the constant severe abdominal pain, but intermittent symptoms have continued. The patient has suffered various abdominal pains for 29 years.

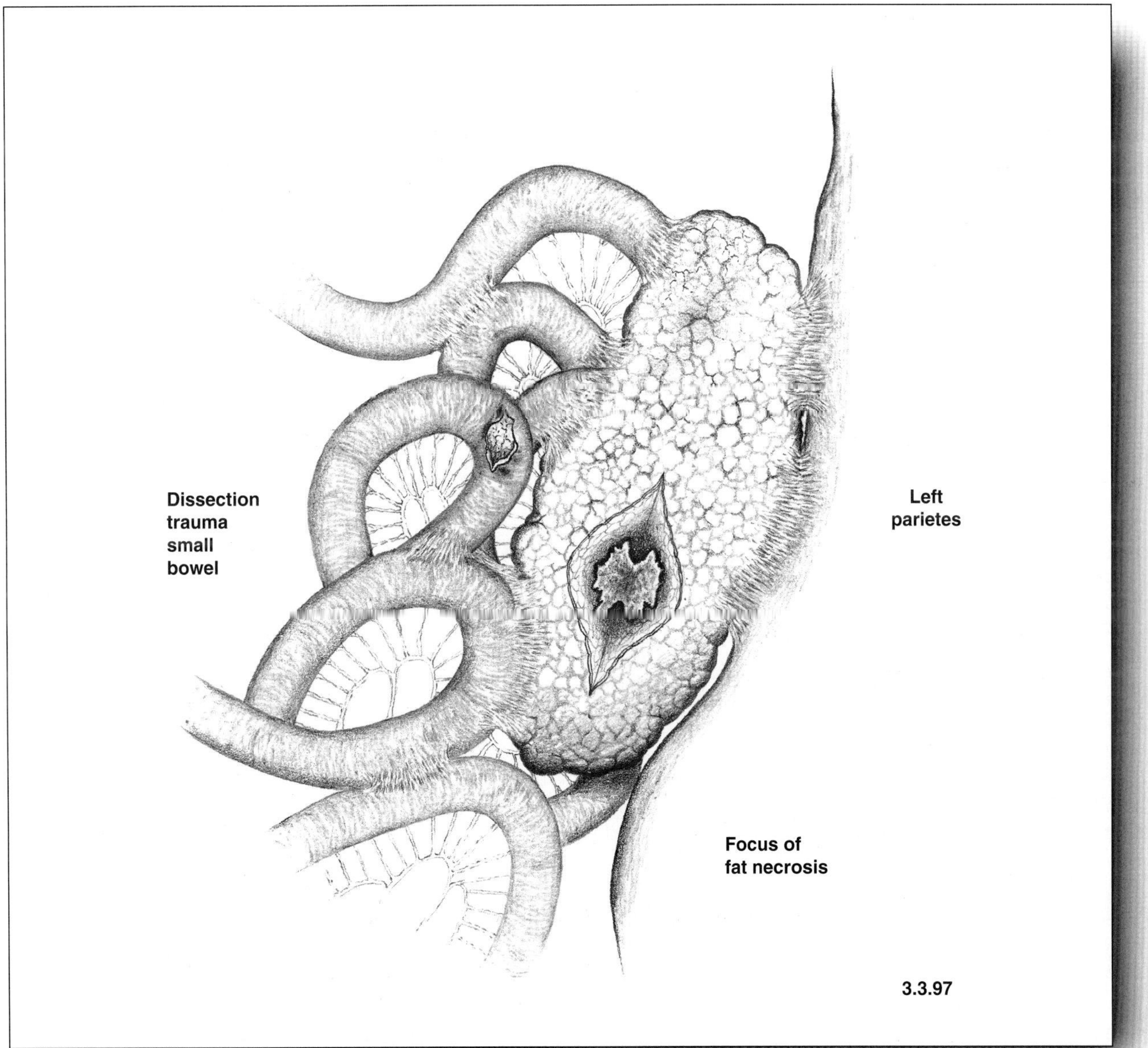

CASE

83 Metastatic Linitis Plastica of thc Colon

Female, 78 Years

History

In October 1996, the patient was admitted to the hospital with acute abdominal pain in the epigastrium and right iliac fossa. Investigations were nonspecific, until a barium enema demonstrated narrowing of the ascending and transverse colon. Colonoscopy was not performed. Six years previously, the patient had a lobular carcinoma of the right breast treated by mastectomy.

Operation (10.18.96)

Elective laparotomy was performed, which revealed extensive carcinomatosis of the large and small bowel, pelvic organs, omentum, and parietal peritoneum. The colon was thickened by infiltration that produced the typical "leather bottle" consistency. There were 2 predominantly affected areas in the colon that corresponded to the strictured areas shown on the barium enema. The terminal ileum was distorted by kinking due to malignant adhesions, with its serosa also markedly affected by the peritoneal nodules of carcinoma. A side:side anastomosis was performed between the ileum and sigmoid colon. The length of small bowel proximal to this anastomosis was 280 cm.

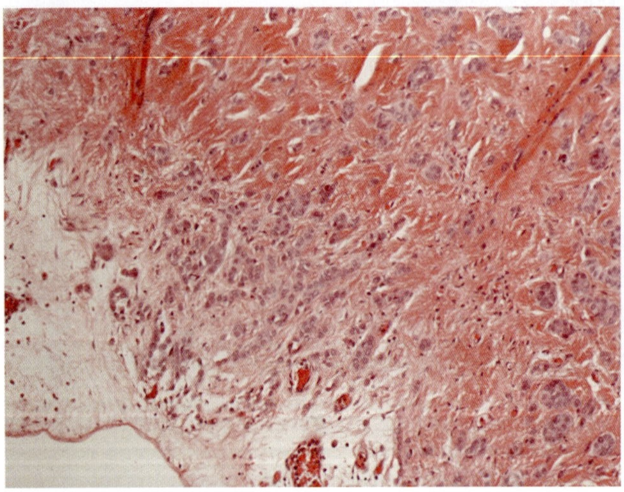

Figure 83.1: Histological appearance of metastatic colon tumor showing cancer cells in "Indian file" typical of lobular breast cancer.

Pathology

Biopsies of peritoneal nodules revealed metastatic adenocarcinoma similar to that seen in the primary breast carcinoma removed in 1990 (Figure 83.1).

Follow-Up (1997)

Recovery from operation was uneventful. An oncologist who treated her with tamoxifen undertook her further management. The response to this treatment was minimal. The patient died of her disseminated malignancy the following year.

Comment

Metastatic linitis plastica of the intestinal viscera due to breast carcinoma is rare. Graham et al reported 7 cases (9.4%) of 75 patients examined at laparotomy or autopsy.[1] The stomach or the colon were the viscera most often affected. The onset of metastatic disease may be delayed for years and may remain confined to the abdomen. It may be that lobular carcinoma has a tendency to metastasize in this fashion.[2] The external appearance of the colon can be confused with chronic inflammatory bowel disease. The intact mucosa, without ulceration, may have a "cobblestone" appearance. This diffuse malignancy affects all layers of the bowel wall. Biopsies of the mucosa or serosal tissue will usually identify the origin of the metastatic disease. Differentiation between a primary bowel cancer and a metastasizing breast cancer can be achieved by the use of immunohistochemical staining to identify primary gastrointestinal cancer (cytokeratin positive) and lobular carcinoma of the breast (estrogen receptor positive).[3]

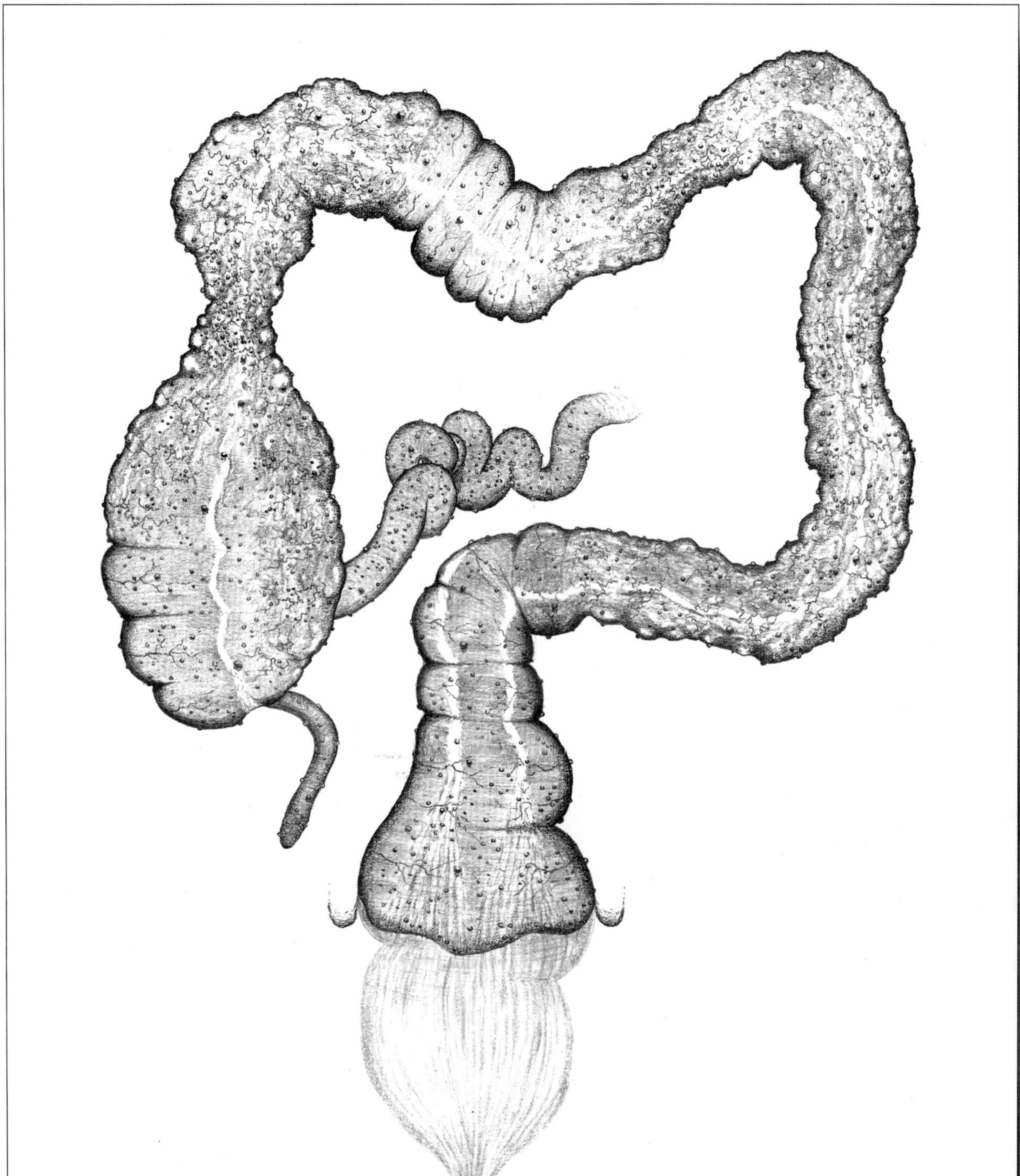

CASE

84 Lipoma Transverse Colon

Male, 65 Years

History

The patient had noticed colicky abdominal pain for 3 weeks. There had been fresh blood on the stool on 3 occasions. A barium enema demonstrated a large polypoidal mass in the mid transverse colon (Figure 84.1). Immediately proximal to the mass there was mucosal irregularity and narrowing of the lumen. Computerized tomography (CT) examination confirmed the lesion and excluded other pathology. A colonoscopy was obstructed in the mid transverse colon by what appeared to be a fungating carcinoma. No biopsy was performed.

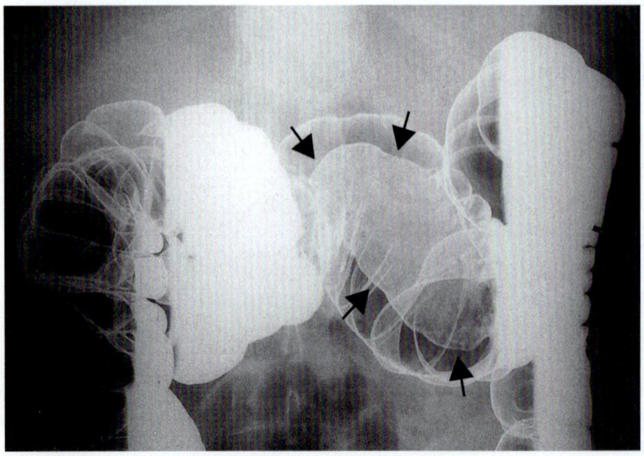

Figure 84.1: The barium enema demonstrates a large lesion in the transverse colon (arrows).

Operation (1.16.98)

A large firm mass was confirmed with no external abnormality of the transverse colon. The lesion was regarded as malignant. An extended right hemicolectomy was performed with anastomosis.

Pathology

The lesion was recognizable as a submucosal lipoma mostly covered by mucosa that had dehisced at the apex and was associated with ischemic necrosis impregnated with barium. It measured 75×45 mm with a broad (20 mm) pedicle. There was ulceration and inflammation in the immediately adjacent mucosa.

Comment

Lipomas of the large bowel are usually asymptomatic until, over a long period, they become large enough to cause obstruction and/or bleeding.[1] The morphology of this lesion suggests that some degree of intussusception was occurring, producing ischemic necrosis at the apex. These changes were interpreted as carcinoma at colonoscopy examination. Confusion with carcinoma is likely only when secondary changes occur to alter the typical smooth surface of a lipoma in the colon. Small lipomas are usually asymptomatic, but lipomas larger than 3.5 cm may become symptomatic[2] and may require removal—most likely by a segmental resection of the bowel or local excision via a colotomy. Colonoscopic removal of a lipoma 50 mm in size, has been reported.[3]

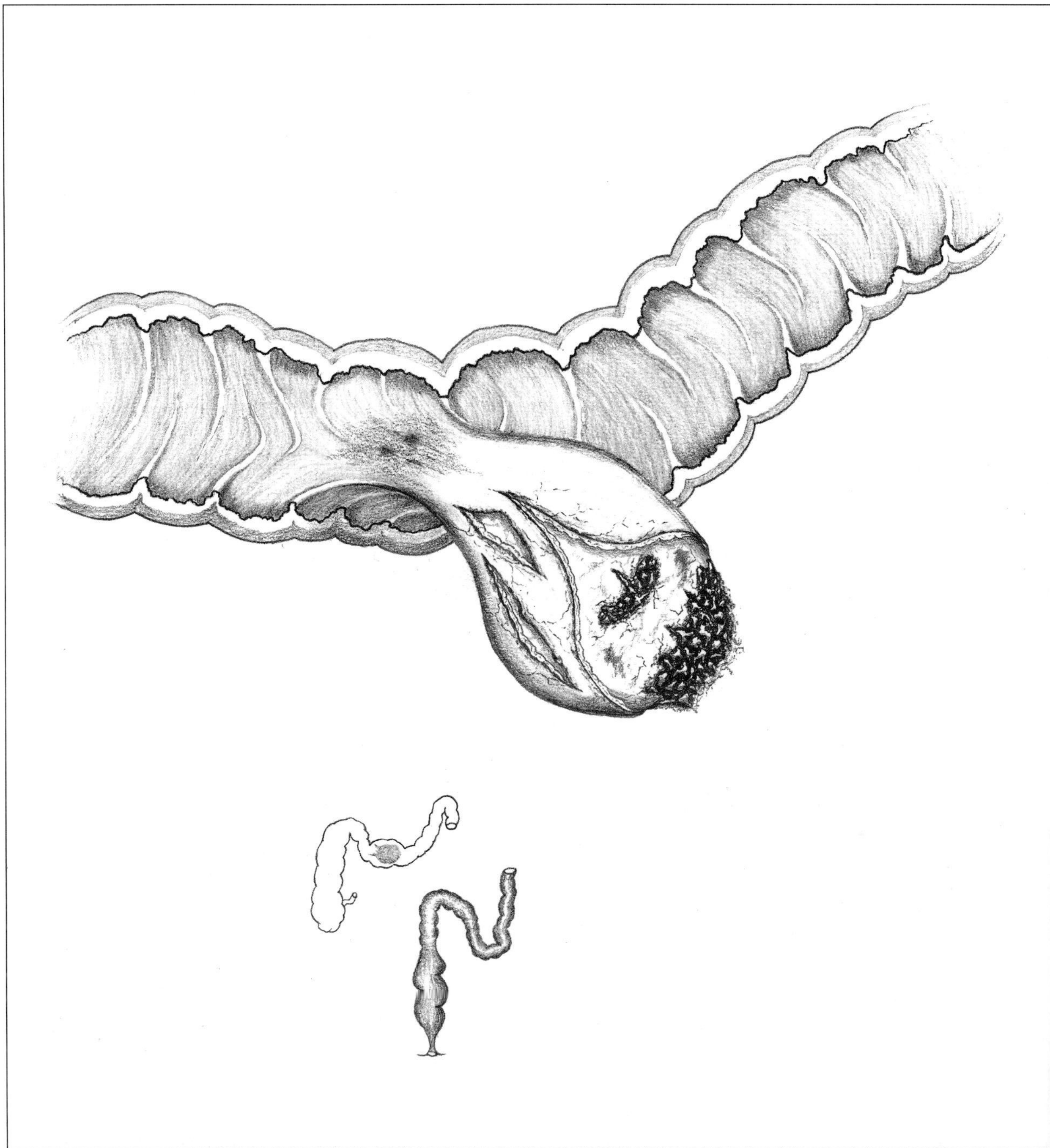

CASE

85 Intestinal Endometriosis

Female, 36 Years

History

The diagnosis of endometriosis had been confirmed some years previously and been treated by ovarian cystectomy and laparoscopic pelvic surgery. In 1987, to investigate chronic lower abdominal pain and constipation, flexible sigmoidoscopy to the splenic flexure revealed dome shaped swellings (Figure 85.1), most obvious in the sigmoid colon, covered with normal mucosa, consistent with endometriomas. A gynecologist supervised a further 5 years of medical treatment until the symptoms were sufficiently disabling to require surgery. Repeat endoscopy showed no extension of the colon lesions, which did not show on a barium enema examination.

Operation (6.4.92)

Laparotomy revealed extensive pelvic endometriosis with widespread adhesions involving ovaries, an enlarged uterus, and upper rectum. There were hard spherical masses involving the sigmoid and lower descending colon causing rotation and constriction, and similar pathology was noted in a short segment of terminal ileum. Hysterectomy with excision of uterine adnexa was performed. The disease in the ileum and colon was removed with a double resection, and the 2 anastomoses were performed with a single layer of interrupted sutures.

Pathology

The left ovary was cystic, 45 × 45 mm in size and densely adherent to the uterus. The right ovary was also cystic, 60 × 40 mm in size, and containing old blood. Both ovaries had smaller cysts associated with the larger cystic lesion. There were fibroids within the body of the uterus and hemorrhagic cysts, 1–5 mm in size within the myometrium. The masses in the ileum and colon were firm and involved the full thickness of the bowel wall. They varied in diameter from 7–30 mm. The serosal surface was indented and the luminal aspect was covered with normal mucosa. The lesions, on section, had a predominantly white appearance with areas of black pigment and small areas of hemorrhage. Histologically, endometriosis was confirmed in the uterus, ovaries, ileum, and colon (Figure 85.2).

Postoperative Course

The patient's recovery in the hospital was satisfactory and uneventful. Unfortunately, 3 weeks after the operation, the patient suddenly collapsed at home and died. Autopsy revealed that a massive pulmonary embolus was the cause of death.

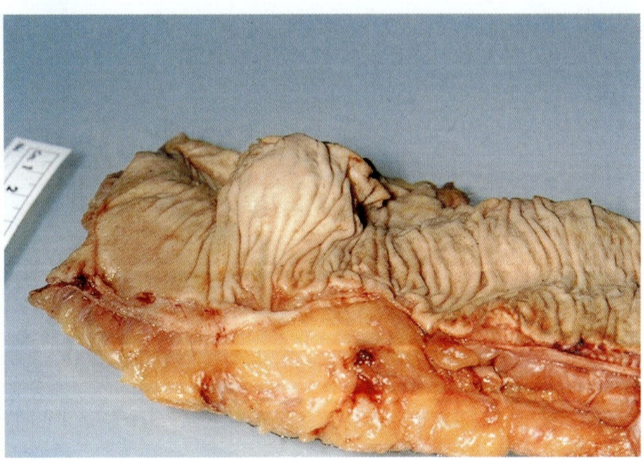

Figure 85.1: The "dome" shaped intramural deposit is covered with intact mucosa.

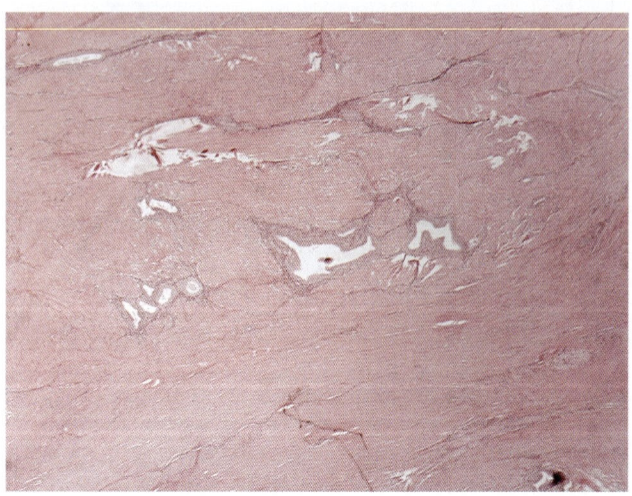

Figure 85.2: A focus of endometriosis is seen within the muscularis propria of the colon.

Comment

This patient illustrates a number of features of intestinal endometriosis, which is reported to occur in 3–18% of patients with endometriosis.[1] The sigmoid and the rectum are most commonly involved (72%).[2] Endoscopy and barium studies may fail to demonstrate endometriosis, even though dome shaped lesions protrude into the lumen. In more extensive disease, transmural fibrosis may cause sufficient deformity to simulate carcinoma. Diagnostic laparoscopy, endorectal ultrasound, computerized tomography (CT) and magnetic resonance imaging (MRI) may more accurately confirm the diagnosis and document the extent of the disease. The long-term results of hormone treatment are disappointing, and, once chronic symptoms of infiltrative intestinal endometriosis are present, surgical treatment is the preferred option. There is a spectrum of surgical treatment available which is determined by the distribution of lesions, the depth, length, and circumferential extent of bowel involvement, and whether future childbearing is hoped for. Woods et al have reported disc excision of the anterior wall of the rectum using the circular stapler.[3] Jatan et al have reviewed the surgical treatment of 95 patients of whom 80% were managed by various laparoscopic procedures, which were: diathermy ablation, shave excision, disc excision, and low anterior resection.[4] Concomitant procedures on other pelvic structures were necessary in 71%. Prior to operation, pain on defecation during menses and previous laparoscopy were predictors that more extensive surgery would be required.[4] The surgical treatment can be complex and is ideally managed by a combined colorectal and gynecological team. The postoperative death in the young patient with benign disease, reported here, was a salutary reminder of the risks of complex pelvic surgery.

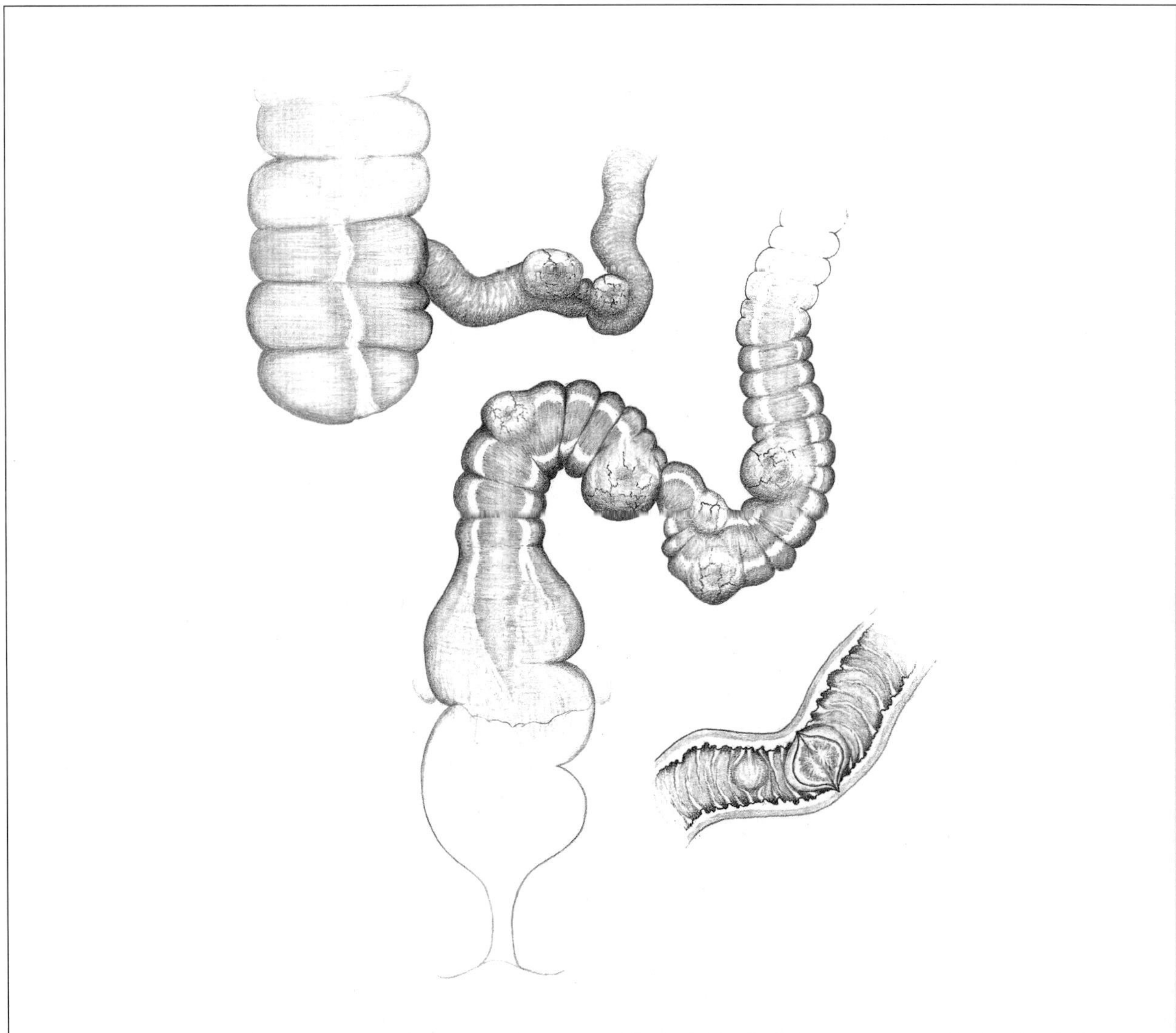

For a full-page image of this figure see the appendix.

CASE

86 Hirschsprung's Disease

Female, 47 Years

History

In 1932, when the patient was a few months old, Hirschsprung's disease was diagnosed. Details of the method of diagnosis are unknown. As a child, constipation was a significant problem, and in 1942, at age 10, bilateral lumber sympathectomy was performed with some relief of symptoms. In adult life, the constipation continued to be a significant disability despite treatment, which included regular self-administered enemas. Periods of absolute constipation for 2 weeks occurred frequently. A barium enema (Figure 86.1) showed a small-caliber rectum with marked dilatation of the sigmoid colon commencing at the recto sigmoid junction, consistent with Hirschsprung's disease. Clinical examination and sigmoidoscopy (15 cm) were normal.

Operation (8.8.80)

Biopsy of the anorectal region revealed absence of ganglia in the myenteric plexus.

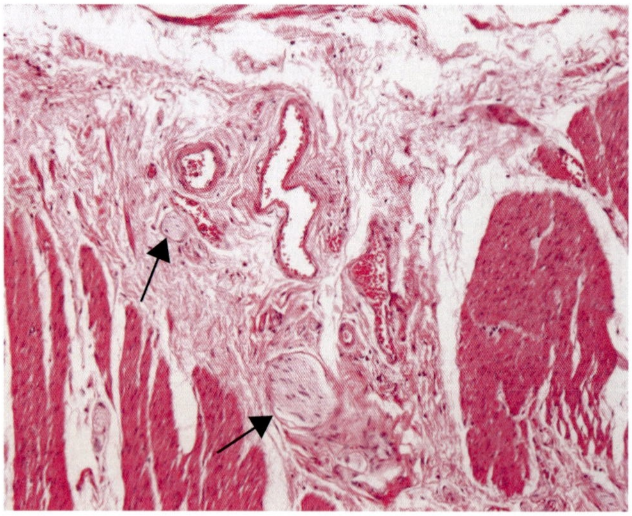

Figure 86.2: In the intermuscular myenteric plexus (low power), nerves were identified, (arrows) but ganglion cells were absent. (This section was close to distal level of resection.)

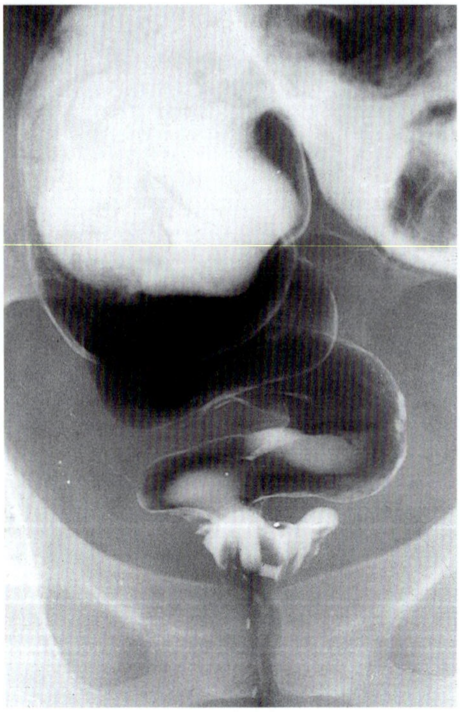

Figure 86.1: Barium enema demonstrates the dilated colon and contracted rectum.

Operation (11.25.80)

Laparotomy revealed gross enlargement of the sigmoid colon, which was 15 cm in diameter with marked prominence of the longitudinal muscle

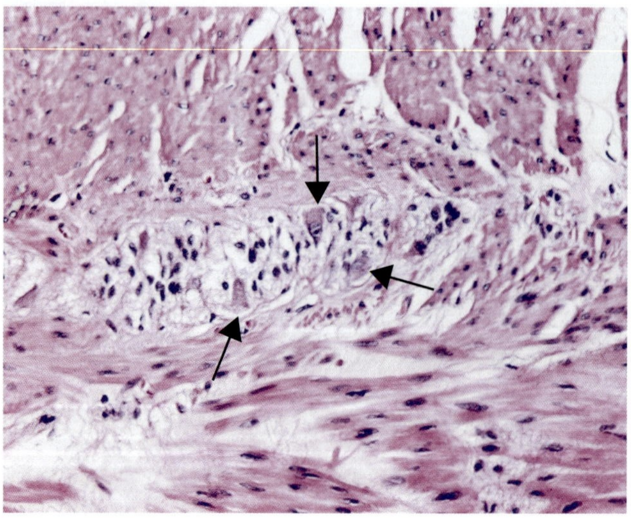

Figure 86.3: Normal ganglion cells in the myenteric plexus (arrows) (proximal resected bowel).

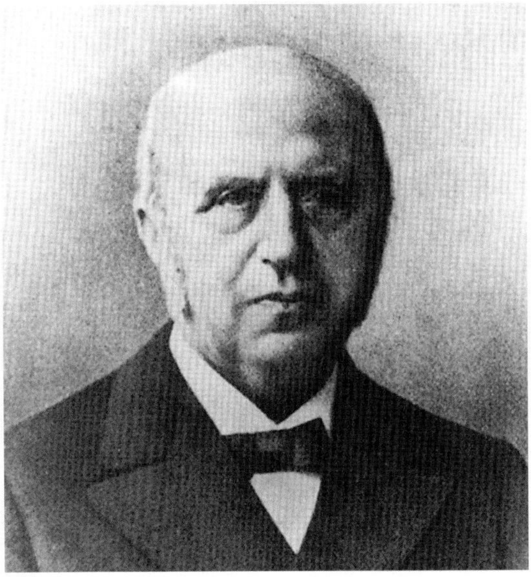

Harald Hirschsprung, 1830–1916 (courtesy of Prof. O. Kronborg).

bundles. The dilatation was relatively abrupt at the level of the sacral promontory. The caliber of the rectum was smaller than normal. The inferior mesenteric vessels were markedly enlarged. Bowel preparation had successfully removed the fecal content of the colon. An extended (ultralow) anterior resection (LARx) was performed with a circular stapler and a loop colostomy made in the transverse colon. At the proximal level of resection in the lower descending colon, the presence of ganglia was confirmed on frozen section.

Pathology

The macroscopic features were a thickened bowel wall and less prominent mucosal folds in a megasigmoid colon. Histological examination revealed an absence of ganglion cells in the distal end of the specimen (Figure 86.2), whereas in the mid and proximal sigmoid colon, a normal population of ganglion cells was present (Figure 86.3).

Follow-Up (2005)

One year after operation, bowel function was 1/24 hrs. The anastomosis level was 5 cm. The patient was not seen for routine follow up examinations after this time. Currently, 25 years since operation, the patient reports that at, 73 years of age, her health is satisfactory. While her bowel habit is irregular with occasional constipation, the result of the operation is satisfactory.

Comment

Hirschsprung's disease presenting in adult life is rare, and such patients are usually young adults. McCready et al reported 50 patients over 10 years of age treated by surgery at the Mayo Clinic over a period of 28 years.[1] The barium enema in the patient reported here was diagnostic (Figure 86.1) but is not always typical of the disease.[2] The x-ray may indicate the likely proximal limit of the aganglionosis.[3] Anal manometry was not available for this patient. The LARx operation, with a long period of follow up, performed in this 47-year-old patient has been successful. Undoubtedly, there remains a small cuff of aganglionic rectum, which has not affected the result. Elliot and Todd reviewed the results of 39 patients from St Mark's Hospital, London, treated by the Duhamel operation with excellent results.[2] Gordon has suggested the Duhamel operation is facilitated by the use of the circular stapler for the colorectal anastomosis and the linear stapler to divide the intervening spur.[4] Wheatley et al. reviewed 199 operations for adult Hirschsprung's disease and concluded that low anterior resection, Duhamel–Martin and Soave operations were the most acceptable methods of treatment.[5]

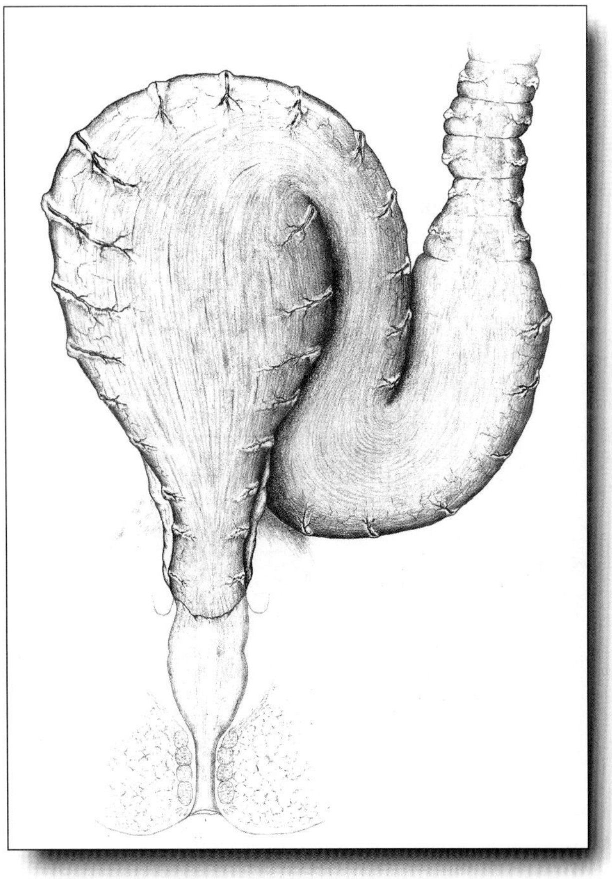

For a full-page image of this figure see the appendix.

CASE

87 Gallstone Obstruction: Sigmoid Colon

Male, 64 Years

History

The patient was admitted to the hospital with a short history of abdominal pain, distention and absolute constipation for some days. Clinical and radiological examinations confirmed the diagnosis of acute large bowel obstruction.

Operation (6.2.86)

The colon was markedly distended due to a hard mass impacted in the lower sigmoid colon. There was a seromuscular tear over this mass and inflammatory changes in the wall of the colon. There was a large inflammatory mass involving the hepatic flexure of the colon, gallbladder, liver, duodenum, and pancreas. Exploration revealed a thickened gallbladder containing a solitary large gallstone with 1 facet surface. There was a large perforation 3 cm in diameter between the gallbladder and the lumen of the colon (Figure 87.1). The stone and the distal half of the gallbladder were removed. Long-term suction drains were placed in its lumen. Abdominal colectomy and a high ileorectal anastomosis were performed, leaving 18 cm of rectum.

Pathology

The stone in the sigmoid colon was tightly wedged in the lumen, causing complete obstruction (Figure 87.2). There was longitudinal and transverse ulceration of the mucosa of the distal colon for a distance of 15 cm. Histological examination of the ulceration, colon fistula, and gallbladder showed nonspecific inflammatory changes. The smooth, dark green gallstones were similar in size and shape to a hen's egg.

Follow-Up

Postoperative recovery was satisfactory. Two months after operation, the drain site from the gallbladder remnant had closed. Four months after operation, bowel function was satisfactory (2/24 hrs). The patient was referred to a hepatobiliary surgeon for follow up but failed to reattend after the initial visit.

Comment

The triad of gallstone ileus : bowel obstruction, air in the biliary tree, and an unusually sited gallstone were not observed in this patient. In the less urgent,

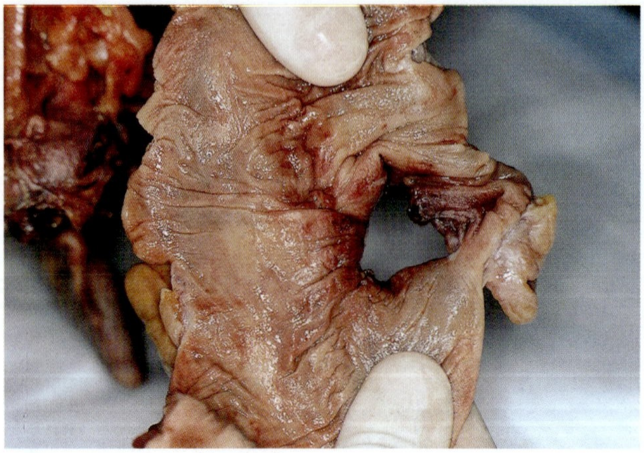

Figure 87.1: The defect in the hepatic flexure of the colon (cholecystocolic fistula).

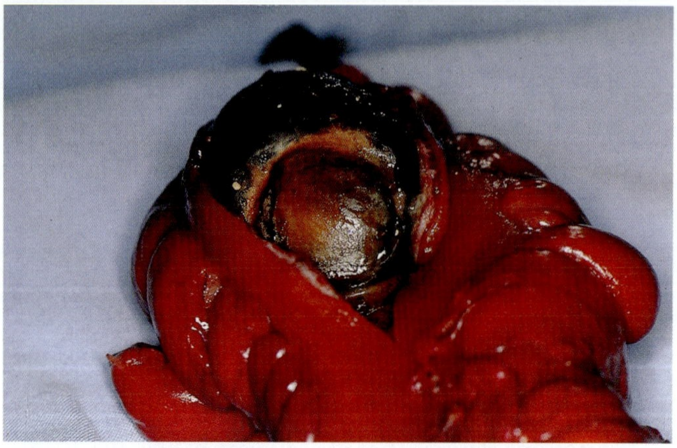

Figure 87.2: Incision in the resected specimen exposes a large gallstone at the point of impaction in the sigmoid colon.

clinical circumstance, barium enema and endoscopic retrograde cholangiopancreatography have been successful radiological investigations.[1] The sigmoid colon is the usual site of impaction, particularly in the presence of sigmoid diverticular disease. The passage of the stone into the colon is more commonly via a cholecystoduodenal fistula.[2] Colotomy, extraction of the obstructing calculus, and proximal stoma may be the optimal treatment if the findings at laparotomy indicate this is appropriate.[3] This patient was treated by resection rather than colotomy–extraction of the stone. Safe repair of the colotomy in the grossly inflamed sigmoid colon was doubtful.

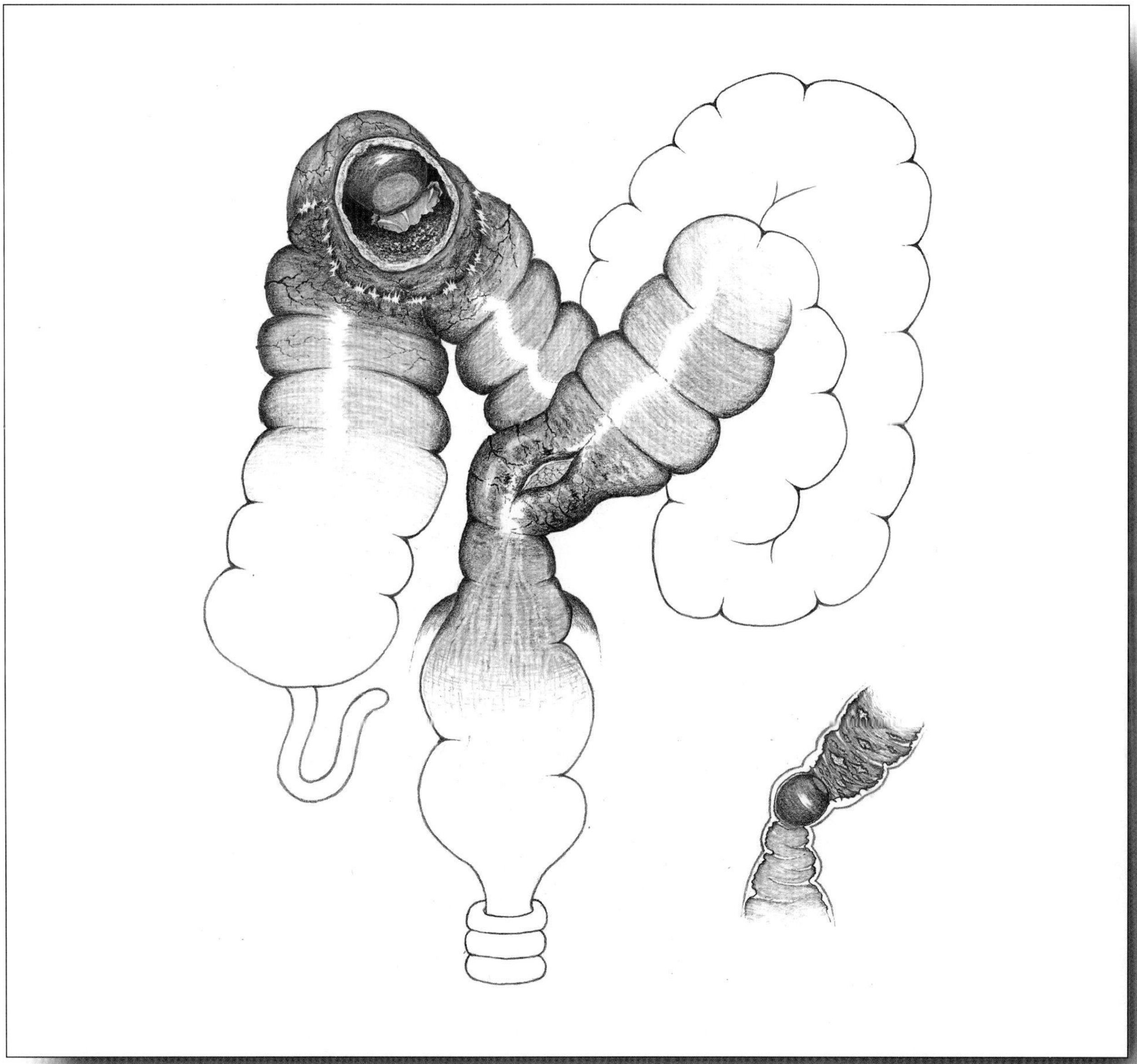

For a full-page image of this figure see the appendix.

CASE

88 Intussusception of the Colon

Male, 90 Years

History

For his age, the patient had been very active until he developed colicky pain in the right iliac fossa associated with loose stools and minor bleeding. These symptoms had been present for 3 weeks. He had lost weight and was found to be anemic (iron deficiency). On examination of the abdomen, there was no abnormality. Ultrasound examination revealed an abdominal mass in the mid abdomen close to the anterior abdominal wall (no description of the mass available). Colonoscopy revealed a large vascular polypoid tumor filling the lumen "in the mid transverse colon" (biopsy showed benign villous adenoma). At the time of the colonoscopy, under sedation, a mass was palpable in the right iliac fossa.

Operation (7.29.92)

The colon, from cecum to the splenic flexure, was thickened and edematous, with marked vascular reaction on its serosal surface. It was initially thought to be Crohn's disease until the diagnosis was realized. There was a large soft polyp occupying the cecum, and the right colon was significantly mobile. There was marked diverticulosis of the left colon. Most of the small bowel was normal in appearance, but the terminal 10–15 cm of the ileum also had a significant vascularity on the serosal aspect. A subtotal colectomy was performed with an end-to-end anastomosis in the mid sigmoid colon.

Pathology

The flat polyp occupying the cecum measured 60 × 60 mm and was deeply hyperemic and soft in consistency. The mucosa of the colon was otherwise normal. Histologically, the polyp contained multiple foci of early invasive, moderately differentiated adenocarcinoma arising in a dysplastic villous adenoma. There were no metastases in the lymph nodes (Dukes A, T_1 N_0 M_0). There was a fibrous reaction on the serosa and in the subserosal tissues of the proximal colon.

Follow-Up

Recovery from operation was satisfactory. In view of the patient's age, routine follow-up visits were not advised and no further clinical details are available.

Comment

This patient's cecal tumor was responsible for intermittent or chronic intussusception, which is often the case in adult intussusception.[1] Its spontaneous reduction caused some initial diagnostic confusion at laparotomy. The diagnosis was supported by the identification of the polyp in the transverse colon at the time of the colonoscopy and the observation of a transient abdominal mass. Adult colonic intussusception is rare: Nagorney et al report 24 cases in 23 years at the Mayo Clinic.[2] The lead point in the colon is likely to be a malignant tumor, and Azar and Berger report an incidence of 43%.[3] Preoperative diagnosis is infrequent[3] and can be best achieved with abdominal computerized tomography (CT) or ultrasound when a target or doughnut sign may be elicited in the transverse view, or a "sausage"-shaped mass or "pseudokidney" may be present in the longitudinal view.[1,3,4,5] If colonic intussusception is encountered at laparotomy, resection, including adequate mesentery, is recommended rather than initial reduction, since malignancy can rarely be excluded and peritoneal contamination with malignant cells could occur on reduction.[1,3,4,5] If the surgeon is unsure that recurrent intussusception has been occurring, the pathologist may identify a number of histological features in the resected specimen that confirm the diagnosis.[6]

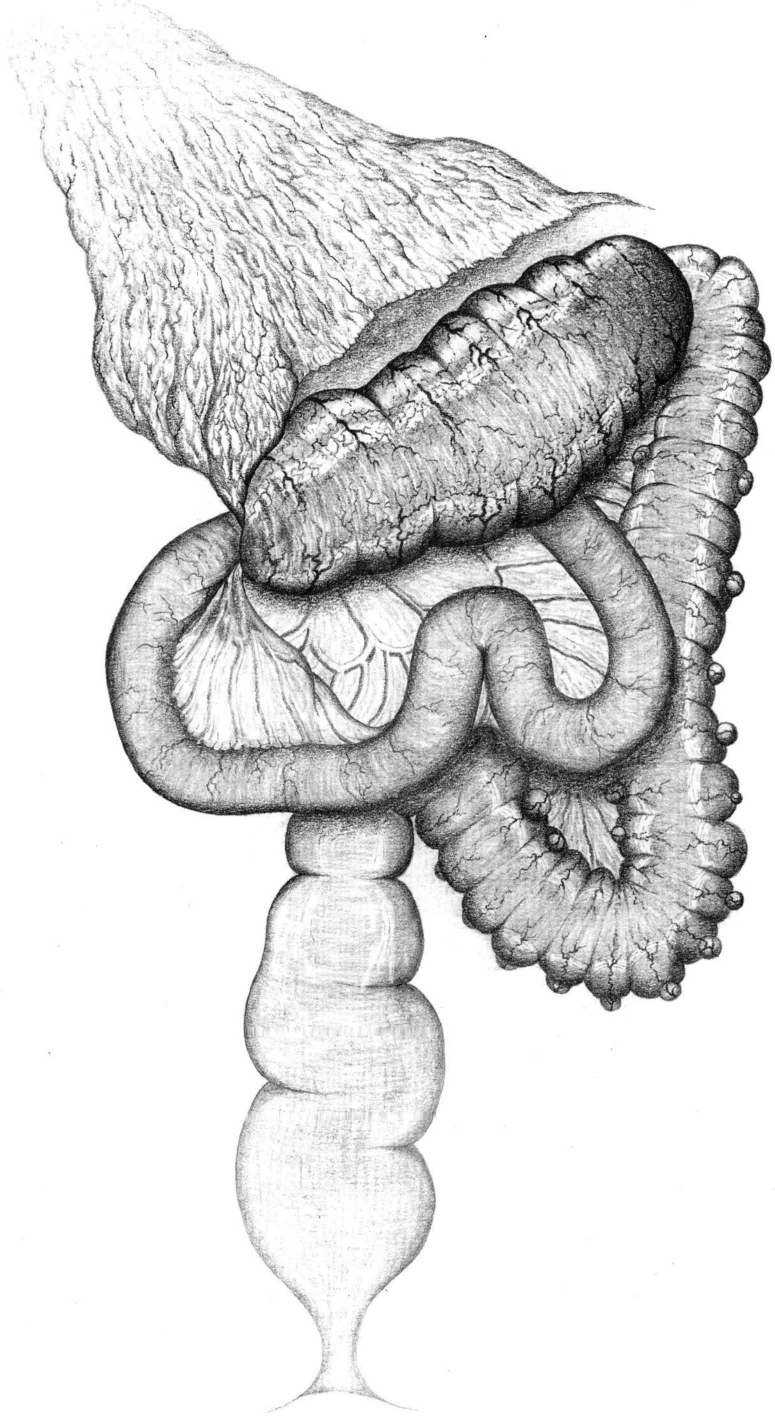

PART X Complications of Investigation and Treatment

CASE

89 Barium Perforation of the Rectum

Male, 58 Years

History

A barium enema was performed to investigate rectal bleeding (10.2.86).

The barium was injected using a "hand pump" technique, continued despite the patient experiencing severe and increasing pain in the rectum. The patient was unable to evacuate the barium. In hospital, sigmoidoscopy revealed marked edema of the lower half of the rectum. Urgent laparotomy revealed no intraabdominal pathology. A left-sided loop colostomy was performed. Two months later, after referral, sigmoidoscopy examination under anesthetic revealed an indurated strictured rectum with intense inflammation of the mucosa and submucosal barium "blebs." A traumatic ulcer was present immediately above the anal canal posteriorly. Plain x-rays showed persistence of a large mass of barium in the pelvis. These clinical and radiological findings showed no resolution over the next 17 months of follow up (Figure 89.1).

Operation (3.31.88)

Resection of the rectum, coloanal anastomosis, and loop ileostomy were performed. Total excision of the internal sphincter and barium deposits on the

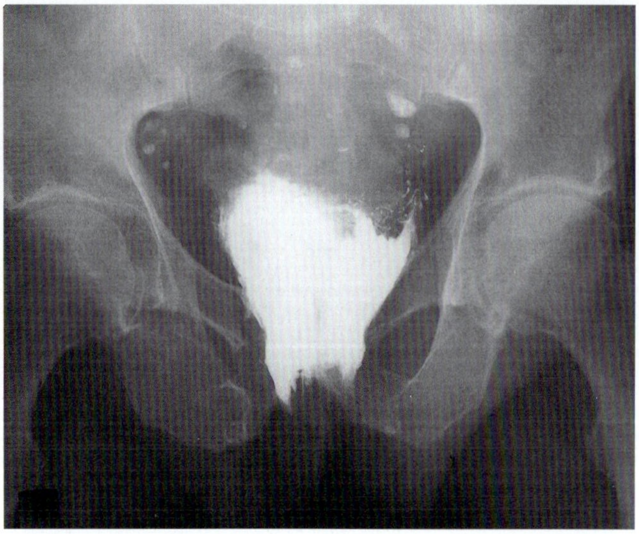

Figure 89.1: Plain x-ray of the pelvis 17 months after perforation shows persistent presence of barium.

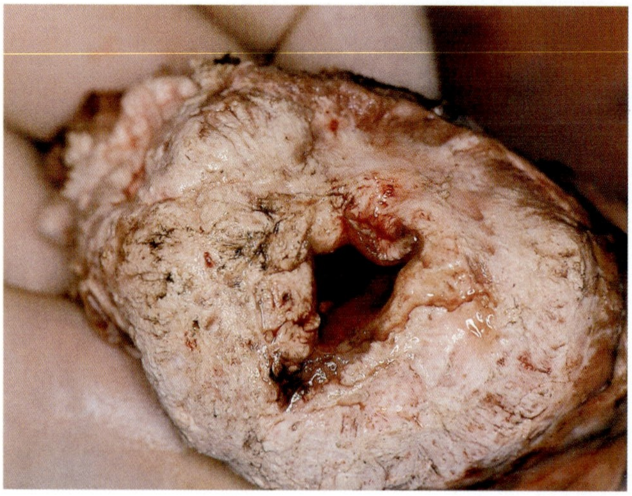

Figure 89.2: Transverse section of the resected specimen shows extensive infiltration of tissues by barium.

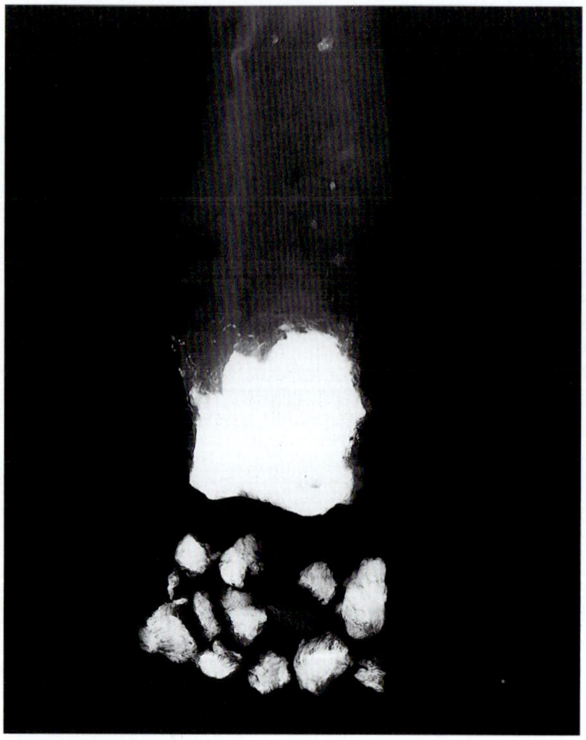

Figure 89.3: An x-ray of resected rectum and fragments of perirectal tissue demonstrates the presence of the barium 17 months after the barium enema.

levator ani were included in the resection. Intense fibrosis was present. There was barium infiltration of all layers of the rectum and perirectal tissues (Figures 89.2 and 89.3).

Follow-Up (1996)

The ileostomy was closed 3 months after resection. Subsequently, bowel function was attenuated but acceptable. There was no evidence of sexual or urinary dysfunction.

Comment

The incidence of this complication has been reported as high as 0.2%.[1] The barium infiltrated all layers of the lower rectum, including the anal sphincter. Examination of the resected specimen illustrates why no resolution was possible after a period of conservative management. The mortality of barium perforation of the rectum has been reported as high as 60%[2] and 100%.[3] Surviving patients frequently require a permanent stoma.

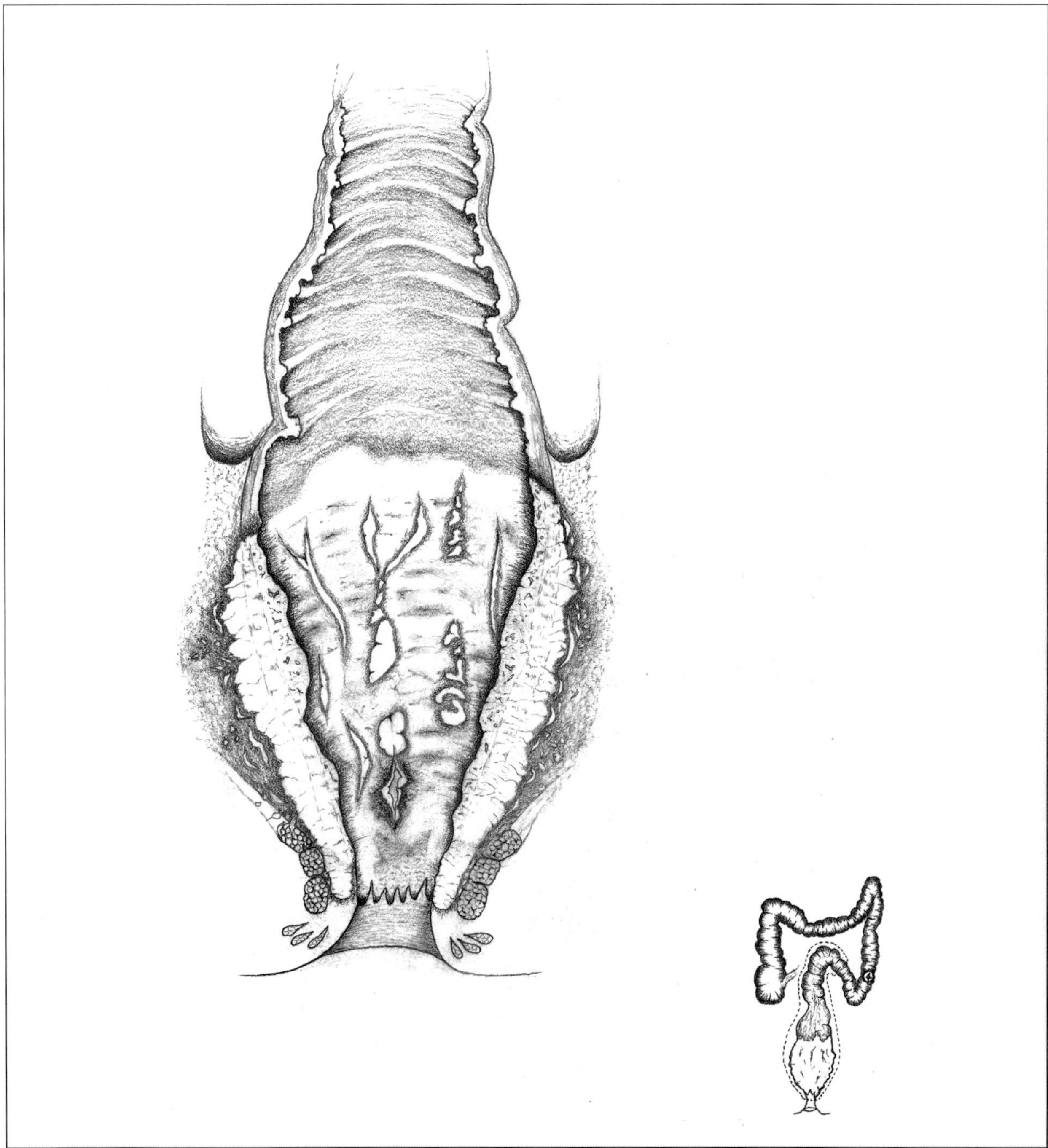

CASE

90 Colonoscopy Injury to the Colon

Male, 67 Years

History

The patient complained of altered bowel habit and rectal bleeding for 6 weeks. He suffered from significant ischemic heart disease. Clinical examination revealed a palpable carcinoma on the left side of the rectum at 5 cm, occupying 50% of the lumen. There was some loss of mobility of the tumor. Colonoscopy was performed to the cecum. The findings were sigmoid diverticulitis and small hyperplastic polyps. No specific difficulty with the examination was recorded. The patient did not complain of any abdominal symptoms subsequent to colonoscopy.

Operation (8.4.89)

Elective laparotomy to resect the rectal cancer was performed 7 days after the colonoscopy. There was an extensive hematoma of the anterior ascending colon, 9 cm in length, disrupting the muscle layers of the bowel wall and associated with free blood (approximately 500 ml) in the peritoneal cavity. A right hemicolectomy was performed. Unusual fragility of the mesenteric blood vessels was noted. There were small metastases in the liver related to the rectal tumor, which was removed by an extended (ultra low) anterior resection without a proximal stoma.

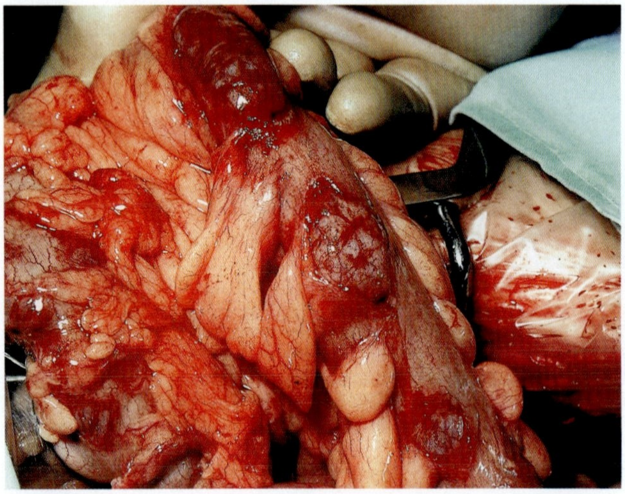

Figure 90.1: Post colonoscopy appearance of sigmoid colon (different patient) showing multiple areas of muscle dehiscence.

Postoperative

The patient's postoperative course was complicated by several episodes of cardiac arrest that responded promptly to resuscitation management. On the 11th day of his recovery, a fecal fistula appeared and this was managed by laparotomy, colon irrigation, and loop ileostomy. Further episodes of cardiac arrest due to his unstable cardiac condition kept him in the hospital for 12 weeks. The patient suffered a further cardiac arrest 5 weeks after discharge, from which he did not recover.

Comment

This complication is very rare following diagnostic colonoscopy, and only one other case has been found in the literature.[1] That patient, reported by Gallo et al, suffered the complication after a difficult colonoscopy without any other procedures such as biopsy. Computer tomography (CT) examination was helpful in diagnosis and in monitoring progress, which continued without the necessity of operation. Trauma to the colon induced by diagnostic colonoscopy is usually located in the sigmoid colon, and injuries less than perforation consist of single or multiple areas of muscle dehiscence (Figure 90.1). The colonoscopist reported that the examination of the patient described here, was not a difficult procedure. The double resection and the anastomotic leak requiring reoperation undoubtedly contributed to the patient's unstable cardiac state, which ultimately caused his death.

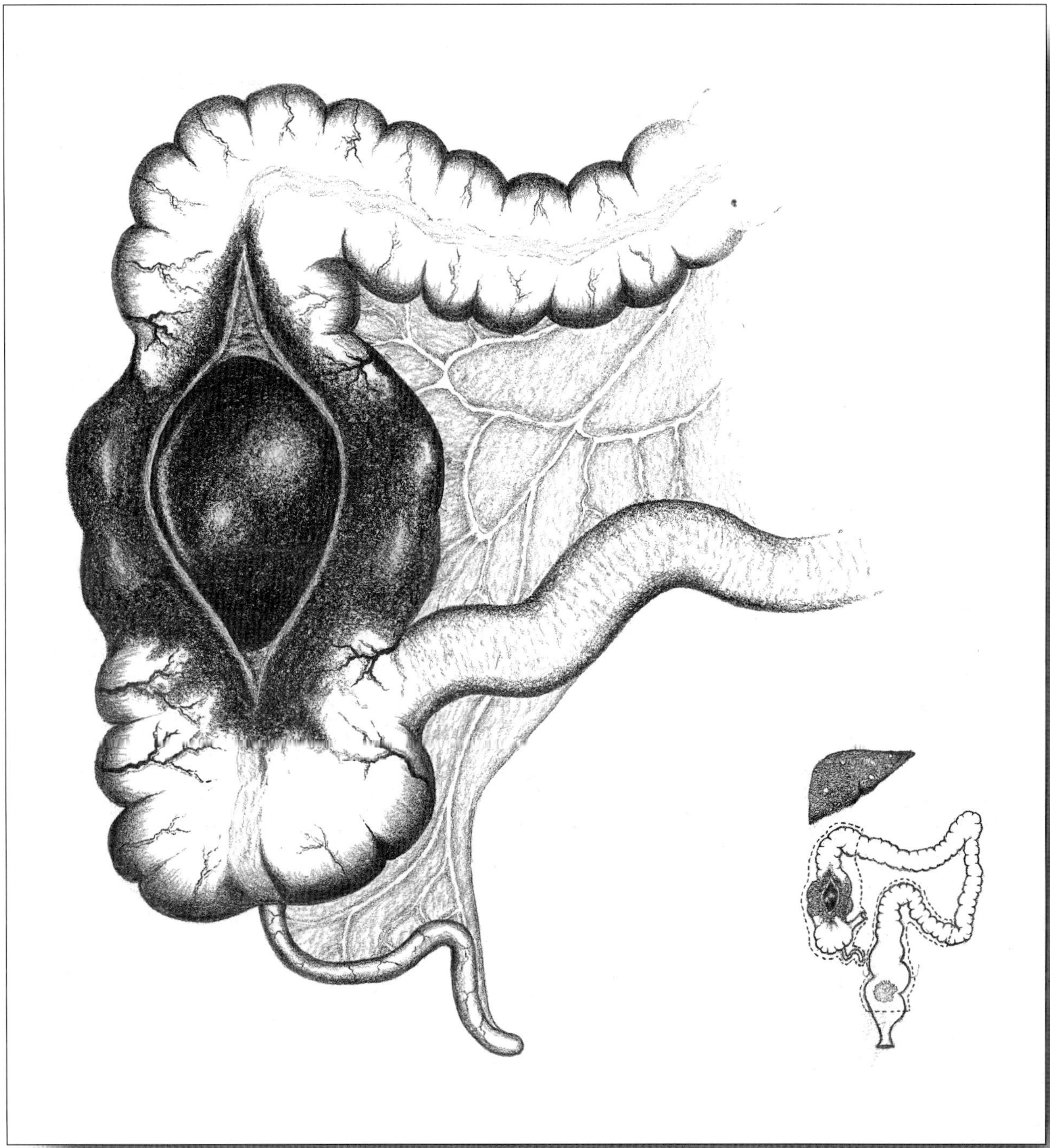

CASE

91 Mesenteric Thrombosis After Colon Resection

Male, 73 Years

History

The patient was investigated for iron deficiency anemia. Colonoscopy revealed a large rectal polyp and a carcinoma of the transverse colon. The ascending colon was not viewed due to the malignant stenosis. The patient's comorbidity included diabetes, asthma, chronic obstructive airways disease, and coronary artery disease. He was declared unsuitable for surgical treatment of his coronary disease.

Operation (7.3.98)

A right hemicolectomy was performed.

Pathology

The resected specimen contained an ulcerating carcinoma of the transverse colon (Dukes B, T3 N0 M0). In the ascending colon, there were 3 polyps. The largest, measuring 30 × 30mm was a benign tubulovillous adenoma. The polyp next to the appendix measured 15 × 15mm and contained a focus of invasive carcinoma (Dukes A, T1 N0 M0) in a tubulovillous adenoma.

Progress

The patient's recovery was satisfactory until the 9th postoperative day, when he complained of severe abdominal pain associated with vomiting. There was generalized abdominal tenderness and a large mass, the size of a rugby football, palpable in the central abdomen.

Operation (7.12.98)

Extensive mesenteric venous thrombosis was present which had caused infarction of the distal half of the small bowel. Resection of the ileum (230cm) and ileocolic anastomosis were performed with an anastomosis of jejunum to the transverse colon. There was 215cm of small bowel remaining. The patient's postoperative recovery was, at times, uncertain but eventually satisfactory.

Operation (1.14.99)

Diathermy snare of the large rectal polyp. It was situated 14cm from the anal margin and filled the lumen at that level. Histological examination revealed a villous adenoma with no evidence of malignancy.

Follow-Up

The patient's cardio-respiratory diseases intensified frequently, requiring repeated admissions to hospital. This caused his death 27 months after his right hemicolectomy.

Comment

Intestinal infarction occurring after elective colon resection for cancer is rare.[1] In a subset of the author's series, the incidence was 3 in 1418 (0.3%),[2] which is less than the 4.8% incidence reported after colectomy for inflammatory bowel disease (IBD).[3] In addition to the surgery, the presence of cancer, diabetes, and severe cardiovascular disease would have been etiological factors of significance. The patient's coagulation profile was normal. The need for urgent reoperation was obvious, and an investigation such as computerized tomography (CT) was not performed. The venous thrombosis was situated in the distal and mid mesenteric veins. The superior mesenteric vein did not contain thrombus. The patient's bowel function subsequently was 2–3 times per day, which was surprising in view of the complete loss of the ileum. Mesenteric vascular occlusion in patients over 70 years of age carries a high mortality rate, and in the series of 74 patients reported by Wadman et al, 28 out of 40 (70%) died within 30 days of the event.[1]

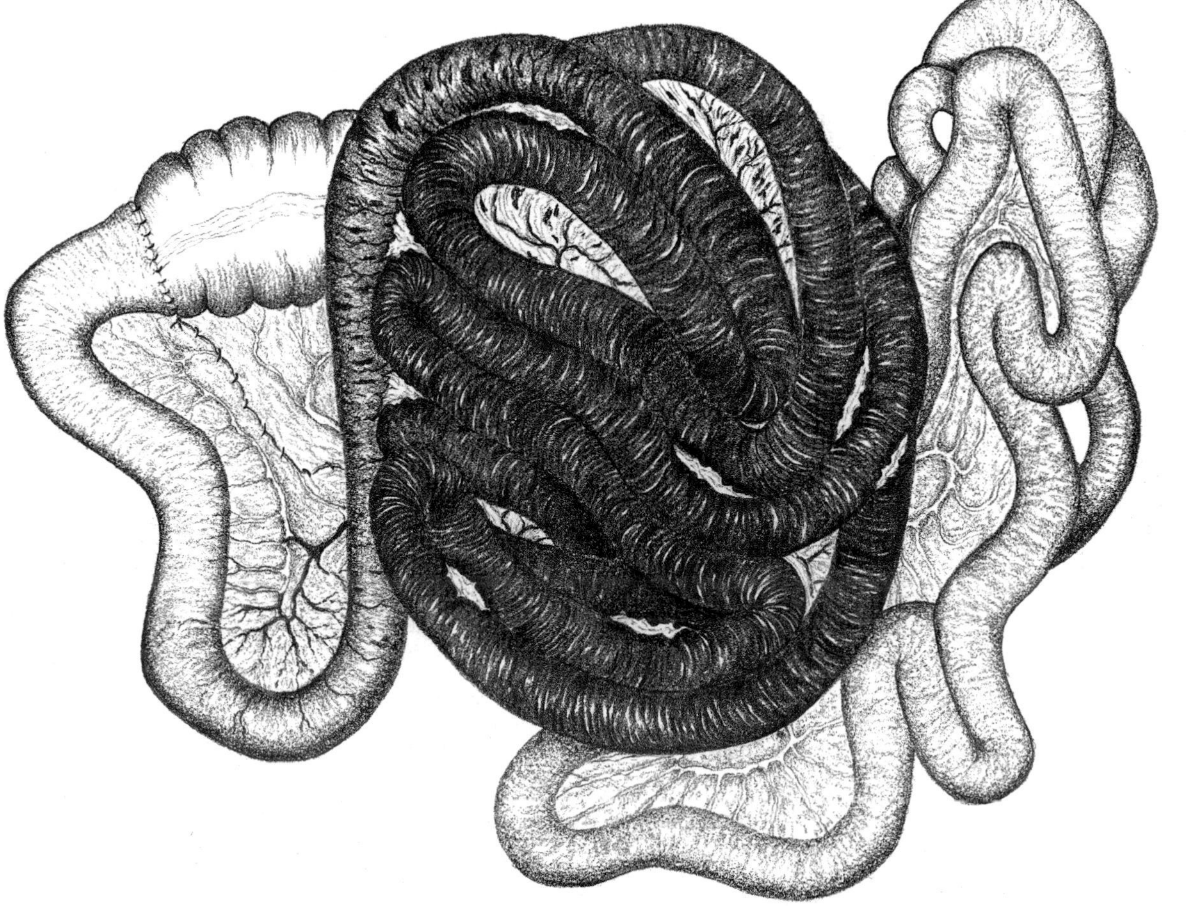

7.12.98

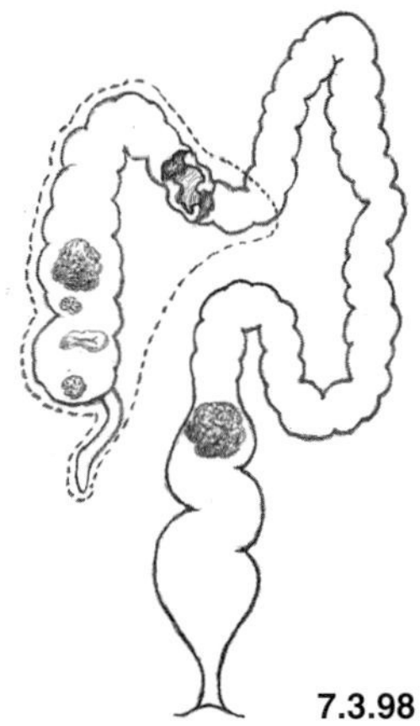

7.3.98

7.12.98

CASE

92 Postoperative Abdominal Apoplexy

Male, 74 Years

History

Investigation of lower abdominal pain and rectal bleeding revealed a carcinoma of the sigmoid colon at 30cm. Apart from well controlled hypertension, the patient was in reasonable health.

Operation (2.20.98)

At laparotomy, the tumor appeared localized with no evidence of metastases. Significant diverticular disease was present in the sigmoid and descending colon. A left hemicolectomy including upper rectum was performed (Figure 92.1).

Pathology

The ulcerating carcinoma was 35 × 35mm in size occupying two-thirds of the lumen. It was a well differentiated lesion that penetrated deeply into the muscularis propria. There were no metastases in the 6 lymph nodes examined (Dukes A, T_2 N_0 M_0).

Postoperative Course

The patient's initial recovery was satisfactory until 48 hrs after operation, when he suddenly developed a tender, distended abdomen, pallor, and hypotension. He was stabilized with resuscitation and transferred to the operative theater.

Operation (2.22.98)

Laparotomy revealed the presence of a profuse hemorrhage filling the abdomen with over 4000ml of blood. The site of bleeding was identified in the upper part of the lesser omentum, where a small artery was still actively bleeding. The lesser omentum and anterior wall of the stomach (subperitoneal) were extensively suffused with blood. The site of the previous colorectal anastomosis was unaffected. The bleeding vessel was ligated.

Postoperative Course/Follow-Up (2004)

Further recovery was uneventful. The patient remains free of recurrent disease 6 years, 7 months after the bowel resection.

Comment

The incidence of intraabdominal bleeding requiring emergency return to the operative theatre is uncommon. In a series of 1418 elective resection-anastomosis for cancer, 4 patients required reoperation for bleeding from the surgical site, and 1 patient (reported here) for bleeding remote from the operation area.[1] Abdominal apoplexy in older patients has been associated with hypertension and atherosclerosis.[2] The most common arteries to be the source of bleeding are the middle colic, left gastric, splenic, and superior mesenteric.[2] The bleeding vessel is not always identifiable, and in such circumstances, a morbidity of 56% has been reported[3] Tan advises that the bleeding vessel is likely to be located at the site of maximum hematoma.[4]

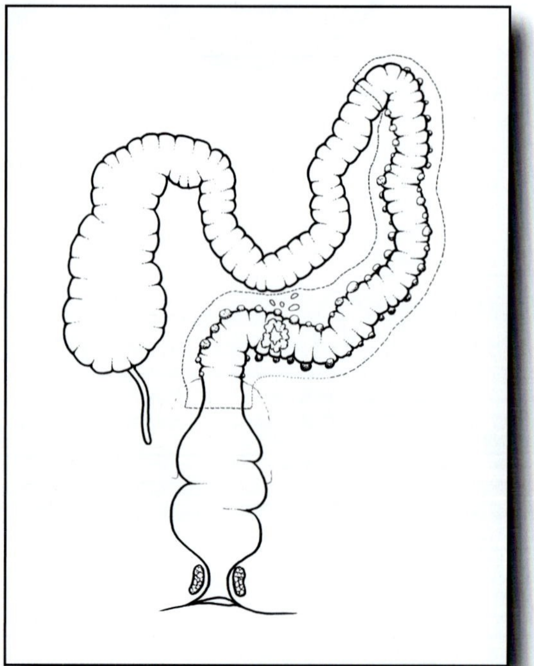

Figure 92.1: Showing the extent of the resection. 2.20.98.

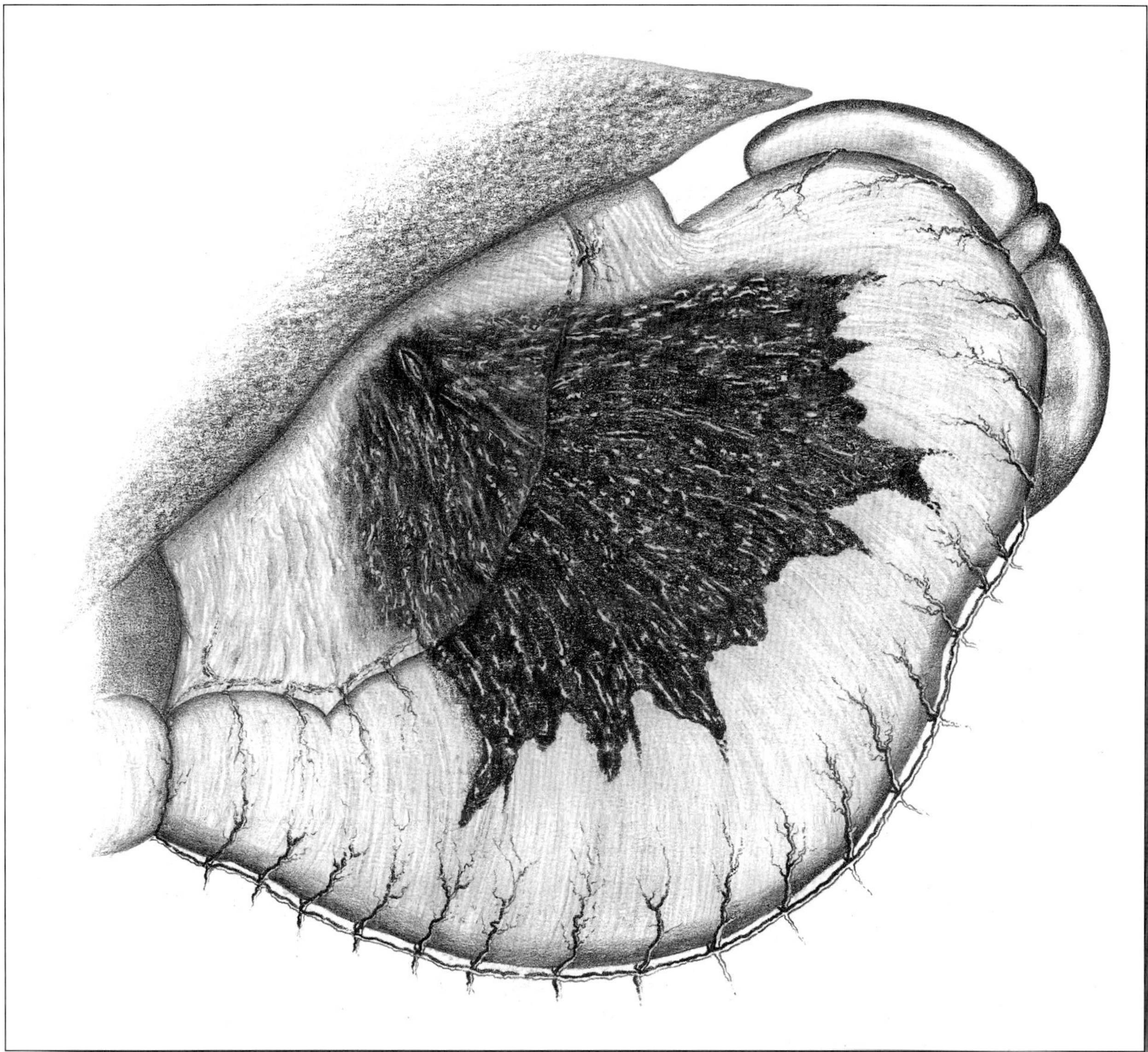

CASE

93 Local Excision of Rectal Cancer and Radiotherapy

Female, 87 Years

History

The patient had noticed dark red rectal bleeding for 5 months accompanied by frequent urge to defecate. Her previous health included mastectomy 51 years previously and stable congestive cardiac failure associated with aortic incompetence. She had borne 12 children and now had 54 grandchildren! She was sprightly physically, but early signs of dementia were present. Examination revealed a carcinoma on the posterior wall of the rectum 6 cm from the anal verge occupying 40% of the lumen. Above the lesion, no pathology was detected on colonoscopy. A computerized tomography (CT) examination showed no evidence of perirectal extension or metastatic disease. A sphincter-saving resection was planned, and the patient was treated with preoperative radiotherapy (37.5 Gy in 15 fractions over 3 weeks).

Operation (10.7.93)

Reexamination of the tumor 4 weeks after completion of radiotherapy revealed increased mobility and a significant decrease in size of the lesion. With underlying concern about the impact of major surgery on the 87-year-old patient, transanal local disc excision (LE) with diathermy was performed instead of the planned resection. The operation was performed 4 weeks after radiotherapy treatment (RT) was completed.

Pathology

The tumor was a flat plaque, 35 mm in diameter. Histologically, it was a moderately well differentiated adenocarcinoma. Its depth occupied the full thickness of the muscular layer but did not extend beyond it (T2). The excision margins were clear by 3 mm.

Postoperative Course/Follow-Up

The immediate postoperative recovery was uneventful. After leaving the hospital, the patient suffered constant rectal pain requiring readmission to hospital. Examination under anesthesia, 5 weeks after the operation, revealed a large necrotic ulcer of the posterior wall of the rectum and upper anal canal 70 mm in length. There was florid granulation tissue present, partly covered by fibrin and slough. Biopsies showed no evidence of carcinoma. There were occasional bizarre cells consistent with radiotherapy effect. The rectal pain continued over a period of 11 months. Healing of the ulcer occurred without specific treatment in 12 months. The referring gastroenterologist in a distant rural area performed further supervision. The patient succumbed to liver metastases 18 months after the local excision. There was no clinical evidence of local recurrence.

Comment

Due to a "last minute" change of treatment plan on the morning of an intended sphincter-saving resection, the patient's sequence of treatment modalities was different from the author's usual practice. For those patients in whom adjuvant radiotherapy has been planned, it has been administered postoperatively when the local excision site has healed. The extensive rectal ulceration is a rare complication of LE and adjuvant RT and may be related to the sequence of the treatment and the method of RT administration. Recent reports of local excision of rectal cancer following preoperative radiotherapy (with doses of RT up to 52.5 Gy) do not document this complication.[1,2] It is now established that, in view of the high risk of local recurrence, T2 tumours[3] are not suitable for local excision unless the operation is a compromise in a frail, high-risk patient. In the case of this 87-year-old patient with early dementia, it would have been better management to select local excision therapy originally. Although the radiotherapy followed by local surgery controlled the pelvic disease, its complication caused 11 of her remaining 18 months of life to be associated with rectal pain.

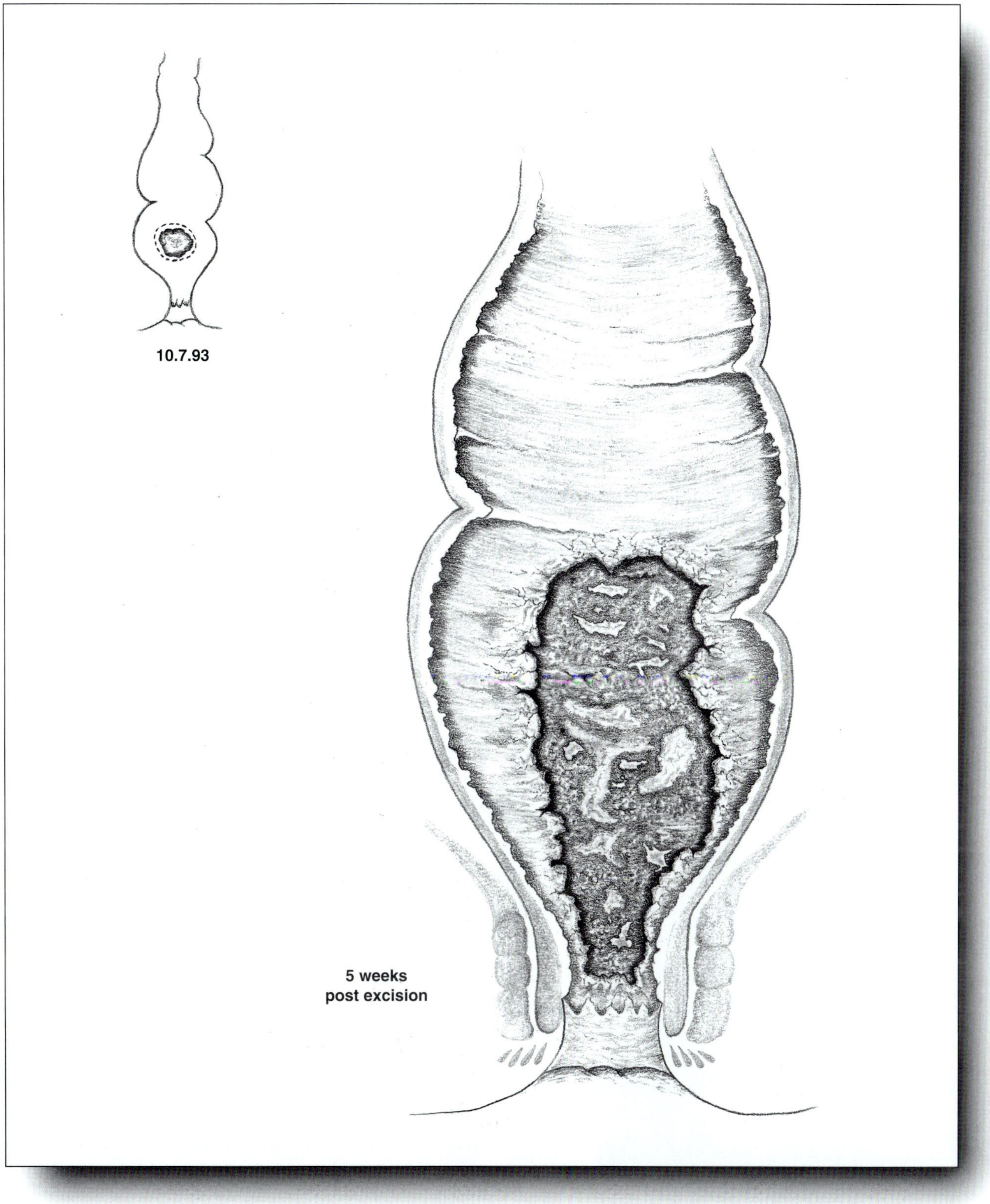
10.7.93
5 weeks
post excision

CASE

94 Residual Diverticulitis After Resection Causing an Elongated Abscess with Prolongated Resolution

Female, 63 Years

History

The patient suffered from asthma, an enormous goiter, obesity (weight, 252 lb), and severe kyphosis of the thoracic spine. In March 1993, a barium enema demonstrated an "apple core" deformity that could not be reached by colonoscopy examination.

Operation (May 1993)

Laparotomy revealed a complex mass involving the sigmoid colon and ovary. A limited resection and anastomosis of the proximal sigmoid and excision of the left ovary was performed in the belief that the operation was a palliative procedure for an ovarian cancer. Pathology examination revealed diverticular disease and no evidence of carcinoma of the colon or ovary. The patient remained unwell with signs of sepsis.

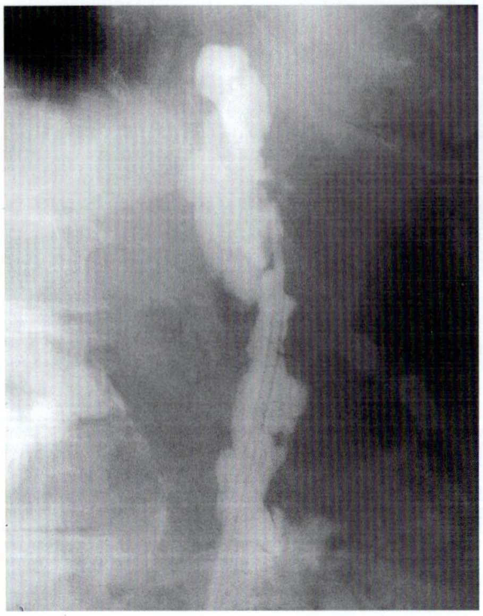

Figure 94.1: Sinogram showing the vertical extent of the retroperitoneal abscess.

Operation (November 1993)

Laparotomy was performed in November 1993 to drain a left subphrenic abscess. The colon was divided above a persistent sigmoid mass, and the proximal end of the colon was established as an end colostomy. A further contrast enema (February 1994) demonstrated extensive diverticular disease and a leak from the colon entering a retroperitoneal abscess, which reached the diaphragm. The patient was referred for further management.

Operation (6.16.94)

Total thyroidectomy was undertaken to obviate any airway difficulties during the anticipated major abdominal surgery. The thyroid was benign and weighed 560 g.

Operation (8.1.94)

A ureteric catheter was inserted on the left side. Laparotomy revealed dense pelvic adhesions in relation to a mass formed by pathology in the distal sigmoid colon, on the surface of which diverticula were obvious. There was a chronic thick-walled abscess in relation to the mass, adherent to the left pelvic brim and related vessels. The abscess involved the intraperitoneal rectum, uterus, and bladder, and extended into the extraperitoneal tissues adjacent to the lower rectum. By intubation, a long retroperitoneal extension of the abscess was identified posteromedial to the left kidney and extending as far as the diaphragm (Figure 94.1). The sigmoid colon was resected to a level immediately distal to the pelvic brim. The abscess in the pelvis was debrided. The unopened cranial extension was irrigated. The colostomy was taken down, the colon was irrigated clear of fecal content via an ileotomy, and a colorectal anastomosis performed. The ileotomy site was converted to a loop ileostomy. Long-term suction drains were placed in the region of the pelvic abscess and the long cranial extension. During the procedure, it was not possible to visualize the left ureter.

Pathology

Examination of the resected colon revealed diverticular disease with stricture formation. Within the stricture, 2 large perforations were present that had previously been in continuity with the complex abscess. The lumen contained pus, the mucosa was inflamed.

Operation (12.2.94)

The ileostomy was closed 4 months after the resection.

Follow-Up

The long retroperitoneal abscess track healed very slowly. Irrigation was complemented by antibiotic therapy. The drainage tube was in situ for a period of 9 months.

Comment

This case highlights the difficulty that can confront the surgeon if preoperative colonoscopy cannot assess the pathology. The surgeon was misled to perform a "palliative debulking procedure" which left perforated the colon in situ. The case also illustrates the tracking potential of a diverticular abscess. The long postoperative period of intubation irrigation was tedious but maintained the patient's health and prevented further surgical treatment. The preoperative preparation included thyroidectomy, which is somewhat unusual.

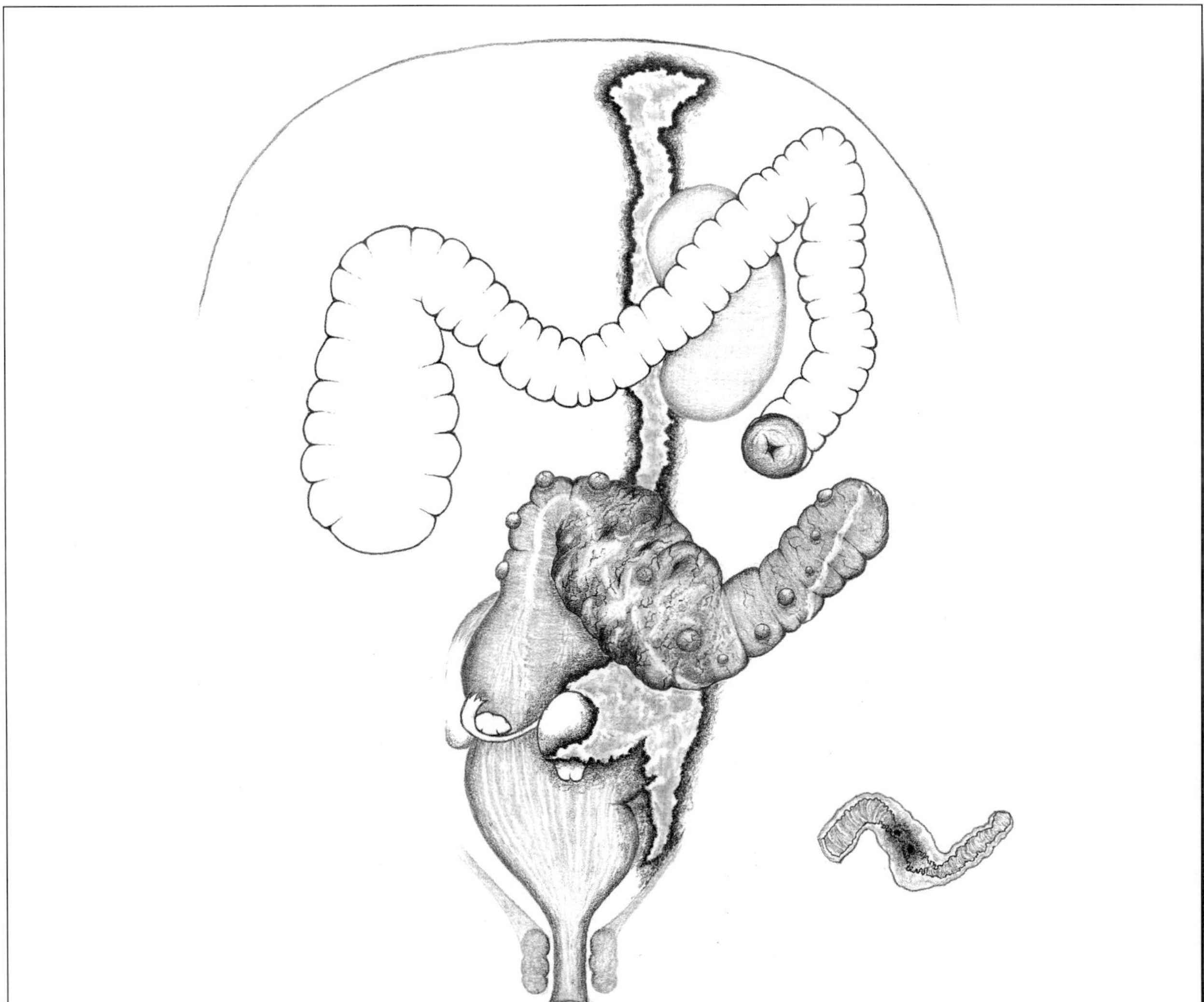

For a full-page image of this figure see the appendix.

CASE

95 Perforated Diverticulitis and Its Consequences

Male, 59 Years

History

In November 1971, this patient suffered a sigmoid colon perforation due to diverticulitis. His general health was very poor due to respiratory insufficiency (heavy smoker), poor nutrition, and homelessness. At laparotomy, fecal peritonitis was present, managed by abdominal irrigation, drainage of the perforation site, and a proximal colostomy. The postoperative course was stormy. A colocutaneous fistula appeared, and radiological investigations diagnosed a colovesical fistula. The patient was referred.

Operation (4.20.72)

At laparotomy, the site of origin of the colocutaneous fistula was identified as the recent perforation in the upper third of the sigmoid colon. The colovesical fistula arose from the mid third of the sigmoid colon and entered the bladder via the trigone. The margins of the defect in the bladder (10 × 15 mm) were densely fibrotic, indicating a long-standing fistula. Closure of this large defect was possible only with more than optimal tension on the sutures. The sigmoid and upper rectum was resected, and a 2-layer anastomosis performed. There was insufficient omentum to place between the bladder repair and the anastomosis.

Postoperative Progress

Although the patient's clinical course appeared satisfactory, contrast radiological studies 21 days after operation demonstrated a subclinical anastomotic leak that was in continuity with the lumen of the bladder.

Operation (11.1.73)

An extended low anterior resection was undertaken to eradicate the persistent anastomotico-vesical fistula (Figures 95.2 and 95.3). A chronic abscess was situated between the rectum and the bladder. The inflammatory changes in the bladder wall had obscured the fistula track, so no repair was attempted. Prior to the anastomosis, the circulation of the small rectal segment was noted to be suspect. The proximal colostomy was maintained.

Early Postoperative Progress

After a difficult operation, it was surprising that recovery appeared to be uncomplicated. Assessment of the anastomosis, however (14 days after operation), revealed complete separation of the colon and rectum. There was purulent discharge per rectum as the only manifestation of this serious complication. In the absence of any clinical evidence of peritoneal infection, it was decided that no further surgical intervention was indicated. It was anticipated that the transverse colostomy would be permanent.

Further Progress

During the next 20 months, the pelvic space between the 2 ends of the bowel healed, and as this occurred, the colon and rectum became approximated with an intervening stricture (Figures 95.1 and 95.5). There appeared to be an adequate lumen for bowel function. The transverse colostomy was closed 20 months after the resection.

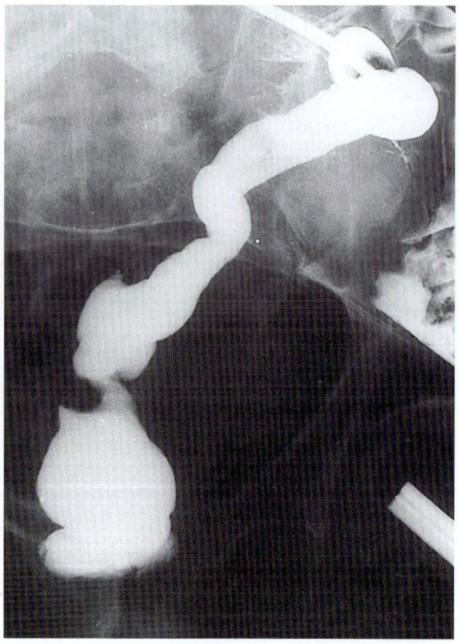

Figure 95.1: The x-ray (6.20.75) demonstrates the bowel continuity, with a stricture, which formed spontaneously, subsequent to anastomotic dehiscence in 1973.

Follow-Up (1976)

Bowel function was variable in frequency but preferred to a stoma 12 months after colostomy closure. Further follow-up was not available as he returned to his homeless existence.

Comment

The first series describing colovesical fistulae (CVF) was published by Harrison Cripps in 1888.[1] Hool et al found an incidence of CVF in 5% of patients requiring surgery for diverticulitis.[2] In the author's series of 206 elective resections for diverticular disease, there were 23 (11.2%) patients with CVF.[3] The trigone of the bladder is an unusual site for CVF, unless the fistula track is extraperitoneal.[4] This location and size of the defect created technical difficulties, which lead to failure of the closure. Although in many patients with a CVF repair of the bladder defect is not required,[5] the size of the fistula in the bladder wall made attempted closure obligatory in this patient. The second rectal anastomosis was a failure, almost certainly due to a vascular problem with the short rectal stump. A coloanal anastomosis would have been a better choice of operation. If a Hartmann operation had been performed, it is unlikely it could have been reversed due to the patient's chronic comorbidity. Remarkably, in the presence of dehiscence the sepsis remained localized, draining per rectum, and without systemic effects. The spontaneous restoration of bowel continuity ("auto-anastomosis") has been seen by the author in only 2 other patient. This unusual sequence permitted closure of the proximal colostomy and acceptable bowel function in a patient whose general health would have contraindicated any further major reconstructive surgery.

Figure 95.2: Shows the anastomotico-vesical/fistula.

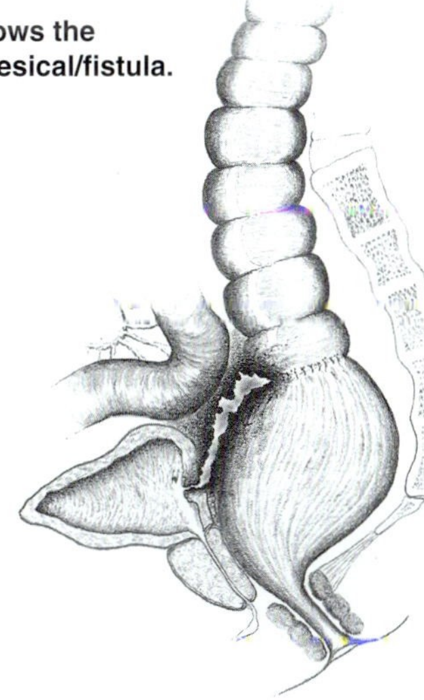

Figure 95.3: The extended low anterior resection (11.1.73).

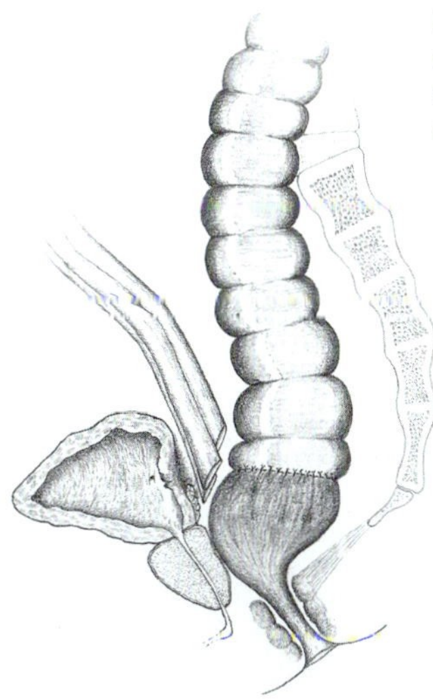

Figure 95.4: Anastomotic dehiscence.

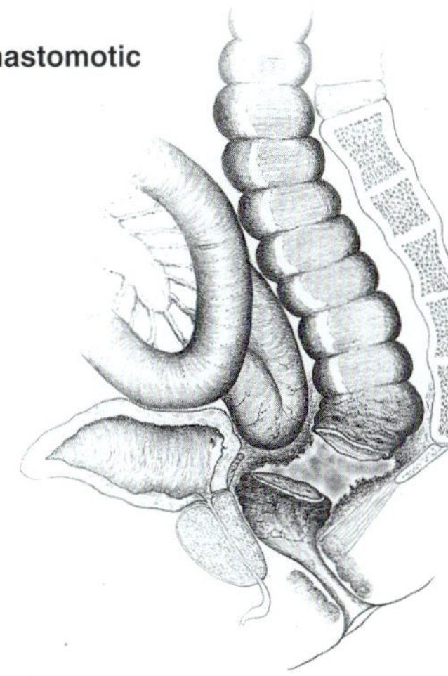

Figure 95.5: Spontaneous auto-anastomosis with stricture.

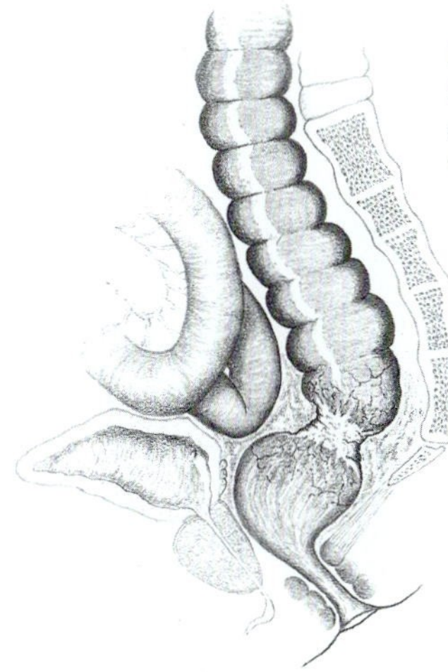

For a full-page image of this figure see the appendix.

CASE

96 Anastomotic Dehiscence After Anterior Resection

Male, 54 Years

History

The patient presented with a 5-month history of rectal bleeding and diarrhea. Colonoscopy revealed a carcinoma at 13 cm and no other significant abnormality to the cecum. The patient's psychological background included depression, aggression, and a tendency towards litigation.

Operation (12.23.88)

The carcinoma was situated in the intraperitoneal rectum. There was no evidence of metastatic spread. The distal two-thirds of the sigmoid and the upper rectum were removed and the extraperitoneal anastomosis performed using an intraluminal stapler. The blood supply to the levels of resection of colon and rectum appeared satisfactory. No proximal stoma was performed. A drain with continuous suction was placed in the presacral space for 48 h.

Pathology

The carcinoma was a polypoidal tumor (6 × 7 cm) of average grade penetrating the muscularis propria without lymph node metastases (Dukes B, T3 No Mo). It was continuous distally, with a soft, flat tubular adenoma (8 × 7 cm).

Postoperative Course

For some days, the patient's temperature remained elevated, and he complained of suprapubic pain. There was minimal abdominal tenderness, and bowel function occurred without delay. He showed no significant signs of intraabdominal sepsis. A routine limited gastrograffin enema revealed a large space in the pelvis with no identification of the anastomosis (Figure 96.1). Sigmoidoscopy revealed that the ends of the bowel were separated by a large cavity (Figure 96.3). Conservative management was pursued with the patient because:

(i) he remained surprisingly free of septic signs;
(ii) bowel function continued;
(iii) the patient was seriously disturbed at the prospect of a stoma; and
(iv) early reoperation would have been a Hartmann procedure.

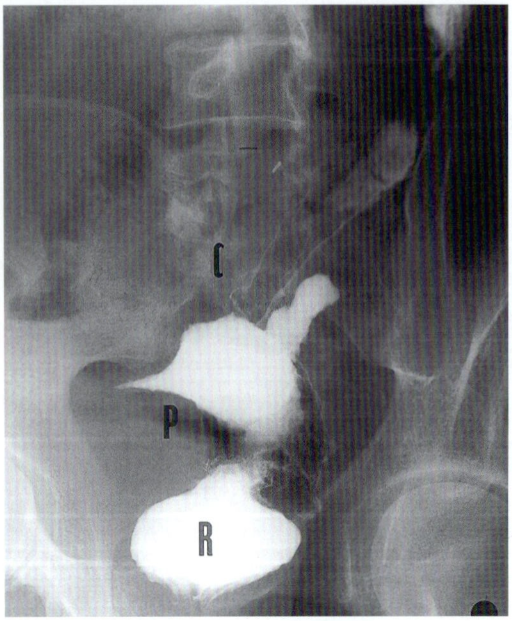

Figure 96.1: Contrast enema 27 days after operation. C: terminal colon; P: pelvic cavity; R: rectum.

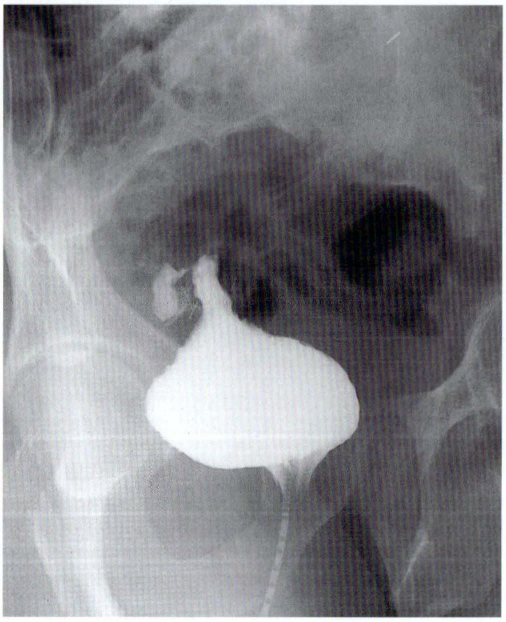

Figure 96.2: Contrast could not pass the anastomotic stricture 9 months after failed anterior resection.

Over a period of 9 months, severe stricture formation occurred that did not respond to dilatation (Figure 96.2).

Operation (9.28.89)

Excision of the anastomotic stricture and distal colon, reanastomosis of colon to rectum, and loop ileostomy. The postoperative course was uneventful.

Pathology

There was a small chronic abscess posterior to the stricture in continuity with the lumen (Figure 96.4). The left colon showed evidence of chronic obstruction. On histological examination, the distal colon adjacent to the persistent defect showed ulceration, and granulation, with submucosal fibrosis, consistent with ischemia.

Operation (12.4.89)

Closure of loop ileostomy.

Comment

A mid rectal (extraperitoneal) anastomosis has a lower incidence of anastomotic leak (1.7%) than an extended (ultra low) anterior resection (5.4%).[1] This difference has been noted in a number of series, including the results of 1014 patients with stapled rectal anastomosis treated at the Cleveland Clinic.[2] Accordingly, complete dehiscence of the anastomosis was not expected in this patient, who was thought to be "risk free." Nevertheless, it is acknowledged that accurate prediction of AL is impossible.[3] There was a concern in this patient that a malfunctioning suction drain may have induced excessive suction pressure, causing damage to the marginal vessels of the terminal colon. In the absence of clinical signs of sepsis, the complication was managed conservatively. Bowel continuity can be gradually established spontaneously in such cases with stricture formation that may allow reasonable bowel function, note Case 95, or require elective reconstructive surgery.

Figure 96.3
Anastomotic dehiscence
(December 1988)

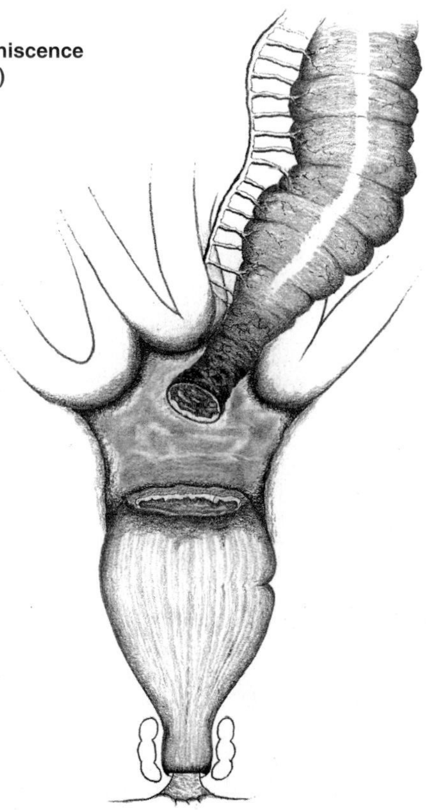

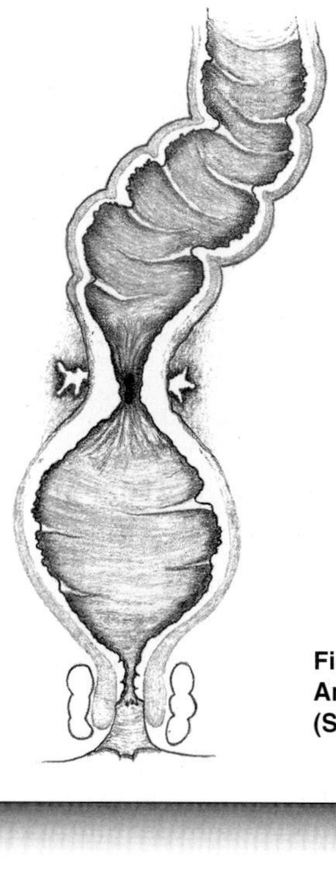

Figure 96.4
Anastomotic stricture
(September 1989)

CASE

97 Postoperative Necrosis of the Left Colon

Female, 35 Years

History

The patient had noticed diarrhea, urgency, and minimal rectal bleeding for 8 months. Until this time, the patient had been in excellent health. Examination revealed a mobile carcinoma of the rectum at 7 cm. It occupied one-third of the lumen circumference in the right lateral quadrant. Colonoscopy revealed no other pathology.

Operation (5.27.94)

Laparotomy revealed no evidence of metastatic disease. The transverse and sigmoid colon was redundant. The bowel was resected from mid sigmoid to lower third of the rectum (3 cm above the pelvic floor). The upper left colic artery was preserved to support the blood flow in the marginal artery, which was found to be excellent at the level of resection of the sigmoid colon. An extended (ultra) low anterior resection (LARx) anastomosis was performed with a single circular stapler. The length of the left colon–sigmoid was more than adequate, and splenic flexure mobilization was not undertaken. No blood transfusion was administered and there were no circulatory abnormalities during the operation. No proximal stoma was performed.

Pathology

The tumor was a flat ulcer, 50 × 40 mm with minimal penetration beyond the muscularis propria (Dukes B, T_3 N_0 M_0). It was a moderately differentiated adenocarcinoma.

Postoperative Progress

Initially, the patient's postoperative state was satisfactory, but by day 7 she was pyrexial with abdominal distention. A limited gastrograffin enema on day 9 (Figure 97.1) suggested ulceration in a narrow distal colon with minimal extravasation of the contrast into the pelvis. The patient was not generally unwell, but remained distended without a bowel action. A rectal examination on day 21 revealed

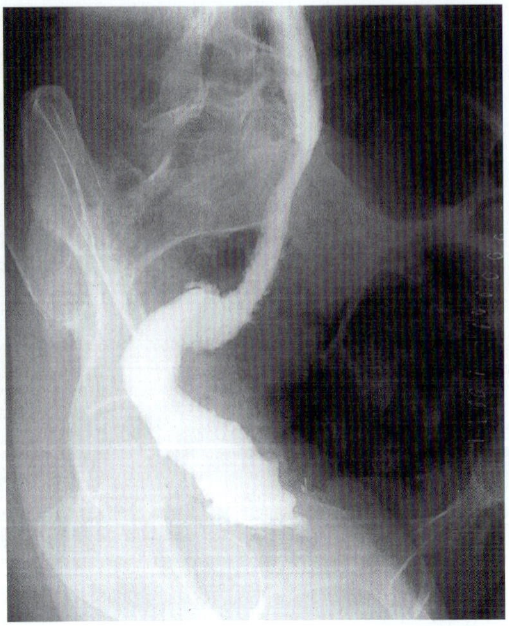

Figure 97.1: Contrast enema on day 9 shows narrowing and ulceration of the colon due to ischemia.

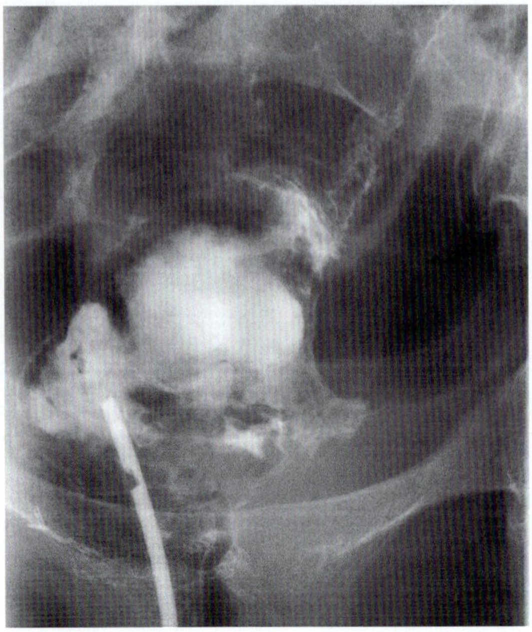

Figure 97.2: Contrast enema on day 21 demonstrates extensive extravasation of contrast into the pelvis due to anastomotic dehiscence. The enema tube is in the pelvic cavity.

complete separation of the anastomosis which was also demonstrated with a further limited contrast enema (Figure 97.2). There were no clinical signs of peritonitis.

Operation (6.18.94)
Laparotomy revealed dehiscence of the anastomosis due to ischemic necrosis of the distal colon. The pelvis was lined by granulation tissue without pus formation or fecal contamination and was effectively sealed off by adherent loops of small bowel. The feces in the dilated colon had not negotiated an ischemic stricture. The pelvic granulation tissue was curetted. The remaining rectum transected at the pelvic floor level and the colon resected to the upper descending colon. The colon was irrigated free of fecal content. After mucosectomy, a straight sleeve coloanal anastomosis was performed with per anal sutures. A loop ileostomy was constructed.

Pathology
The resected bowel showed mucosal ulceration, stricture formation, areas of full thickness necrosis, and thrombus within arteries consistent with an ischemic process.

Follow-Up (2004)
The patient's recovery was uneventful. The ileostomy was closed three months after the reoperation. Bowel function is sporadically frequent ("clustering"), but continence is normal. The patient's colorectal cancer (CRCa) follow up has been satisfactory for 10 years and 2 months.

Comment
This catastrophic complication was unexpected in an otherwise healthy 35-year-old patient. During the operation, the marginal blood flow to the sigmoid colon was seen to be satisfactory. Thrombosis in the postoperative period must have supervened. The clinical presentation of complete separation of the anastomosis was that of obstruction and not peritonitis. The "clean" pelvis facilitated an immediate reconstruction to be performed with a coloanal anastomosis, which is an unusual opportunity in the presence of this serious complication.

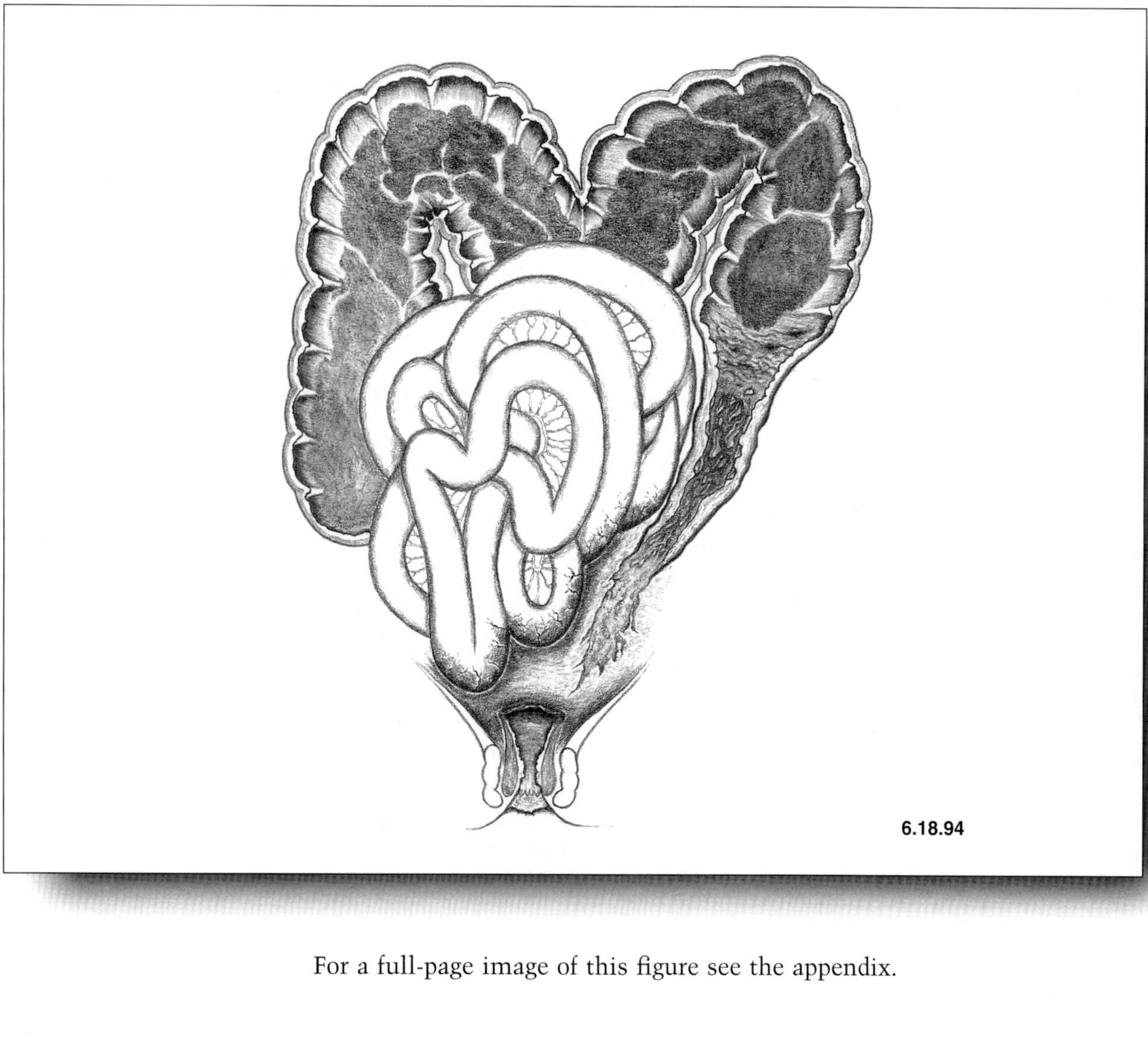

For a full-page image of this figure see the appendix.

CASE

98 Ileostomy Closure: An Impasse Due to Adhesions

Male, 69 Years

History

In 1975, cholecystectomy was performed for gallstones. In 1982, appendectomy for gangrenous appendicitis was followed by several operations for a pelvic abscess. During 1996, episodes of acute small bowel obstruction necessitated 3 admissions to the hospital. Laparotomy (9.19.96) revealed small bowel obstruction due to extensive adhesions. Complete adhesiolysis of small bowel was performed with repair to several sites of the bowel wall. The obstruction failed to settle over the subsequent 17 days and reoperation was necessary. Laparotomy (10.6.96), revealed a "mass of matted bowel with adhesions rock solid, like concrete." Extensive dissection resulted in ischemia to segments of small bowel and the left colon. A "massive" resection of ileum was performed (leaving 100 cm of small bowel), and the left colon was resected as a Hartmann operation. Subsequent to this operation, a small bowel fistula presented in the lower part of the abdominal wound. It failed to heal with conservative treatment. The patient was referred for further management.

Operation (1.13.97)

The small bowel fistula was attached to the lower end of the incision. Dense fibrous adhesions involved the total length of the small bowel. Ten centimeters of small bowel containing the fistula was resected with anastomosis. The patient was discharged from the hospital 28 days after operation, when nutritional support was stabilized.

Operation (4.20.98)

Reversal of Hartmann operation. The shortened colon was brought through the mesentery of the jejunum. Adhesions in the right iliac fossa were left undisturbed, which meant the loop stoma was more proximal than was ideal. (Figure 98.1).

Operation (5.4.98)

Closure of the ileostomy was performed by resection 14 days after the preceding surgery. This was well prior to the usual 3-month delay for this operation. Phlegmonous adhesive changes were maximal, with dense fibrosis obscuring the small bowel. The usual trephine wound required significant extension. The distal limb of the small bowel was fixed by adhesions that could not be safely dissected. Fortunately, the proximal ileum could be mobilized for a satisfactory single layer anastomosis. Two denuded areas of the seromuscular layer could not be closed without tension due to the fixation of the ileum by adhesions.

Follow-Up (October 2004)

The patient's nutritional state requires continued support. Investigations have demonstrated a degree of malabsorption. Bowel function is: Day/Night: 2-5/0. There have been no further episodes of bowel obstruction.

Comment

The adhesion pathology encountered in the ileostomy closure in this patient made it difficult to progress or "back off" to another day. The tough reactive adhesions caused the dissection to dangerously denude the exposed small bowel. The patient

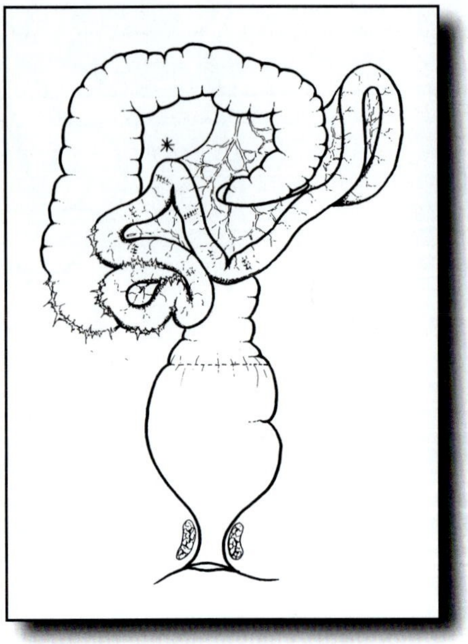

Figure 98.1: Reversal of Hartmann Operation (4.20.98).*:Indicates the site selected for loop ileostomy.

was known to form difficult adhesions, as observed at previous surgery, and attempting ileostomy closure at 14 days postoperatively almost certainly increased the operative difficulties. The author's preference has been to close stomas after 12 weeks but was persuaded otherwise in this case. Bakx et al, however, have reported early closure of ileostomies, during the same admission as the initial operation, and found this was associated with a low incidence of morbidity.[1] Trials with adhesion-preventing substances have not as yet established their efficacy beyond doubt. Tang et al, in a randomized trial, studied early closure of ileostomies in which an adhesion barrier membrane had been previously wrapped around the limbs of the ileostomy. They concluded that the technique reduced peristomal adhesions and facilitated early closure of the ileostomies.[2] Tjandra and Ng, in a randomized controlled trial, assessed the use of a spray gel when creating an ileostomy and found there were fewer adhesions at the closure of the ileostomy in those cases where spray gel was used.[3]

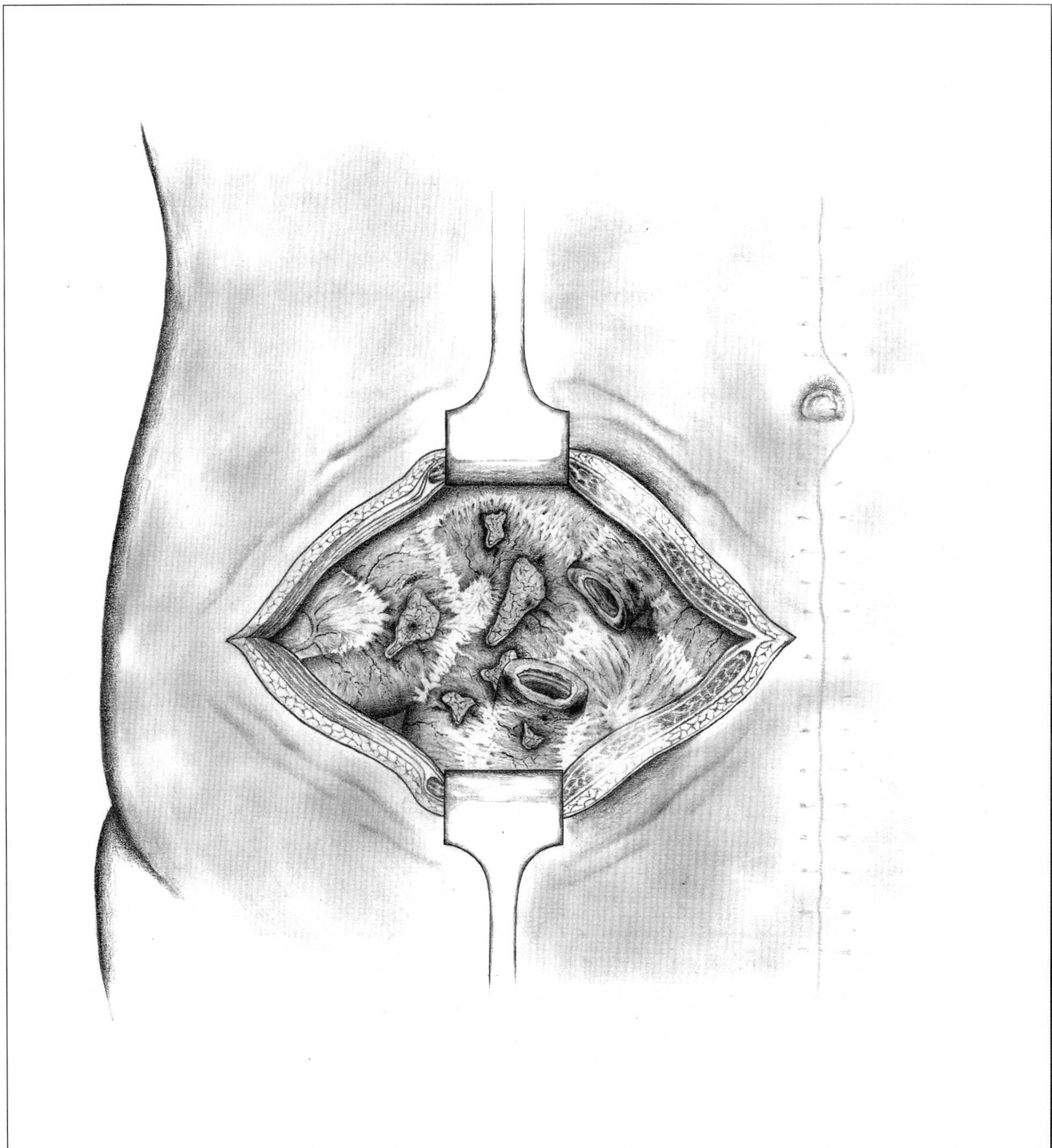

CASE

99 Perforation of the Sigmoid Colon Due to Radiation Injury

Female, 72 Years

History

In April 1996, the patient was urgently admitted to the hospital, with severe abdominal pain. Clinical examination revealed evidence of peritonitis, indicating the need for immediate operation. Her relevant past history was:

1965 Removal of ovarian tumor and postoperative radiotherapy (RT) to the pelvis (diagnosis and dose of RT not known).

1993 Stroke followed by full recovery.

1994 Left femoropopliteal bypass.

1995 (Aug.) External beam radiotherapy (60 Gy) to the pelvis for a high-grade transitional cell carcinoma of the bladder.

1996 (Feb.) Flexible sigmoidoscopy to investigate pelvic pain revealed stenosis at 20 cm and evidence of irradiation proctocolitis.

Operation (4.26.96)

Laparotomy revealed a purulent generalized peritonitis due to a perforation in the mid sigmoid colon. The perforation was situated on the antemesenteric border of the colon, 7–8 mm in diameter with a thin necrotic edge. The sigmoid colon was shortened in length, contracted in diameter with absence of haustra. The bowel wall felt thickened. There were acute and chronic inflammatory changes on the serosal surface. The small bowel was adherent to the sigmoid colon, and dense adhesions had "welded" together adjacent loops. There was pallor and an abnormal vascularity on the serosal aspect of the sigmoid colon and small bowel, typical of an irradiation reaction. The left colon was dilated and impacted with solid feces. There was a 2 cm metastasis in the anterior aspect of the right lobe of the liver. A Hartmann resection was performed after thorough irrigation of the abdominal cavity.

Pathology

The mucosa of the opened specimen showed hemorrhagic inflammation and ulceration. The perforation had occurred in the base of a radionecrotic ulcer. The bowel wall was thickened and the lumen stenosed. Histologically, there were changes due to the radiation (Figures 99.1 and 99.2).

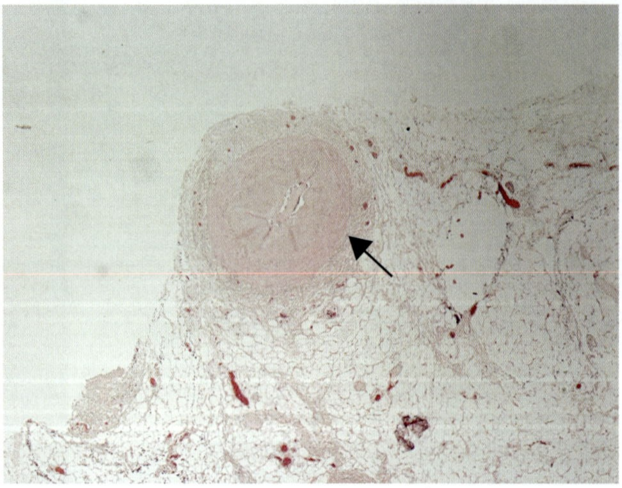

Figure 99.1: Endarteritis typical of radiation effect (arrow).

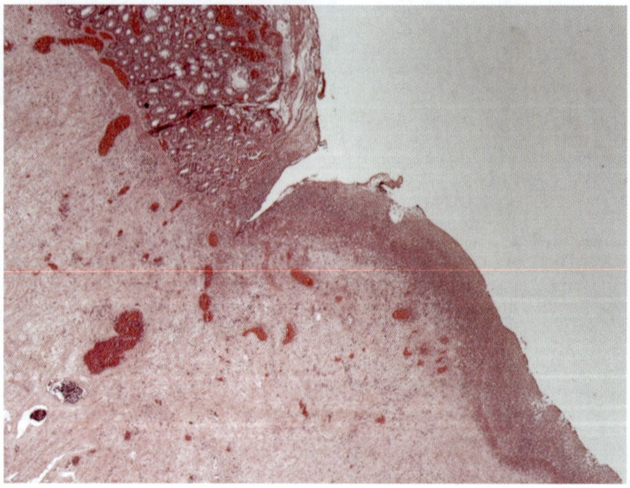

Figure 99.2: Section shows complete loss of mucosa with edema and granulation in the submucosa.

Postoperative Course

On day 2 after operation, an urgent left iliac endarterectomy was performed for acute arterial obstruction. Although bowel function returned satisfactorily, reestablishing oral feeding failed and total parenteral nutrition was commenced. The patient remained anorexic, lethargic, and depressed, and continued to decline until her death on day 14 after operation. No autopsy was performed.

Comment

Radiotherapy was selected for treatment of the bladder tumor, because the patient was regarded as unfit for cystectomy. The radiotherapist discussed with the patient his concern about the potential morbidity of radical radiotherapy in relation to the unknown dose of pelvic radiotherapy 30 years previously, her age, and general health. Schellhammer et al state that preexisting arteriosclerotic vascular disease is important in determining the degree of early and late radiation injuries.[1] The patient's demise occurred in the absence of any obvious abdominal complications. This mode of postoperative decline has been noted previously in the frail elderly patient undergoing surgery for the complications of radiotherapy.

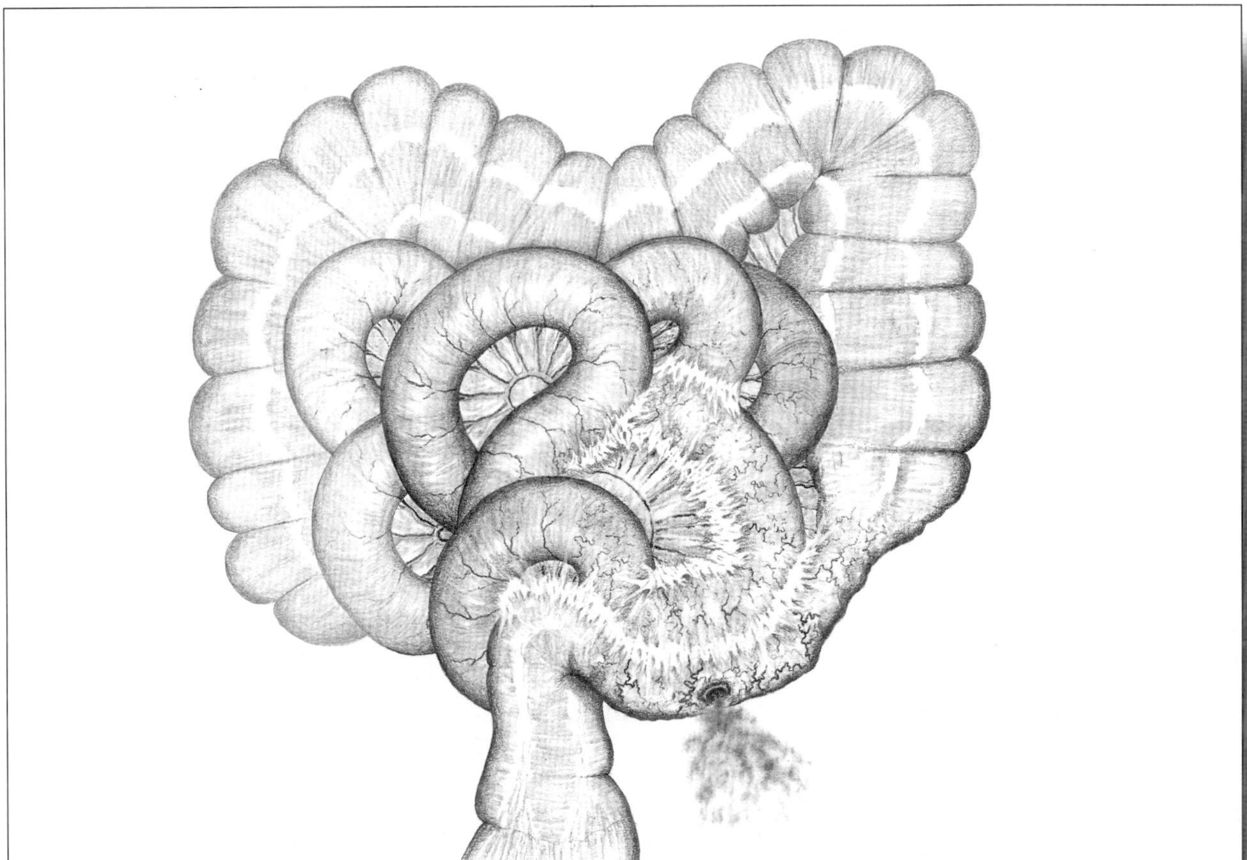

CASE

100 Radiation Rectovaginal Fistula

Female, 30 Years

History

In 1974, the patient, aged 28 years, was diagnosed with chorionic carcinoma. Local spread had formed a large pelvic mass and lung metastases were present. The latter disappeared after treatment with methotrexate. Laparotomy was performed in August 1974 when extensive pelvic spread was found beyond surgical excision. This pelvic disease was successfully treated with external beam radiotherapy (58.6 Gy) and actinomycin D. Eighteen months after completing this treatment, the patient was referred for the surgical management of a stricture (6 mm in diameter) of the rectum and a rectovaginal fistula discharging into the posterior fornix. Investigations revealed no evidence of recurrent tumor. The skin of the perineum showed evidence of tissue reaction to radiotherapy (Figure 100.1).

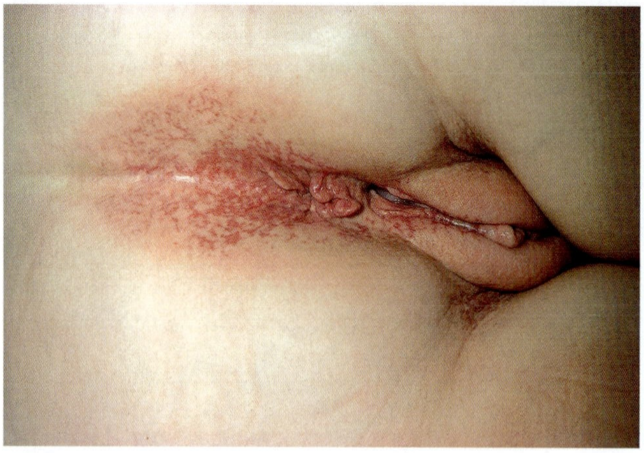

Figure 100.1: The perineum shows permanent telangiectasia due to radiotherapy.

Operation (9.7.76)

Laparotomy–loop ileostomy. The rectovaginal fistula subsequently appeared to heal.

Operation (10.18.77)

Laparotomy revealed no evidence of recurrent tumor. There was dense pelvic fibrosis, particularly in the rectovaginal septum. The bowel was resected from proximal sigmoid to mid rectum. After mucosectomy of the rectum and anal canal, the colon was "sleeved" within the rectum and a coloanal anastomosis performed (Soavé operation).

Pathology

The site of the rectovaginal fistula was not identified. There were 2 rectal strictures present. The rectal mucosa was pale and atrophic, with telangiectases prominent on its surface. The rectal wall was thickened due to fibrosis. Histologically, there was mucosal ulceration, chronic inflammation, and fibrosis in the submucosa and the muscle wall (Figure 100.2). There were vascular changes consistent with a radiation effect. There was no evidence of recurrent tumor.

Operation (2.7.78)

Closure of the ileostomy.

Follow-Up (2000)

The coloanal anastomosis remained well healed and supple, but bowel function was unsatisfactory with poor control of flatus, rectal discomfort, and prolonged efforts to evacuate stool. A permanent ileostomy was established 5/26/81. The patient was last assessed, 26 years after the diagnosis of chorionic carcinoma. There was no evidence of recurrent disease.

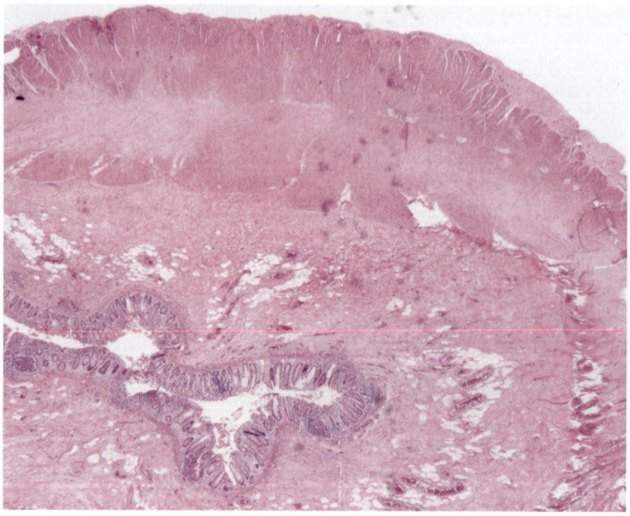

Figure 100.2: Histology of the rectum showing fibrosis in the muscularis propria and fibrous thickening of the submucosa.

Comment

Currently, the cure rate for chorionic carcinoma has been reported to be 86.4%.[1] This patient appears to have been cured but at the cost of serious postradiation morbidity. The high dose of radiotherapy administered in 1974 was 58.6 Gy in 29 fractions, but severe complications are not always dose related.[2] The operative technique in this patient avoided the difficult, if not hazardous, deep pelvic dissection. Unfortunately, the technical success was a functional failure due to poor compliance caused by the rigid rectal remnant. Parks et al, however, demonstrated in 4 patients that the Soavé procedure has a role in treating this difficult problem.[3]

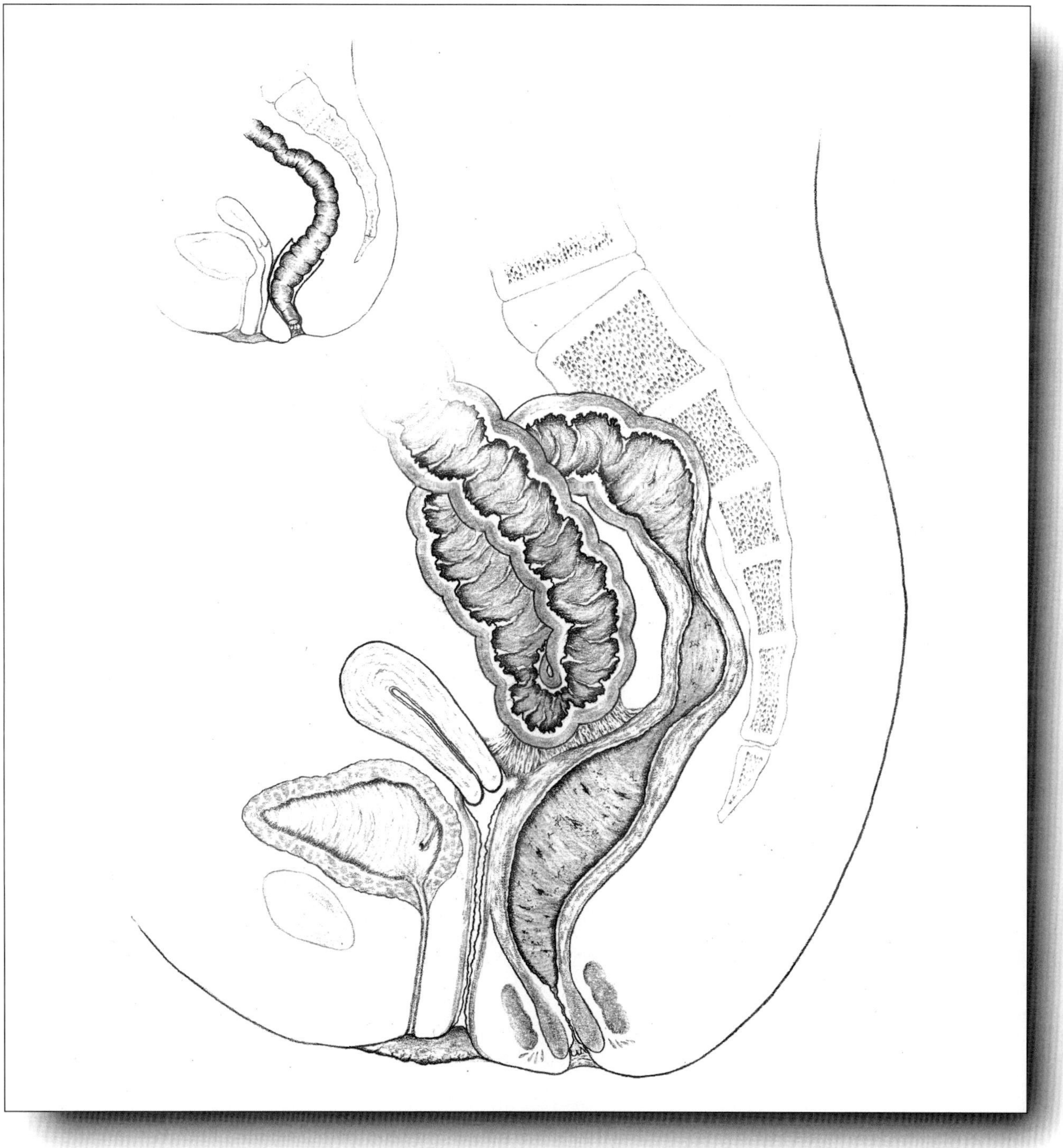

For a full-page image of this figure see the appendix.

References

CASE 1

1. Minardi AJ Jr, Zibari GB, Aultman DF, McMillan RW, McDonald JC. Small bowel tumors. *J. Am. Coll. Surg.* 1998;**186**:664–668.
2. Pan Y, Kuo H, Lai H, Chuang S, Liu C. Solitary ileal lipoma presenting with ileocolic intussusception: an unusual cause of enteritis cystica profunda. *J. Formos. Med. Assoc.* 1997;**96**:469–472.
3. Chong AK, Taylor AC, Miller AM, Desmond PV. Initial experience with capsule endoscopy at a major referral hospital. *Med. J. Aust.* 2003;**178**: 537–540.

Case 2

1. Thompson GB, van Heeden JA, Martin Jr JK, Schutt AJ, Ilstrup DM, Carney JA. Carcinoid tumors of the gastrointestinal tract: presentation, management and prognosis. *Surgery* 1985;**98**: 1054–1063.
2. Vinik AI, McLeod MK, Fig LM, Shapiro B, Lloyd RV, Cho K. Clinical features, diagnosis and localization of carcinoid tumors and their management. *Gastroenterol. Clin. North Am.* 1989;**18**:865–896.
3. Memon MA, Nelson H. Gastrointestinal carcinoid tumors. *Dis. Colon Rectum* 1997;**40**:1101–1118.

Case 3

1. Tse V, Lochhead A, Adams W, Tindal D. Concurrent colonic adenocarcinoma and two ileal carcinoids in a 72-year-old male. *Aust. N.Z. J. Surg.* 1997;**67**:739–741.
2. Thompson GB, van Heerden JA, Martin JK Jr., Schutt AJ, Ilstrup DM, Carney JA. Carcinoid tumors of the gastrointestinal tract: presentation, management, and prognosis. Surgery 1985;**98**: 1054–1063.
3. Chong AK, Taylor AC, Miller AM, Desmond PV. Initial experience with capsule endoscopy at a major referral hospital. *Med. J. Aust.* 2003;**178**: 537–540.

Case 4

1. Rangiah DS, Co M, Richardson M, Tompsett E, Crawford M. Small bowel tumors: a 10 year experience in four Sydney teaching hospitals. *Aust. N.Z. J. Surg.* 2004;**74**:788–792.
2. Huilgol RL, Young CJ, Solomon MJ. The GIST of it: case reports of a gastrointestinal stromal tumor and a leiomyoma of the anorectum. *Aust. N.Z. J. Surg.* 2003;**73**:167–169.
3. Skandalakis J. Smooth muscle tumors of the gastrointestinal tract. Introduction. *World J. Surg.* 2000;**24**:389–390.
4. Wolber RA, Scudamore CH. The gastrointestinal tract. In: Banks PM, Kraybill WG, eds. *Pathology for the Surgeon.* Philadelphia: Saunders, 1996:176.
5. Clary BDE, Matteo R, Lewis J. Gastrointestinal stromal tumors and leiomyosarcomas of the abdomen and retro peritoneum: a clinical comparison. *Ann. Surg. Oncol.* 2001;**8**:290–299.

Case 5

1. Hutchins RR, Bani Hani A, Kojodjojo P, Ho R, Snooks SJ. Adenocarcinoma of the small bowel. *Aust. N.Z. J. Surg.* 2001;**71**:428–437.
2. Kusumoto H, Takahashi I, Yoshida M, Maehara Y, Watanabe A, Oshiro T. Primary malignant tumors of the small intestine: analysis of 40 Japanese patients. *J. Surg. Oncol.* 1992;**50**:139–143.
3. Howe JR, Karnell LH, Menck HR, Scott-Conner C. Adenocarcinoma of the small bowel. Rev. Nat. Cancer Data Base 1985–1995. *Cancer* 1999;**86**:2693–2706.

Case 6

1. Walfish J, Frankel A. Chronic pseudo-obstruction secondary to side-to-side intestinal anastomosis. *Arch. Surg.* 1979;**114**:1075–1078.
2. Whitaker Jr WG, Shepard D. Late complications of side-to-side intestinal anastomosis: case reports. *Ann. Surg.* 1965;**161**:824–831.
3. Frank P, Batzenschlager A, Philippe E. Blind-pouch syndrome after side-to-side intestinal anastomosis. *Chirurgie.* 1990;**116**:586–596.
4. Clawson DK. Side-to-side intestinal anastomosis complicated by ulceration, dilatation, and anemia: a physiologically unsound procedure. Review of the literature and presentation of a case. *Surgery* 1953;**34**:254–257.

Case 7

1. Black BM, McEachern CG. Redundant blind segments of intestine following side-to-side

anastomosis with division of the bowel. *Surg. Gynecol. Obstet.* 1948;**86**:177–182.

2. Bucknall TE, Wastell C. Ileo-colic blind loop following side-to-side anastomosis. *J. R. Soc. Med.* 1980;**73**:882–884.
3. Frank P, Batzenschlager A, Phillippe E. Blind-pouch syndrome after side-to-side intestinal anastomosis. *Chirurgie*. 1990:**116**:586–596.

Case 9

1. Kahn M, Friedman IH. Mucocele of the appendix: diagnosis and surgical management. *Dis. Colon Rectum* 1979;**22**:267–269.
2. Woodruff R, McDonald JR. Benign and malignant cystic tumors of the appendix. *Surg. Gynecol. Obstet.* 1940;**71**:750–755.
3. Ponsky JL. An endoscopic view of mucocele of the appendix. *Gastroint. End.* 1976;**23**:42–43.

Case 10

1. Iswariah H, Metcalfe M, Lituri D, Maddern GJ. Mucinous cystadenoma of the appendix. *Anz. J. Surg.* 2004;**74**:918–919.
2. Khan SL, Novell JR. An unusual pelvic mass. *J. Royal Soc. Med.* 2001;**94**:353–354.
3. Rutledge RH. Primary appendiceal malignancies. In: Morris PJ, Malt RA, eds. *Oxford Textbook of Surgery* Vol 1, Oxford: Oxford University Press, 1994:1118.
4. Ronnett BM, Zahn CM, Kurman RJ, Kass ME, Sugarbaker PH, Shmookler BM. Disseminated peritoneal adenomucinosis and peritoneal mucinous carcinomatosis. A clinicopathologic analysis of 109 cases with emphasis on distinguishing pathologic features, site of origin, prognosis and relationship to "pseudomyxoma peritonei." *Am. J. Surg. Pathol.* 1995;**19**:1390–1408.

Case 11

1. Nitecki SS, Wolff BG, Schlinkert R, Sarr MG. The natural history of surgically treated primary adenocarcinoma of the appendix. *Ann. Surg.* 1994;**219**:51–57.
2. Hiromichi I, Osteen RT, Bleday R, Zinner MJ, Ashley SW, Whang EE. Appendiceal adenocarcinoma: long term outcomes after surgical therapy. *Dis. Colon Rectum* 2004;**47**:474–480.

Case 12

1. Fielding LP, Arsenault PA, Chapuis PH, Dent O, Gathright B, Hardcastle JD, Hermanek P, Jass JR, Newland RC. Clinicopathological staging for colorectal cancer: an international documentation system (IDS) and an international comprehensive anatomical terminology (ICAT). *J. Gastroenterol. Hepatol.* 1991;**6**:325–344.
2. Morson BC, Dawson IMP, Day DW, Jass JR, Price AB, Williams GT. Benign epethelial tumours and polyps. In: Morson BC, Dawson IMP, eds. *Morson and Dawson's Gastrointestinal Pathology*. 3rd ed. London: Blackwell Scientific Publications, 1990;Ch 29, pp. 563–596.
3. Sakamoto GD, MacKeigan JM, Senagore AJ. Transanal excision of large villous adenomas. *Dis. Colon Rectum* 1991;**34**:880–885.

Case 13

1. Galandiuk S, Fazio VW, Jagelman DG, Lavery IC, Weakley FA, Petras RE, Badhwar K, McGonagle B, Eastin K, Sutton T. Villous and tubulovillous adenomas of the colon and rectum. A retrospective review, 1964–1985. *Am. J. Surg.* 1987:**153**:41–47.
2. Nivatvongs S, Balcos EG, Schottler JL, Goldberg SM. Surgical management of large villous tumours of the rectum. *Dis. Colon Rectum* 1973;**16**: 508–514.
3. Featherstone JM, Grabham JA, Fozard JB. Per-anal excision of large rectal villous adenomas. *Dis. Colon Rectum* 2004;**47**:86–89.
4. Cripps WH. *Cancer of the Rectum*. London: Churchill, 1880.
5. Whitlow CB, Beck DE, Gathright JB. Surgical excision of large rectal villous adenomas. *Surg. Oncol. Clin. North Am.* 1996;**5**:723–734.

Case 15

1. Oliver GC, Vachon D, Eisenstat TE, Rubin RJ, Salvati EP. Delorme's procedure for complete rectal prolapse in severely debilitated patients. An analysis of 41 cases. *Dis. Colon Rectum* 1994;**37**: 461–467.
2. Tobin SA, Scott IH. Delorme operation for rectal prolapse. *Br. J. Surg.* 1994; **81**:1681–1684.

Case 16

1. McColl I, Bussey HJR, Veale AMO, Morson BC. Juvenile polyposis coli. *Proc. R. Soc. Med.* 1964;**57:** 896–897.
2. Smilow PC, Pryor CA, Swinton NW. Juvenile polyposis coli. *Dis. Colon Rectum* 1966;**9**:248–254.
3. Howe JR, Mitros FA, Summers RW. The risk of gastrointestinal carcinoma in familial juvenile polyposis. *Ann. Surg. Oncol.* 1998;**5**:751–756.

Case 17

1. Platell C, Levitt S. Juvenile polyposis: a premalignant condition? *Anz. J. Surg.* 1990;**60**:481–482.

2. Reed K, Vose PC. Diffuse juvenile polyposis of colon: a premalignant condition? *Dis. Colon Rectum* 1981:**24**:205–210.

3. Jass JR, Williams CB, Bussey HJR, Morson BC. Juvenile polyposis—a precancerous condition. *Histopathology* 1988;**13**:619–630.

4. Desai DC, Neale KF, Talbot IC, Hodgson SV, Phillips RKS. Juvenile polyposis. *Br. J. Surg.* 1995;**82**:14–17.

5. Howe JR, Ringold JC, Summers RW, Mitros FA, Nishimura DY, Stone EM. A gene for familial juvenile polyposis maps to chromosome 18q21.1. *Am. J. Hum. Genet.* 1998;**62**:1129–1136.

6. Oncel M, Church JM, Remzi FH, Fazio VW. Colonic surgery in patients with juvenile polyposis syndrome: a case series. *Dis. Colon Rectum* 2005;**48**:49–56.

Case 18

1. McGarrity TJ, Kulin HE, Zaino RJ. Peutz-Jeghers syndrome. *Am. J. Gastroenterol.* 2000;**95**:596–604.

2. Spigelman AD, Murday V, Phillips RKS. Cancer and the Peutz-Jeghers syndrome. *Gut.* 1989;**30**: 1588–1590.

3. Oncel M, Remzi FH, Church JM, Connor JT, Fazio VW. Benefits of "clean sweep" in Peutz-Jeghers patients. *Colorectal Dis.* 2004;**6**:332–335.

4. Parsi MA, Burke CA. Utility of capsule endoscopy in Peutz-Jeghers syndrome. *Gastrointest. Endosc. Clin. N. Am.* 2004:**14**:159–167.

5. Schulmann K, Hollerbach S, Kraus K, Willert J, Vogel T, Moslein G, Pox C, Reiser M, Reinacher-Schick A, Schmiegel W. Feasibility and diagnostic utility of video capsule endoscopy for the detection of small bowel polyps in patients with hereditary polyposis syndromes. *Am. J. Gastroenterol.* 2005: **100**:27–37.

6. von Herbay A, Arens N, Friedl W, Vogt-Moykopf I, Kayser K, Muller KM, Back W. Bronchioloalveolar carcinoma: a new cancer in Peutz–Jeghers syndrome. *Lung Cancer* 2005;**47**:283–288.

Case 19

1. Keighley MRB, Williams NS. Intestinal fistulas. *Surgery of the Anus, Rectum and Colon.* London:WB Saunders, 1993;Ch 63, pp. 2013–2102.

2. Kropilak M, Jagelman DG, Fazio VW, Lavery IC, McGannon E. Brain tumors in familial adenomatous polyposis. *Dis. Colon Rectum* 1989;**32**: 778–782.

Case 20

1. Bussey HJ, Eyers AA, Ritchie SM, Thomson JP. The rectum in adenomatous polyposis: the St Mark's policy. *Br. J. Surg.*1985;**72**:S29–S31.

2. Church J, Burke C, McGannon E, Pastean O, Clark B. Risk of rectal cancer in patients after colectomy and ileorectal anastomosis for familial adenomatous polyposis. *Dis. Colon Rectum* 2003;**46**: 1175–1181.

3. De Cosse JJ, Bülow S, Neale K, Järvinen H, Alms T, Hultcrantz R, Moesgaard F, Costello C. Rectal risk in patients treated for familial adenomatous polyposis. *Br. J. Surg.* 1992;**79**:1372–1375.

4. Bess MA, Adson MA, Elveback LR, Moertel CG. Rectal cancer following colectomy for polyposis. *Arch. Surg.* 1980;**115**:460–467.

Case 21

1. Kunakemakon P, Ontai G, Balin H. Pelvic inflammatory pseudotumor: a case report *Am. J. Obstet. Gynecol.* 1976;**126**:286–287.

2. Ramtrez JM, Ortego J, Deus J, Bustamante E, Lozano R, Dominguez M. Lipomatous polyposis of the colon. *Br. J. Surg.* 1993;**80**:349–350.

3. Swain VAJ, Young WF, Pringle EM. Hypertrophy of the appendices epiploicae and lipomatous polyposis of the colon. *Gut* 1969;**10**:587–589.

4. Catania G, Petralia GA, Migliore M, Cardi F. Diffuse colonic lipomatosis with giant hypertrophy of the epiploic appendices and diverticulosis of the colon. *Dis. Colon Rectum* 1995;**38**: 769–775.

5. Brouland J-Ph, Poupard B, Nemeth J, Valleur P. Lipomatous polyposis of the colon with multiple lipomas of peritoneal folds and giant diverticulosis. *Dis. Colon Rectum* 2000;**43**:1767–1769.

Case 22

1. Schnyder P, Moss AA, Thoen RF. A double-blind study of radiologic accuracy in diverticulitis, diverticulosis and carcinoma of the sigmoid colon. *J. Clin. Gastroenterol.* 1979;**1**:55–66.

Case 23

1. Thompson GB, van Heerden JA, Martin JK Jr., Schutt AJ, Ilstrup DM, Carney JA. Carcinoid tumors of the gastrointestinal tract: presentation, management, and prognosis. *Surgery* 1985;**98**: 1054–1063.

2. Memon MA, Nelson H. Gastrointestinal carcinoid tumors. *Dis. Colon Rectum* 1997;**40:**1101–1118.

3. Lotlikar U, Fogler R, Novetsky AD, Yoon NY. Concurrent colonic carcinoma and small bowel

carcinoid tumor: Case reports and review of the literature. *Dis. Colon Rectum* 1982;**25:**375–382.

Case 24

1. Killingback M, Barron PE, Dent OF. Elective surgery for diverticular disease: an audit of surgical pathology and treatment. *ANZ J. Surg.* 2004;**74**: 530–536.

Case 25

1. Sasson L. Metastatic neoplasm of esophagus simulating primary carcinoma. *JAMA* 1960;**174**: 2075–2076.
2. Segalin A, Bonavina L, Ruol A, Boccasanta P, Salamina G, Peracchia A. Secondary esophageal tumors: treatment and outcome in 115 consecutive patients. *Dis. Esoph.* 1994;**7**:118–122.

Case 28

1. Okuno M, Ikehara T, Nagayama M, Kato Y, Umeyama K. Mucinous colorectal carcinoma: clinical pathology and prognosis. *Ann. Surg.* 1988;**54**:681–685.
2. Mayer R, Wong WD, Rothenberger DA, Goldberg SM, Madoff RD. Colorectal cancer in inflammatory bowel disease. A continuing problem. *Dis. Colon Rectum* 1999;**42**:343–347.
3. Umpleby HC, Ranson DL, Williamson RCN. Peculiarities of mucinous colorectal carcinoma. *Br. J. Surg.* 1985;**72**:715–718.
4. Sugarbaker PH, Kern K, Lack E. Malignant pseudomyxoma peritonei of colonic origin. Natural history and presentation of a curative approach to treatment. *Dis. Colon Rectum* 1987;**30**:772–779.
5. Ronnett BM, Zahn CM, Kurman RJ, Kass ME, Sugarbaker PH, Shmookler BM. Disseminated peritoneal adenomucinosis and peritoneal mucinous carcinomatosis. A clinicopathologic analysis of 109 cases with emphasis on distinguishing pathologic features, site of origin, prognosis and relationship to "pseudomyxoma peritonei." *Am. J. Surg. Pathol.* 1995;**19**:1390–1408.

Case 29

1. Shirouzu K, Isomoto H, Morodomi T, Ogata Y, Akagi Y, Kakegawat T. Primary linitis plastica carcinoma of the colon and rectum. *Cancer* 1994;**74**:1863–1868.

Case 30

1. Nissan A, Guillem JG, Paty PB, Wong WD, Cohen AM. Signet-ring cell carcinoma of the colon and rectum. *Dis. Colon Rectum* 1999;**42**:1176–1180.
2. Nakahara H, Ishikawa T, Itabashi M, Hirota T. Diffusely infiltrating primary colorectal carcinoma of linitis plastica and lymphangiosis types. *Cancer* 1992;**69**:901–906.
3. Rao TR, Hambrick E, Abcarian H, Salgia K, Recant WM. Colorectal linitis plastica. *Dis. Colon Rectum* 1982;**25**:239–244.
4. Ooi BS, HoYH, Eu KW, Seow-Choen F. Primary colorectal signet-ring carcinoma in Singapore. *ANZ J. Surg.* 2001;**71**:703–706.

Case 32

1. Dha DK, Yoshimura H, Kinukawa N, Maruyama R, Tachibana M, Kohno H, Kubota H, Nagasue N. Metastatic lymph node size and colorectal cancer prognosis. *J. Am. Coll. Surg.* 2005;**200**:20–28.

Case 34

1. Abulafi AM, Williams NS. Local recurrence of colorectal cancer: the problems, mechanisms, management and adjuvant therapy. *Br. J. Surg.* 1994;**81**:7–19.
2. Phillips RK, Hittinger R, Blesovsky L, Fry JS, Fielding LP. Local recurrence following "curative" surgery for large bowel cancer: I. The overall picture. *Br. J. Surg.* 1984;**71**:12–16.
3. Harris GJ, Church JM, Senagore AJ, Lavery IC, Hull TL, Strong SA, Fazio VW. Factors affecting local recurrence of colonic adenocarcinoma. *Dis. Colon Rectum* 2002;**45**:1029–1034.
4. Read TE, Mutch MG, Chang BW, McNevin MS, Fleshman JW, Birnbaum EH, Fry RD, Caushaj PF, Kodner IJ. *J. Am. Coll. Surg.* 2002;**195**:33–40.
5. Rieger N, Tjandra J, Solomon M. Endoanal and endorectal ultrasound: applications in colorectal surgery. *ANZ J. Surg.* 2004;**74**:671–675.
6. Robinson P, Carrington BM, Swindell R, Shanks JH, O'Dwyer ST. Recurrent or residual pelvic bowel cancer: accuracy of MRI local extent before salvage surgery. *Clin. Radiol.* 2002;**57**:514–522.
7. Caplin S, Cerottini JP, Bosman FT, Constanda MT, Givel JC. For patients with Dukes' B (TNM Stage II) colorectal carcinoma, examination of six or fewer lymph nodes is related to poor prognosis. *Cancer* 1998;**83**:666–672.
8. Burdy G, Panis Y, Alves A, Nemeth J, Lavergne-Slove A. Identifying patients with T3–T4 node-negative colon cancer at high risk of recurrence. *Dis. Colon Rectum* 2001;**44**:1682–1688.
9. Goldberg RM, Fleming TR, Tangen CM, Moertel CG, MacDonald JS, Haller DG, Laurie JA. Surgery for recurrent colon cancer: strategies for identifying resectable recurrence and success rates after

resection. Eastern Cooperative Oncology, the North Central Cancer Treatment Group, and the Southwest Oncology Group. *Ann. Intern. Med.* 1998;**129**:27–35.

Case 35

1. Lennard-Jones JE, Melville DM, Morson BC, Ritchie JK, Williams CB. Precancer and cancer in extensive ulcerative colitis: findings among 401 patients over 22 years. *Gut* 1990;**31**:800–806.
2. Mayer R, Wong WD, Rothenberger DA, Goldberg SM, Madoff RD. Colorectal cancer in inflammatory bowel disease. A continuing problem. *Dis. Colon Rectum* 1999;**42**:343–347.
3. Landmann DD, Fazio VW, Lavery IC, Weakley FL, Jagelman DG. En Bloc resection for contiguous upper abdominal invasion by adenocarcinoma of the colon. *Dis. Colon Rectum* 1989;**32**:669–672.
4. Lehnert T, Methner M, Pollok A, Schaible A, Hinz U, Herfath C. Multivisceral resection for locally advanced primary colon and rectal cancer: an analysis of prognostic factors in 201 patients. *Ann. Surg.* 2002;**235**:217–225.
5. Nakafusa Y, Tanaka T, Tanaka M, Kitajima Y, Sato S, Miyazaki K. Comparison of multivisceral resection and standard operation for locally advanced colorectal cancer: analysis of prognostic factors for short-term and long-term outcome. *Dis. Colon Rectum* 2004;**47**:2055–2062.
6. Hunter JA, Ryan JA, Schultz P. En bloc resection of colon cancer adherent to other organs. *Am. J. Surg.* 1987;**145**:67–71.
7. Gall FP, Tonak J, Altendorf A. Multivisceral resections in colorectal cancer. *Dis. Colon Rectum* 1987;**30**:337–341.
8. Johnson WR, McDermott FT, Hughes ESR, Pihl EA, Milne BJ, Price AB. Carcinoma of the colon and rectum in inflammatory disease of the intestine. *Surg. Gynecol Obstet.* 1988;**156**:193–197.
9. Walfisch S, Stern H. Use of thoracoabdominal incision for cancer of the splenic flexure in the obese patient. *Dis. Colon Rectum* 1989;**32**:169–170.

Case 36

1. Morson BC. The muscle abnormality in diverticular disease of the colon. *Proc. R. Soc. Med.* 1963a;**56**:798–800.
2. Killingback M, Barron PE, Dent OF. Elective surgery for diverticular disease: an audit of surgical pathology and treatment. *ANZ J. Surg.* 2004;**74**:530–536.
3. Le Moine MC, Falore JM, Varcher C, Navarro F, Picot MC, Domergue J. Factors and consequences of conversion in laparoscopic sigmoidectomy for diverticular disease. *Br. J. Surg.* 2003;**90**:232–236.

Case 37

1. Kelly JK. Polypoid prolapsing mucosal folds in diverticular disease. *Am. J. Surg. Pathology.* 1991; **15**:871–878.
2. Gore S, Shepherd NA, Wilkinson SP. Endoscopic crescentic fold disease of the sigmoid colon: the clinical and histopathological spectrum of a distinct endoscopic appearance. *Int. J. Colorectal Dis.* 1992;**7**:76–81.

Case 38

1. Gooszen AW, Tollenaar RA, Geelkerken RH, Smeets HJ, Bemelman WA, van Schaardenburgh P, Gooszen HG. Prospective study of primary anastomosis following sigmoid resection for suspected acute complicated diverticular disease. *Br. J. Surg.* 2001;**88**:693–697.
2. Ravo B, Metawally N, Castera P, Polansky PJ, Ger R. The importance of intraluminal anastomotic fecal contact and peritonitis in colonic anastomotic leakages. An experimental study. *Dis. Colon Rectum* 1988;**31**:868–871.
3. Zorcolo L, Covotta L, Carlomagno N, Bartolo DCC. Safety of primary anastomosis in emergency colorectal surgery. *Colorectal Dis* 2003;**5**:262–269.
4. Salem L, Flum D. Primary anastomosis or Hartmann's procedure for patients with diverticular peritonitis? A systemic review. *Dis. Colon Rectum* 2004;**47**:1953–1964.

Case 39

1. Killingback M, Barron PE, Dent OF. Elective surgery for diverticular disease: an audit of surgical pathology and treatment. *Aust. N. Z. J. Surg.* 2004;**74**:530–536.
2. Pheils MT, Duraiappah B, Newland RC. Chronic phlegmonous diverticulitis. *Aust. N. Z. J. Surg.* 1973;**42**:337–341.
3. Whelan RL, Umana JP. Colon cancer versus diverticulitis. In: Welch JP, Cohen JL, Sardella WV, Vignati PV, eds. *Diverticular Disease: Management of the Difficult Case.* Baltimore: Williams and Wilkins, 1998;Ch 4, pp. 55–66.

Case 41

1. Fazio VW, Church JM, Jagelman DG, Weakley FL, Lavery IC, Tarazi R, van Hillo M. Colocutaneous fistulas complicating diverticulitis. *Dis. Colon Rectum* 1987;**30**:89–94.

2. Parks AG, Gordon PH. Perineal fistula of intra-abdominal or intrapelvic origin simulating fistula in ano:report of 7 cases. *Dis. Colon Rectum* 1976;**19**:500–506.

Case 43

1. Del Pino A, Abcarian H. Colovesical fistula. In: Welch JP, Cohen JL, Sardella WV, Vignati PV, eds. *Diverticular Disease: Management of the Difficult Surgical Case.* Baltimore:Williams and Wilkins, 1998;Ch 10, pp. 151–166.
2. Killingback M, Barron PE, Dent OF. Elective surgery for diverticular disease: an audit of surgical pathology and treatment. *ANZ J. Surg.* 2004;**74**:530–536.
3. Woods RJ. Diverticulitis and fistula. In: Fazio VW, Church JM, Delaney CP, eds. *Current Therapy in Colon and Rectal Surgery.* 2nd ed. Philadelphia: Elsevier Mosby, 2005;Ch 52, pp. 297–300.
4. Killingback M. Elective surgery for sigmoid diverticular disease. In: Fielding LP, Goldberg SM, eds. *Rob and Smiths Operative Surgery. Surgery of the Colon Rectum and Anus.* 5th ed. Oxford: Butterworth-Heinemann, 1993:369–386.

Case 45

1. Killingback M, Barron PE, Dent OF. Elective surgery for diverticular disease: an audit of surgical pathology and treatment. *ANZ J. Surg.* 2004;**74**:530–536.

Case 46

1. Heimann T, Aufses AH Jr. Giant sigmoid diverticula. *Dis. Colon Rectum* 1981;**24**:468–470.
2. Ellerbroek CJ, Lu CC. Unusual manifestations of giant colonic diverticulum. *Dis. Colon Rectum* 1984;**27**:545–547.
3. Altaf N, Geary S, Ahmed I. Giant colonic diverticulum. *J. R. Soc. Med.* 2005;**98**:169–170.
4. Choong CK, Frizelle FA, Giant colonic diverticulum. Report of 4 cases and review of the literature. *Dis. Colon Rectum* 1998;**41:**1178–1186.

Case 47

1. Choong CK, Frizelle FA. Giant colonic diverticulum. Report of 4 cases and review of the literature. *Dis. Colon Rectum* 1998;**41**:1178–1186.
2. Killingback M, Barron PE, Dent OF. Elective surgery for diverticular disease: an audit of surgical pathology and treatment. *ANZ J. Surg.* 2004;**74**:530–536.
3. Gallagher JJ, Welch JP. Giant diverticula of the sigmoid colon. *Arch. Surg.* 1979;**114**:1079–1083.

Case 49 Recommended Reading List

Morson BC, Dawson IMP, Day DW, Jass JR, Price AB, Williams GT. Inflammatory disorders. In: Morson BC, Dawson IMP, eds. *Morson and Dawson's Gastro Intestinal Pathology.* 3rd ed. London: Blackwell Scientific Publications, 1990;Ch 37, pp. 477–549.

Keighley MRB, Williams NS. Crohn's disease: pathology, diagnosis and differential diagnosis. *Surgery of the Anus, Rectum, and Colon.* London:WB Saunders, 1993;Ch 50, pp. 1631–1659.

Kleer CG, Appelman HD. Surgical pathology of Crohn's disease. *Surg. Clin. North Am.* 2001;**81**: 13–30.

Case 51

1. Yamamoto T, Allan RN, Keighley MR. An audit of gastroduodenal Crohn's disease: clinicopathologic features and management. *Scand. Gastroenterol.* 1999;**34**:1019–1024.

Case 52

1. Keighley MRB, Williams NS. Surgical treatment of small bowel Crohn's disease. *Surgery of the Anus, Rectum, and Colon.* 1st ed. London: W.B. Saunders, 1993;Ch 55, pp. 1710–1756.
2. Simonowitz DA, Rusch VW, Stevenson JK. Natural history of incidental appendectomy in patients with Crohn's disease who required subsequent bowel resection. *Am. J. Surg.* 1982;**143**:171–173.
3. Nakano H, Miyachi I, Kitagawa Y, Saito H, Yamauchi M, Horiguchi Y, Nakajima S, Itoh M, Miyagawa S, Iwase K, et al. Crohn's disease associated with giant inflammatory polyposis. *Endoscopy.* 1987;**9**:246–248.

Case 55

1. Morson BC, Dawson IMP, Day DW, Jass JR, Price AB, Williams GT. Inflammatory disorders. In: Morson BC, Dawson IMP, eds. *Morson and Dawson's Gastrointestinal Pathology.* 3rd ed. London:Blackwell Scientific Publications, 1990; Ch 22, pp. 240–302.
2. Keighley MRB, Williams NS. Crohn's disease: pathology, dignosis and differential diagnosis. *Surgery of the Anus, Rectum and Colon.* London: WB Saunders, 1993;Ch 50, pp. 1631–1659.

Case 56

1. Dietz DW, Lauretti S, Strong SA, Hull TL, Church J, Remi FH, Lavery IC, Fazio VW. Safety and long term efficacy of strictureplasty in 314 patients with obstructing small bowel Crohn's disease. *J. Am. Coll. Surg.* 2001;**192**:330–337.

2. Strong SA. Crohn's disease of the small bowel. In: Fazio VW, Church JM, Delaney CP, eds. *Current Therapy in Colon and Rectal Surgery*. 2nd ed. Philadelpia: Elsevier Mosby, 2004;Ch 77, pp. 459–464.

Case 57

1. van Hogezand RA, Bemelman WA. Management of recurrent Crohn's disease. *Neth. J. Med.* 1998;**53**:S32–S38.
2. Fazio VW, Marchetti F, Church M, Goldblum JR, Lavery IC, Hull TL, Milsom JW, Strong SA, Oakley JR, Secic M. Effect of resection margins on the recurrence of Crohn's disease in the small bowel. A randomized controlled trial. *Ann. Surg.* 1996; **224**:563–573.
3. Borley NR, Mortensen NJ, Chaudry MA, Mohammed S, Warren BF, George BD, Clark T, Jewell DP, Kettlewell MG. Recurrence after abdominal surgery for Crohn's disease: relationship to disease site and surgical procedure. *Dis. Colon Rectum* 2002;**45**:377–383.
4. Poritz LS, Gagliano GA, McLeod RS, MacRae H, Cohen Z. Surgical management of entero and colocutaneous fistulae in Crohn's disease: 17 year's experience. *Int. J. Colorectal Dis.* 2004:**19**: 481–486.

Case 58

1. Fisher J, Mantz F, Calkins WG. Colonic perforation in Crohn's disease. *Gastroenterol.* 1976;**71**: 385–388.
2. Connell WR, Sheffield JP, Kamm MA, Ritchie KJ, Hawley PR, Lennard-Jones JE. Lower gastrointestinal malignancy in Crohn's disease. *Gut* 1994;**35**:347–352.
3. Gillen CD, Andrews HA, Prior P, Allan RN. Crohn's disease and colorectal cancer. *Gut* 1994;**35**:651–655.
4. Ribeiro MB, Greenstein AJ, Sachar DB, Barth J, Balasubramanian S, Harpaz N, Heimann TM, Aufses AH Jr. Colorectal adenocarcinoma in Crohn's disease. *Ann. Surg.* 1996;**223**:186–193.

Case 59

1. Gan IS, Beck PL. A new look at toxic megacolon: an update and review of incidence, etiology, pathogenesis and management. *Am. J. Gastroenterol.* 2003;**98**:2363–2371.
2. Turnbull RB Jr., Hawk WA, Weakley FL. Surgical treatment of toxic megacolon. Ileostomy and colostomy to prepare patients for colectomy. *Am. J. Surg.* 1971;**122**:325–331.
3. Khoo REH, Rothenberger DA, Wong WD, Buls JG, Najarian JS. Tube decompression of the dilated colon. *Am. J. Surg.* 1988;**156**:214–216.
4. Remzi FH, Oncel M, Hull TL, Strong SA, Lavery IC, Fazio VW. Current indications for blow-hole colostomy:ileostomy procedure. A single center experience. *Int. J. Colorectal Dis.* 2003;**18**:361–364.

Case 60

1. Goligher JC. Ulcerative colitis. *Surgery of the Anus, Rectum and Colon.* 4th ed. London: Baillière Tindall, 1980;Ch 21, pp. 689–826.
2. Joffe N. Localised giant pseudopolyps secondary to ulcerative colitis or granulomatous colitis. *Clin. Radiol.* 1977;28:609–616,
3. Fenoglio-Preiser CM, Noffsinger AE, Stemmermann GN, Lantz PE, Listrom MB, Rilke FO. Inflammatory bowel disease. *Gastrointestinal Pathology. An Atlas and Text.* 2nd ed. Philadelphia: Lipincott-Raven, 1999;Ch 16, pp. 631–716.
4. Dukes CE. The surgical pathology of ulcerative colitis. *Ann. Roy. Coll. Surg.* 1954;14:389–400.
5. Keighley MRB, Williams NS. Pathology and diagnosis of ulcerative colitis. *Surgery of the anus, rectum and colon.* London: WB Saunders, 1993;Ch 39, pp. 1274–1303.

Case 61

1. Johnson WR, Hughes ESR, McDermott FT, Katrivessis H. The outcome of patients with ulcerative colitis managed by subtotal colectomy. *Surg. Gynecol. Obstet.*1986:**162**:421–425.

Case 62

1. Mayer R, Wong WD, Rothenberger DA, Goldberg SM, Madoff RD. Colorectal cancer in inflammatory bowel disease. A continuing problem. *Dis. Colon Rectum* 1999;**42**:343–347.
2. Lennard-Jones JE, Melville DM, Morson BC, Ritchie JK, Williams CB. Precancer and cancer in extensive ulceration colitis: findings among 401 patients over 22 years. *Gut* 1990;**31**:800–806.
3. Morson BC, Pang LSC. Rectal biopsy as an aid to cancer control in ulcerative colitis. *Gut* 1967;**8**:423–434.
4. Connell W. Endoscopic surveillance minimizes the risk of cancer. *Am. J. Gastroenterol* 2004;**99**: 1631–1633.

Case 63

1. Payne JE, Killingback M. Carcinoma complicated by colitis. *Med. J. Aust.* 1972;1:985–987.

2. Feldman PS. Ulcerative disease of the colon proximal to partially obstructive lesions: report of two cases and review of the literature. *Dis. Colon Rectum* 1975:**18**:601–612.

3. Toner M, Condell D, Obriain DS. Obstructive colitis. Ulceroinflammatory lesions occurring proximal to colonic obstruction. *Am. J. Surg. Pathol.* 1990;**14**:719–728.

4. Morson BC, Dawson IMP, Day DW, Jass JR, Price AB, Williams GT. Vascular disorders. In: Morson BC, Dawson, IMP. Morson *and Dawson's Gastrointestinal Pathology*. 3rd ed. London: Blackwell Scientific Publications, 1993;Ch 38, pp. 550–562.

5. Boley SJ, Agrawal G, Warren A. Pathophysiologic effects of bowel distention on intestinal blood flow. *Am. J. Surg.* 1969;**117**:228–234.

6. Teasdale C, Mortensen NJ. Acute necrotising colitis and obstruction. *Br. J. Surg.* 1983;**70**:44–47.

Case 64

1. Bradbury AW, Barrett S. Surgical aspects of clostridium difficile colitis. *Brit. J. Surg.* 1997;**84:**150–159.

2. Longo WE, Mazuski JE, Virgo KS, Lee P, Bahadursingh AN, Johnson FE. Outcome after colectomy for clostridium difficile colitis. *Dis. Colon Rectum* 2004;**47**:1620–1626.

3. Gan SI, Beck PL. A new look at toxic megacolon: an update and review of incidence, megacolon eitiology, pathogenesis and management. *Am. J. Gastroenterol.* 2003;**98**:2363–2371.

4. Prendergast TM, Marini CP, D'Angelo AJ, Sher ME, Cohen JR. Surgical patients with pseudomembranous colitis: factors affecting prognosis. *Surgery* 1994;**116**:768–774.

5. Lipsett PA, Samantaray DK, Tam ML, Bartlett JG, Lillemoe KD. Pseudomembranous colitis: a surgical disease? *Surgery* 1994;**116**:491–496.

Case 65

1. Findlay JA, Addison NV, Stevenson BK, Mirza ZA. Tuberculosis of the gastrointestinal tract in Bradford 1967–1977. *J. R. Soc. Med.* 1979;**72**:587–590.

2. Keighley MRB, Williams NS. Tropical coloproctology. *Surgery of the Anus, Rectum and Colon.* London: WB Saunders Company Ltd., 1993;Ch 68, pp. 2223–2261.

3. Crohn BB, Ginzberg L, Oppenheimer GD. Regional ileitis. A pathologic and clinical entity. *J. Am. Med. Assoc.* 1932;**99**:1323–1329.

Case 66

1. Ioachim HL, Ratech H. Burkitt lymphoma. *Ioachim's Lymph Node Pathology*. 3rd ed., Philadelphia: Lippincott, Williams, and Wilkins, 2002;Ch 69, pp. 428–434.

Case 67

1. Morson BC, Dawson IMP, Day DW, Jass JR, Price AB, Williams GT. Non-epithelial tumours. In: Morson BC, Dawson IMP, eds. *Morson and Dawson's Gastrointestinal Pathology*. 3rd ed. London: Blackwell Scientific Publications, 1990;Ch 27, pp. 372–387.

2. Lin KM, Penney DG, Mahmoud A, Chae W, Kolachalam RB, Young SC. Advantage of surgery and adjuvant chemotherapy in the treatment of primary gastrointestinal lymphoma. *J. Surg. Oncol.* 1997;**64**:237–241.

Case 68

1. Bargen JA. Chronic ulcerative colitis associated with malignant disease. *Arch. Surg.* 1928;**17**:561–576.

2. Baker D, Chiprut RO, Rimer D, Lewin KJ, Roseberg MZ. Colonic lymphoma in ulcerative colitis. *J. Clin. Gastroenterol.* 1985;**7**:379–386.

3. Fan CW, Changchien CR, Wang JY, Chen JS, Hsu KC, Tang R, Chiang JM. Primary colorectal lymphoma. *Dis. Colon Rectum* 2000;**43**:1277–1282.

4. Wagonfeld JB, Platz CE, Fishman FL, Sibley RK, Kirsner JB. Multicentric colonic lymphoma complicating ulcerative colitis. *Am. J. Dig. Dis.* 1977;**22**:502–508.

Case 69

1. Au E, Ang PT, Tan P, Sng I, Fong CM, Chua EJ, Ong YW. Gastrointestinal lymphoma–a review of 54 patients in Singapore. *Ann. Acad. Med. Singap.* 1997;**26**:758–761.

2. Crump M, Gospodarowicz M, Shepherd FA. Lymphoma of the gastrointestinal tract. *Semin. Oncol.* 1999;**26**:324–337.

Case 70

1. Tan GY, Chong CK, Eu KW, Tan PH. Gastrointestinal stromal tumor of the anus. *Tech. Coloproctol.* 2003;**7**:169–172.

2. Robb JA, Jones RA. Spindle cell lipoma in a perianal location. *Hum. Pathol.* 1982;**13**:1052.

3. Frick EJ Jr, Lapos L, Vargas HD. Solitary neurofibroma of the anal canal: report of two cases. *Dis. Colon Rectum* 2000;**43**:109–112.

4. Cohen MG, Greenwald ML. Garbus JE, Zager JS. Granular cell tumor—a unique neoplasm of the internal anal sphincter: report of a case. *Dis. Colon Rectum* 2000;**43**:1444–1447.

5. Bacher H, Schweiger W, Cerwenka H, Mischinger H. Use of anal endosonography in diagnosis of endometriosis of the external anal sphincter. *Dis. Colon Rectum* 1999;**42**:680–682.

6. Rieger N, Tjandra J, Solomon M. Endoanal and endorectal ultrasound: applications in colorectal surgery. *ANZ J. Surg.* 2004;**74**:671–675.

Case 71

1. Tsang WY, Chan JK, Lee KC, Fisher C, Fletcher CD. Aggressive angiomyxoma. A report of four cases occurring in men. *Am. J. Surg. Pathol.* 1992;**11**:1059–1065.
2. Wilson E. Ischiorectal tumor. *Med. J. Aust.* 1969;**2**:402–403.
3. Nyam DCNK, Pemberton JH. Large aggressive angiomyxoma of the perineum and pelvis: an alternative approach. *Dis. Colon Rectum* 1998;**41**: 514–516.

Case 72

1. Guiss RL. The implantation of cancer cells with a fistula-in-ano. *Surgery* 1954;**36**:136–139.
2. Keynes WM. Implantation from the bowel lumen in cancer of the large intestine. *Ann. Surg.* 1961;**153**:357–364.
3. Killingback M, Wilson TE, Hughes ESR. Anal metastases from carcinoma of the rectum and colon. *ANZ J. Surg.* 1965;**34**:178–187.
4. Hyman N, Kida M. Adenocarcinoma of the sigmoid colon seeding a chronic anal fistula. *Dis. Colon Rectum* 2003;**46**:835–836.
5. Kline RJ, Spencer RJ, Harrison Jr. EG. Carcinoma associated with fistula-in-ano. *Arch. Surg.* 1964;**89**:989–994.

Case 74

1. Stuart M. Proctitis cystica profunda. *Dis. Colon Rectum* 1984;**27**:153–156.
2. Nagasako K, Nakee Y, Kitao Y, Aoki G. Colitis cystica profunda: report of a case in which differentiation from rectal cancer was difficult. *Dis. Colon Rectum* 1977;**20**:618–624.
3. Valenzuela M, Martin-Ruiz JL, Alvarez-Cienfuegos E, Caballero AM, Gallego F, Carmona I, Rodriguez-Tellez M. Colitis cystica profunda: imaging diagnosis and conservative treatment: report of two cases. *Dis. Colon Rectum* 1996;**39**:587–590.

Case 75

1. Madigan MR, Morson BC. Solitary ulcer of the rectum. *Gut* 1969;**10**:871–881.
2. Keighley MRB, Williams NS. Solitary rectal ulcer syndrome. *Surgery of the Anus, Rectum and Colon*. London: WB Saunders, 1993;Ch 25, pp. 720–738.
3. Nicholls RJ, Simson JNL. Anterior posterior rectopexy in the treatment of the solitary ulcer syndrome without overt prolapse. *Br. J. Surg.* 1986;**73**:222–224.

Case 76

1. Parks AG, Gordon PH, Hardcastle JC. A classification of fistula in ano. *Br. J. Surg.* 1976;**63:**1–12.

Case 78

1. Weiss S, Goldblum J. Fibromatoses. *Enzinger and Weiss's Soft Tissue Tumors*. 4th ed. St Louis: Mosby Inc., 2001;Ch 10, pp. 309–346.
2. Church JM. Desmoid tumors. In Fazio VW, Church JM, Delaney CP, eds. Current Therapy in Colon and Rectal Surgery. 2nd ed. Philadelphia: Elsevier Mosby, 2005;Ch 61 pp. 355–358.
3. Clarke SK, Neale KF, Landgrebe JC, Phillips RK. Desmoid tumours complicating familial adenomatous polyposis. *Br. J. Surg.* 1999;**86**:1185–1189.

Case 79

1. Gagliardi G, Thompson IW, Herhsman MJ, Forbes A, Hawley PR, Talbot IC. Pneumatosis coli: a proposed pathogenesis based on study of 25 cases and review of the literature. *Int. J. Colorectal. Dis.* 1996;**11**:111–118.
2. Galandiuk S and Fazio VW. Pneumatosis cystoides intestinalis. A review of the literature. *Dis. Colon Rectum* 1986;**29**:358–363.
3. Forgacs P, Wright PH, Wyatt AP. Treatment of intestinal gas by oxygen breathing. *Lancet* 1973; **1**:579.

Case 80

1. Maurer CA, Renzulli P, Mazzucchelli L, Egger B, Seiler CA, Büchler MW. Use of accurate diagnostic criteria may increase the incidence of stercoral perforation of the colon. *Dis. Colon Rectum* 2000;**43**:991–998.
2. Serpell JW, Nicholls RJ. Stercoral perforation of the colon. *Br. J. Surg.* 1990;**77**:1325–1329.
3. Haddad R, Bursle G, Piper B. Stercoral perforation of the sigmoid colon. *ANZ J. Surg.* 2005;**75**:244–246.

Case 81

1. Marston A, Pheils MT, Thomas ML, Morson BC. Ischemic colitis. *Gut* 1966;**7**:1–15.

2. Brown AR. Non-gangrenous ischaemic colitis: a review of 17 cases. *Br. J. Surg* 1972;**59**:463–473.

3. Longo WE, Ballantyne GH, Gusberg RJ. Ischemic colitis: patterns and prognosis. *Dis. Colon Rectum* 1992;**35**:726–730.

Case 83

1. Graham WP, Goldman L. Gastrointestinal metastases from carcinoma of the breast. *Ann. Surg.* 1964;**159**:477–480.

2. Rabau MY, Alon RJ, Werbin N, Yossipov Y. Colonic metastases from lobular carcinoma of the breast. *Dis. Colon Rectum* 1988;**31**:401–402

3. Tot T. The role of cytokeratins 20 and 7 and estrogen receptor analysis in separation of metastatic lobular carcinoma of the breast and metastatic signet ring cell carcinoma of the gastrointestinal tract. *Acta Pathol. Microbiol. Scand.* 2000;**108**: 467–472.

Case 84

1. Taylor BA, Wolff BG. Colonic lipomas. *Dis. Colon Rectum* 1987;**30**:888–893.

2. Chung YFA, Ho Y-H, Nyam DCNK, Leong AFPK, Seow-Choen F. Management of colonic lipomas. *ANZ J. Surg.* 1998;**68**:133–135.

3. Church JM. Experience in the endoscopic management of large colonic polyps. *ANZ J. Surg.* 2003;**73**:988–995.

Case 85

1. Tran KTC, Kuijpers HC, Willemsen WNP, Bulten H. Surgical treatment of symptomatic rectosigmoid endometriosis. *Eur. J. Surg.* 1996;**162**: 139–141.

2. Macafee CHG, Greer HLH. Intestinal endometriosis: a report of 29 cases and a survey of the literature. *J. Obstet. Gynaecol Br. Commonw.* 1960;**67**:539–555.

3. Woods RJ, Herior AG, Chen FC. Anterior wall excision for endometriosis using circular stapler. *ANZ J. Surg.* 2003;**73**:647–648.

4. Jatan AK, Solomon MJ, Young J, Cooper M, Pathma-Nathan N. Laparoscopic management of rectal endometriosis. *Dis. Colon Rectum* 2005 Dec 8; [pub ahead of print].

Case 86

1. McCready RA, Beart RW. Adult Hirschsprung disease. Results of surgical treatment in the Mayo Clinic. *Dis. Colon Rectum* 1980;**23**:401–407.

2. Elliot MS, Todd IP. Adult Hirschsprung's disease: results of the Duhamel procedure. *Br. J. Surg.* 1985;**72**:884–885.

3. Keighley MRB, Williams NS. Adult Hirschsprung's disease, megacolon and megarectum. *Surgery of the Anus, Rectum and Colon*. London: WB Saunders, 1993;Ch 23, pp. 639–674.

4. Gordon PH. An improved technique for the Duhamel operation using the EEA stapler. *Dis. Colon Rectum* 1983;**26**:690–692.

5. Wheatley MJ, Wesley JR, Coran AG, Polley TZ Jr. Hirschsprung's disease in adolescents and adults. *Dis. Colon Rectum* 1990;**33**:622–629.

Case 87

1. Hession PR, Rawlinson J, Hall JR, Keating JP, Guyer PB. The clinical and radiological features of cholecystocolic fistulae. *Brit. J. Radiol.* 1996;**69**: 804–809.

2. Milson JW, MacKeighan JM. Gallstone/obstruction of the colon. Report of two cases and review of management. *Dis. Colon Rectum* 1985;**28**:367–370.

3. Anseline P. Colonic gallstone ileus. *Postgrad. Med. J.* 1981;**57**:62–65.

Case 88

1. Begos DG, Sandor A, Modlin IM. The diagnosis and management of adult intussusception. *Am. J. Surg.* 1997;**173**:88–94.

2. Nargoney DM, Sarr MG, McIlrath DC. Surgical management of intussusception in the adult. *Ann. Surg.* 1981;**193**:230–236.

3. Azar T, Berger DL. Adult intussusception. *Ann. Surg.* 1997;**226**:134–138.

4. Takeuchi K, Tsuzuki Y, And T, Sekihara M, Har T, Takayuki K, Kuwano H. The diagnosis and treatment of adult intussusception. *J. Clin. Gastroenterol.* 2003;**36**:18–21.

5. Tan KY, Tan SM, Tan AG, Chen CY, Chng HC, Hoe MN. Adult intussusception: experience in Singapore. *ANZ J. Surg.* 2003;**73**:1044–1047.

6. Fenoglio-Preiser CM, Noffsinger AE, Stemmermann GN, Lantz PE, Listrom MB, Rilke FO. Nonneoplastic lesions of the colon. *Gastrointestinal Pathology. An Atlas and Text.* 2nd ed. Philadelphia: Lippencott-Raven, 1999;Ch 19, pp. 763–908.

Case 89

1. Fry RD, Shemesh EI, Kodner IJ, Fleshman JW, Timmcke AE. Perforation of the rectum and sigmoid colon during barium enema examination. *Dis. Colon Rectum* 1986;**32**:759–764.

2. Rosenklint A, Buemann B, Hansen P, Baden H. Extraperitoneal perforation of the rectum during barium enema. *Scand J Gastroenterol.* 1975;**10**: 87–90.

3. Nelson RN, Abcarian H, Prasad ML. Iatrogenic perforation of the colon and rectum. *Dis. Colon Rectum* 1982;**25**:305–308.

Case 90

1. Gallo D, Tebrock C, Rivera D. Intramural cecal hematoma: an unusual complication of colonoscopy. *Gastrointest. Endosc.* 2003;**57**:254–257.

Case 91

1. Wadman M, Syk I, Elmståhl S. Survival after operation for ischaemic bowel disease. *Eur. J. Surg.* 2000;**166**:872–877.

2. Killingback M, Barron P, Dent O. Elective resection and anastomosis for colorectal cancer: a prospective audit of mortality and morbidity 1976–1998. *ANZ J. Surg.* 2002;**72**:689–698.

3. Fichera A, Cicchiello LA, Mendelson DS, Greenstein AJ, Heimann TM. Superior mesenteric vein thrombosis after colectomy for inflammatory bowel disease. A not uncommon cause of postoperative acute abdominal pain. *Dis. Colon Rectum* 2003;**46**:643–648.

Case 92

1. Killingback M, Barron P, Dent O. Elective resection and anastomosis for colorectal cancer: a prospective audit of mortality and morbidity 1976–1998. *ANZ. J. Surg.* 2002;**72**:689–698.

2. Stevenson IM, Mansfield AO, Temple JG. Abdominal apoplexy. *Br. J. Surg.* 1978;**65**:318–320.

3. Kleinsasser IJ. Abdominal apoplexy. *Am. J. Surg.* 1970;**120**:623–628.

4. Tan YM, Tan BKT, Chow PKH. Abdominal apoplexy: a potentially fatal enigma. *ANZ. J. Surg.* 2003;**73**:461–462.

Case 93

1. Kim CJ, Yeatman TJ, Coppola D, Trotti A, Williams B, Barthel JS, Dinwoodie W, Karl RC, Marcet J. Local excision of T2 and T3 rectal cancers after downstaging chemoradiation. *Ann. Surg.* 2001;**234**:352–358; discussion 358–359.

2. Bonnen M, Crane C, Vauthey JN, Skibber J, Delclos ME, Rodriguez-Bigas M, Hoff PM, Lin E, Eng C, Wong A, Janjan NA, Feig BW. Long-term results using local excision after preoperative chemoradiation among selected T3 rectal cancer patients. *Int. J. Radiat. Oncol. Biol. Phys.* 2004;**60**:1098–1105.

3. Paty PB, Nash GM, Baron P, Zakowski M, Minsky BD, Blumberg D, Nathanson DR, Guillem JG, Enker WE, Cohen AM, Wong WD. Long-term results of local excision for rectal cancer. *Ann. Surg.* 2002;**236**:522–529; discussion 529–530.

Case 95

1. Cripps WH, *The Passage of Air and Faeces from Urethra.* London: JA Churchill Ltd., 1888.

2. Hool GJ, Bokey EL, Pheils MT. Diverticular coloenteric fistulae. *Aust. N. Z. J. Surg.* 1981;**51**: 358–359.

3. Killingback M, Barron PE, Dent OF. Elective surgery for diverticular disease: an audit of surgical pathology and treatment. *ANZ J. Surg.* 2004;**74**:530–536.

4. Del Pino A, Abcarian H. Colovesical fistulas. In: Welch JP, Cohen JL, Sardella WV, Vignati PV, eds. *Diverticular disease. Management of the Difficult Case.* Baltimore: Williams and Wilkins, 1998;Ch 10, pp. 151–166.

5. Woods RJ, Lavery IC, Fazio VW, Jagelman DG, Weakley FL. Internal fistulas in diverticular disease. *Dis. Colon Rectum* 1988;**31**:591–596.

Case 96

1. Killingback M, Barron P, Dent O. Elective resection and anastomosis for colorectal cancer: a prospective audit of mortality and morbidity 1976–1998. *ANZ J. Surg.* 2002;**72**:689–698.

2. Vignali A, Fazio VW, Lavery IC, Milsom JW, Church JM, Hull TL, Strong SA, Oakley JR. Factors associated with the occurrence of leaks in stapled rectal anastomoses: a review of 1014 patients. *J. Am. Coll. Surg* 1997,**185**:105–113.

3. Alberts JCJ, Parvaiz A, Moran BJ. Predicting risk and diminishing the consequences of anastomotic dehiscence following rectal resection. *Colorectal Dis.* 2003;**5**:478–482.

Case 98

1. Bakx R, Busch OR, van Geldere D, Bemelman WA, Slors JF, Lanschot JJ. Feasibility of early closure of loop ileostomies: a pilot study. *Dis. Colon Rectum* 2003;**46**:1680–1684.

2. Tang CL, Seow-Choen F, Fook-Chong S, Eu KW. Bioresorbable adhesion barrier facilitates early closure of the defunctioning ileostomy after rectal excision: a prospective randomized trial. *Dis. Colon Rectum* 2003;**46**:1200–1207.

3. Tjandra JJ, Ng KH. A sprayable hydrogel adhesion barrier facilitates closure of defunctioning loop ileostomy: a randomized trial. *Dis. Colon Rectum* 2004;**47**:640.

Case 99

1. Schellhammer PF, Jordan GH, El-Mahdi AM. Pelvic complications after interstitial and external beam irradiation of urologic and gynecologic malignancy. *World J. Surg.* 1986;**10**:259–268.

Case 100

1. Rodabaugh KJ, Bernstein MR, Goldstein DP, Berkowitz RS. Natural history of postterm choriocarcinoma. *J. Reproductive Med.* 1998;**43**:75–80.
2. Anseline PF, Lavery IC, Fazio VW, Jagelman DG, Weakley FL. Radiation injury to the rectum. *Ann. Surg.* 1981;**194**:716–724.
3. Parks AG, Allen CLO, Frank JD, McPartlin JF. A method of treating post-irradiation rectovaginal fistulas. *Br. J. Surg.* 1978;**65**:417–421.

Appendix

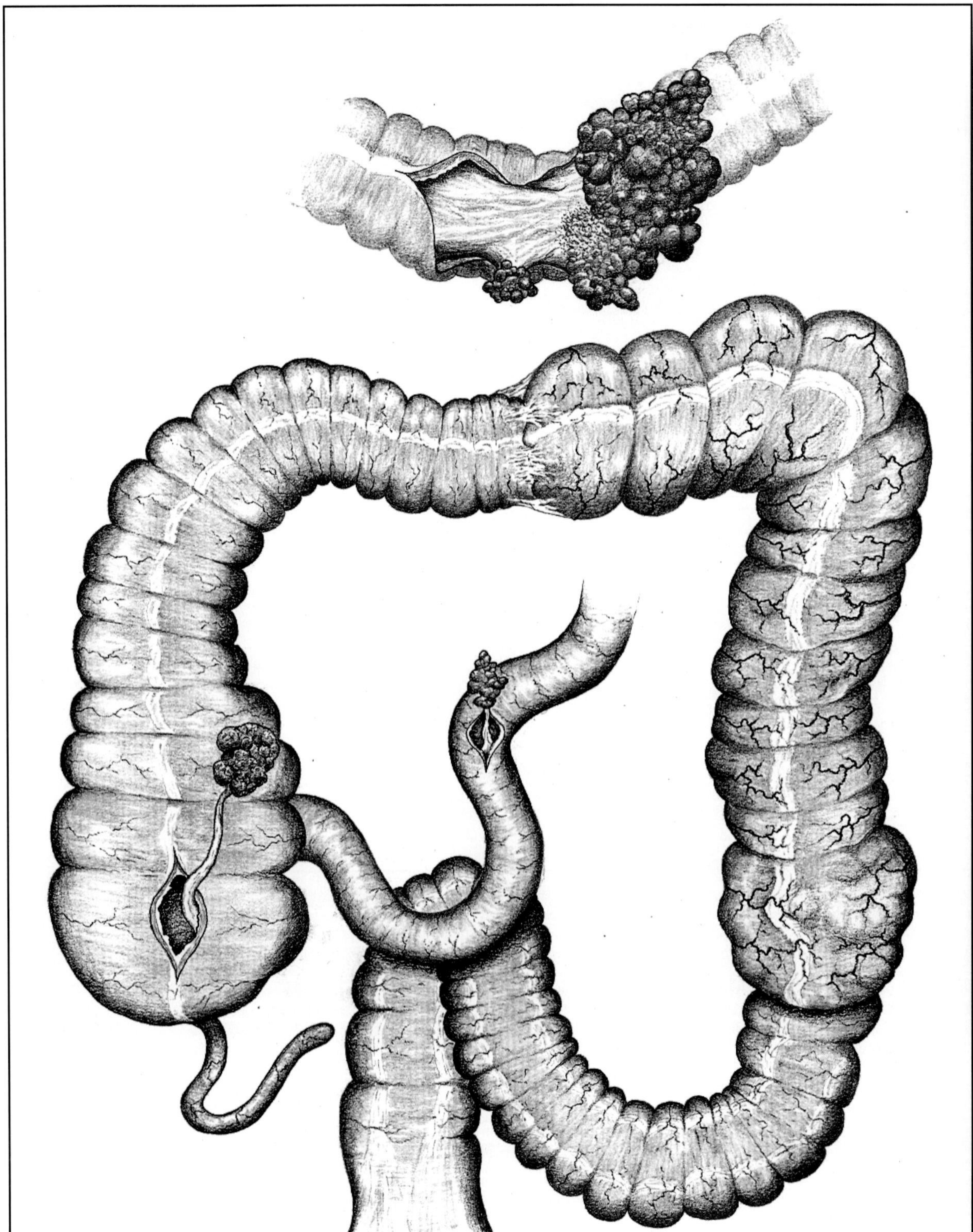

Case 18 (pp. 40–41)

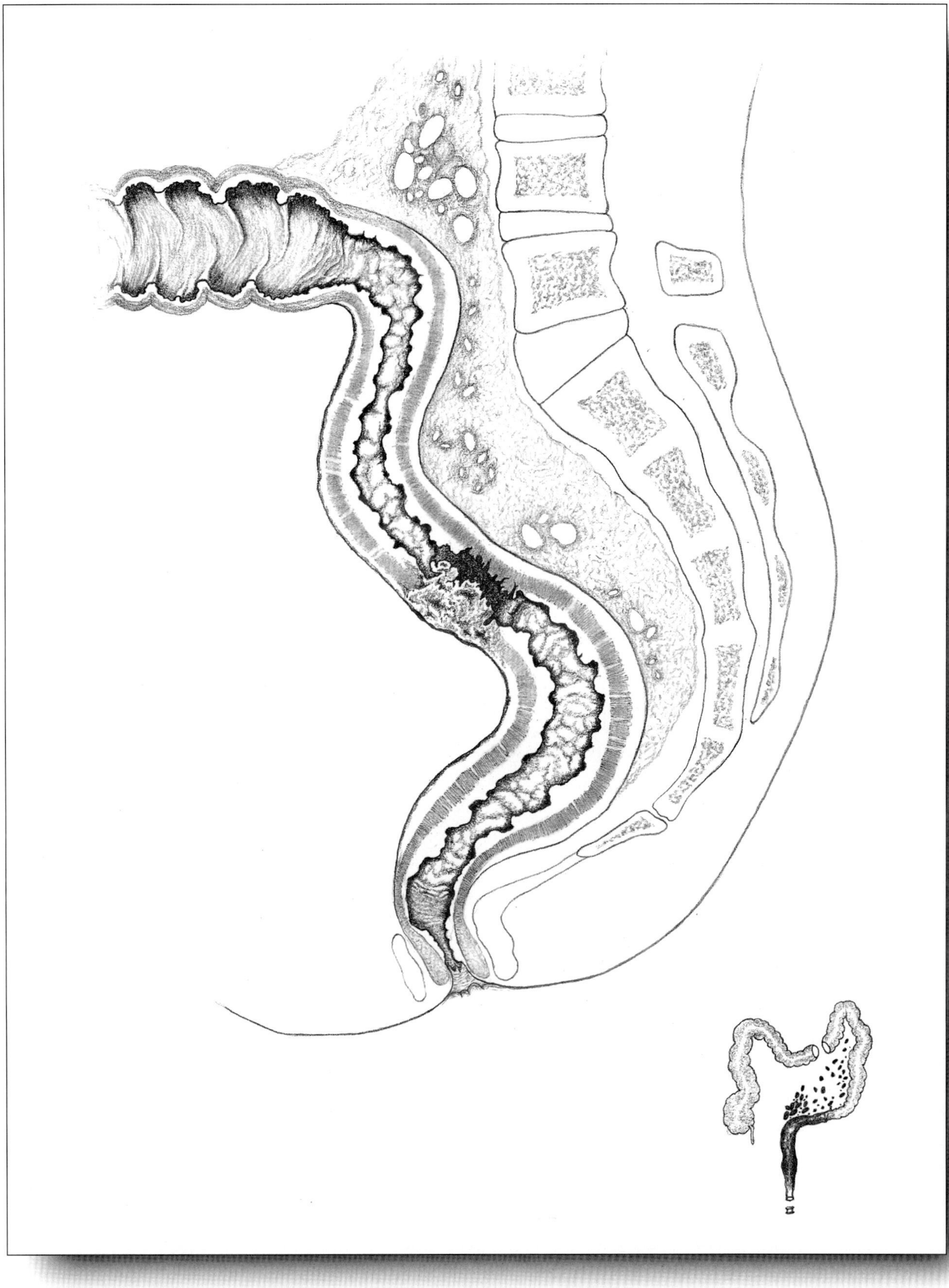

Case 30 (pp. 66–67)

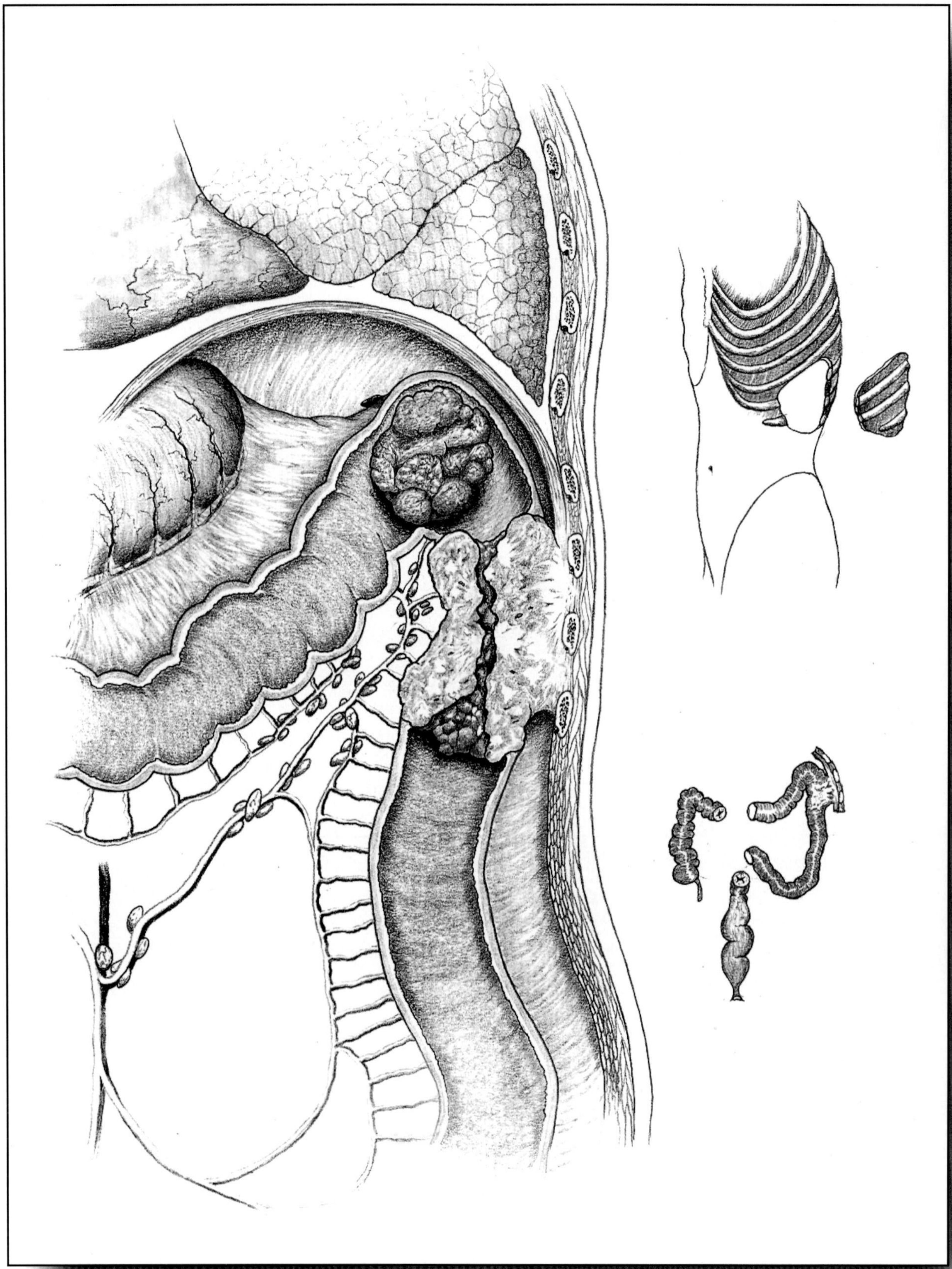

Case 35 (pp. 76–77)

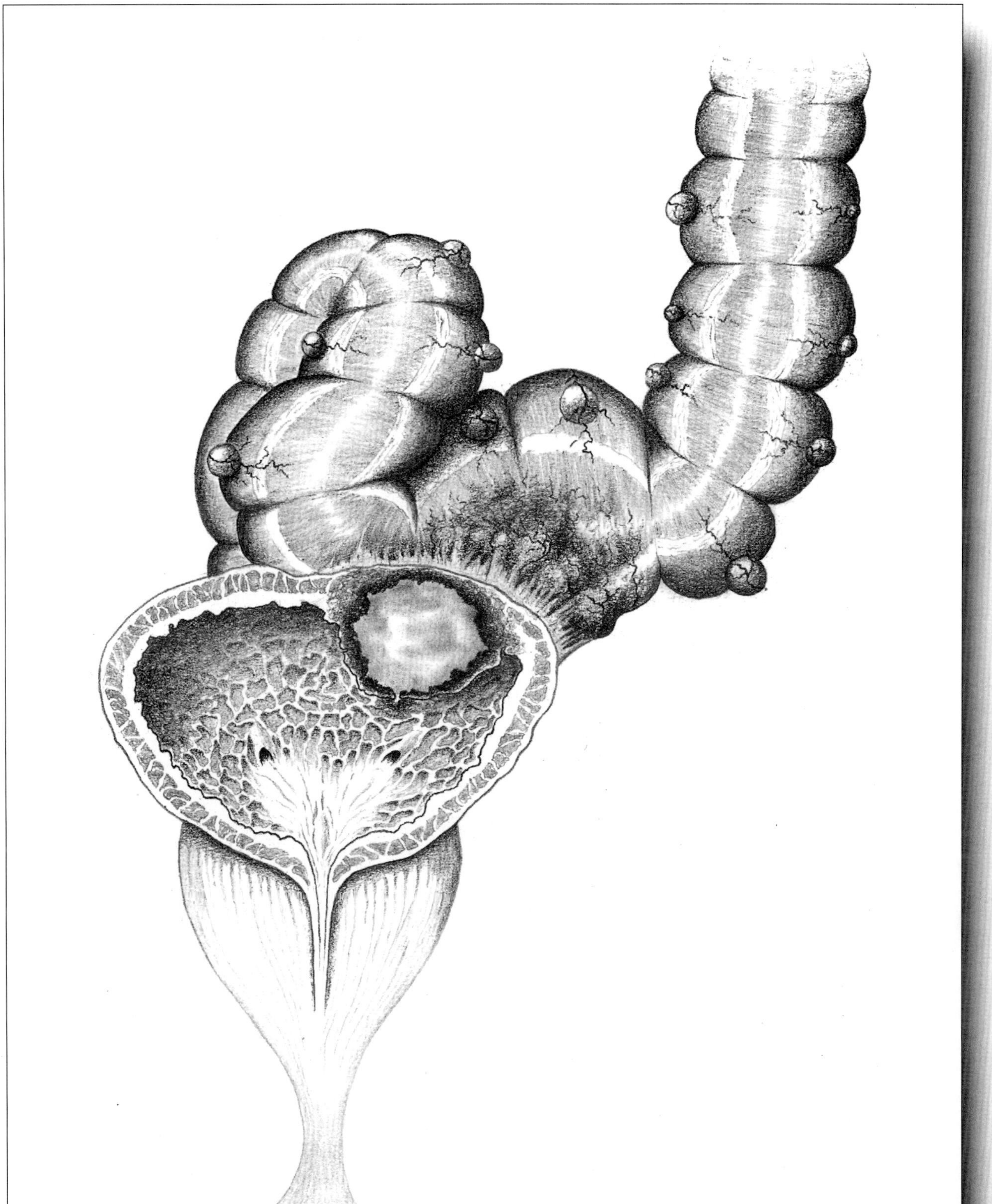

Case 43 (pp. 94–95)

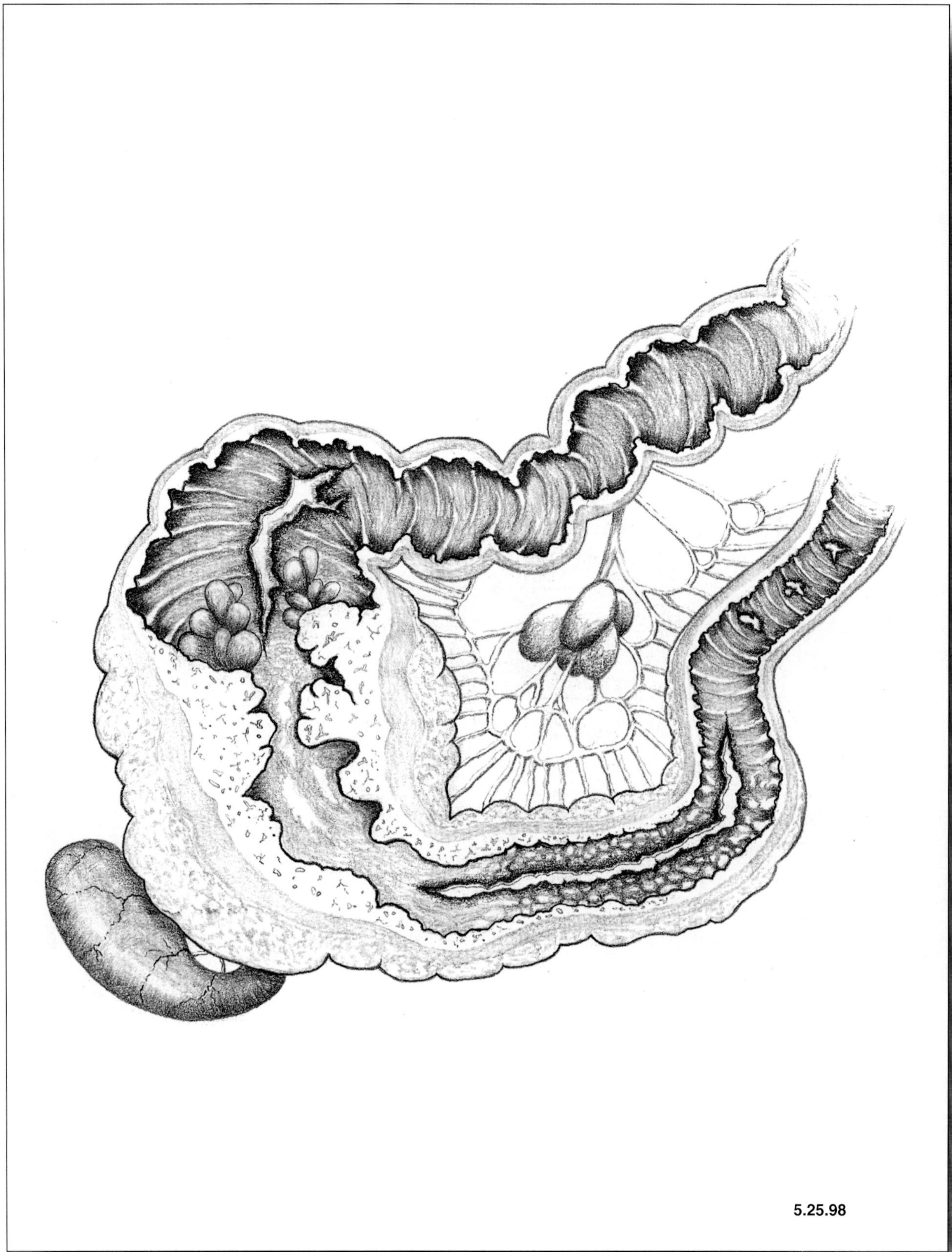

Case 51 (pp. 112–113)

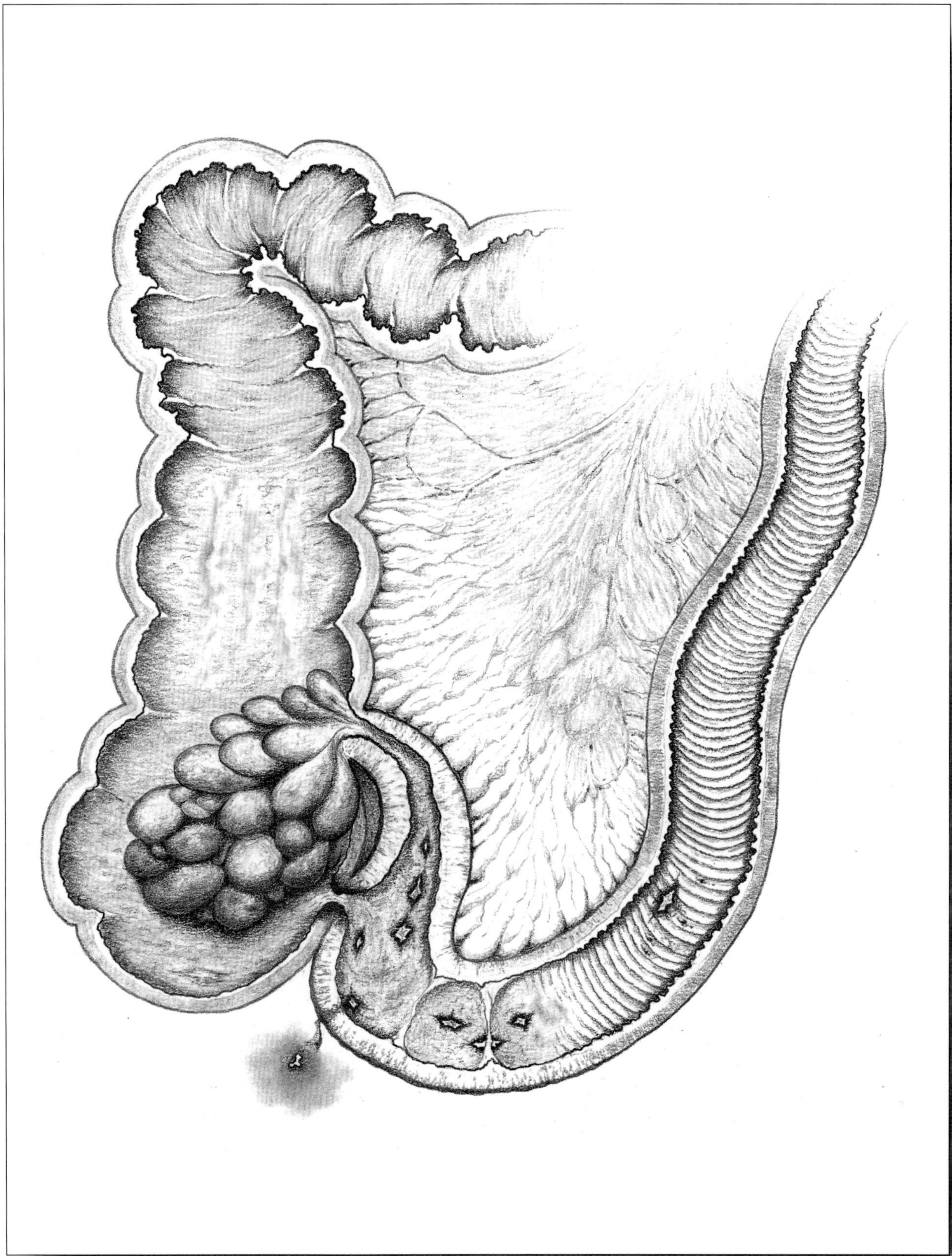

Case 52 (pp. 114–115)

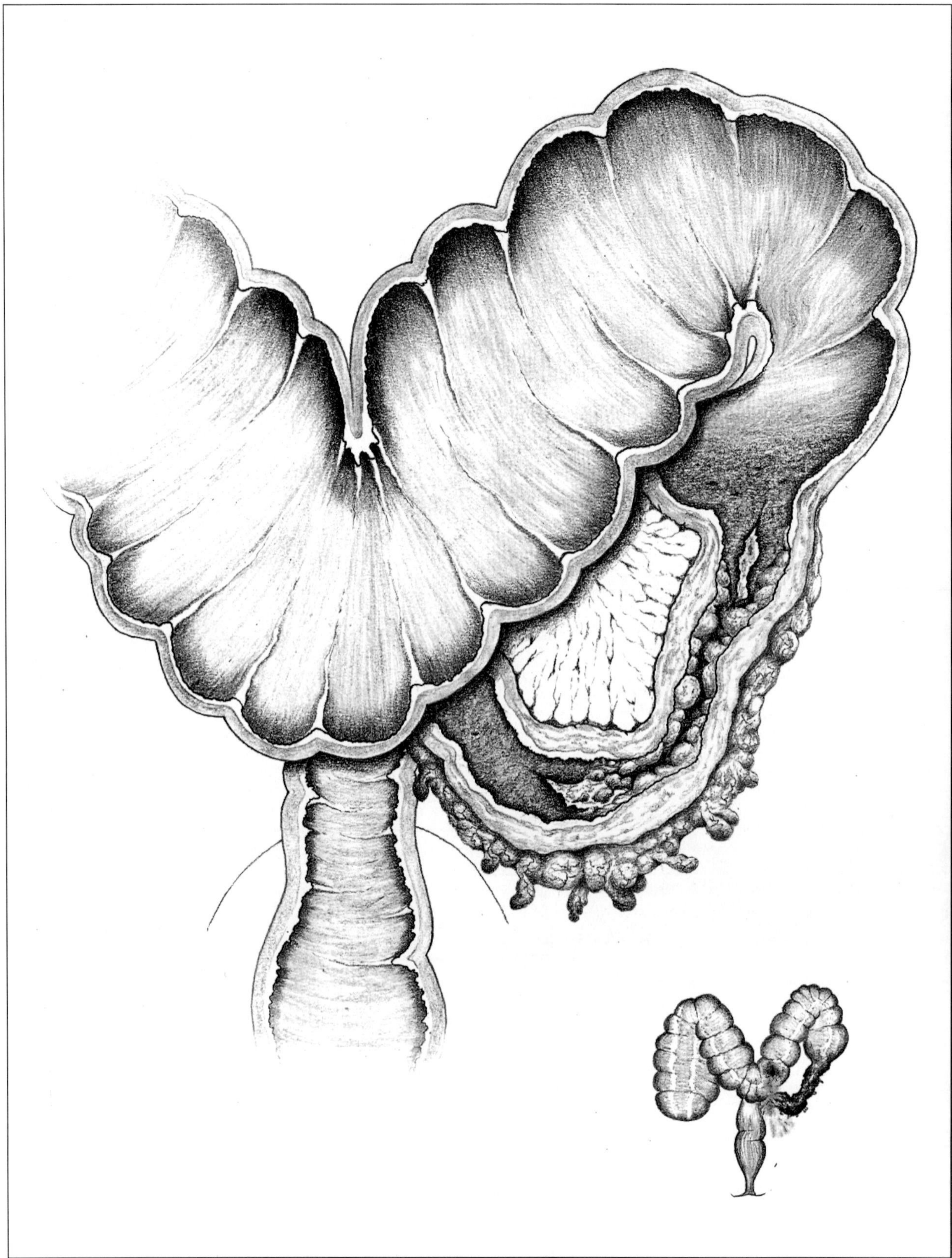

Case 58 (pp. 126–127)

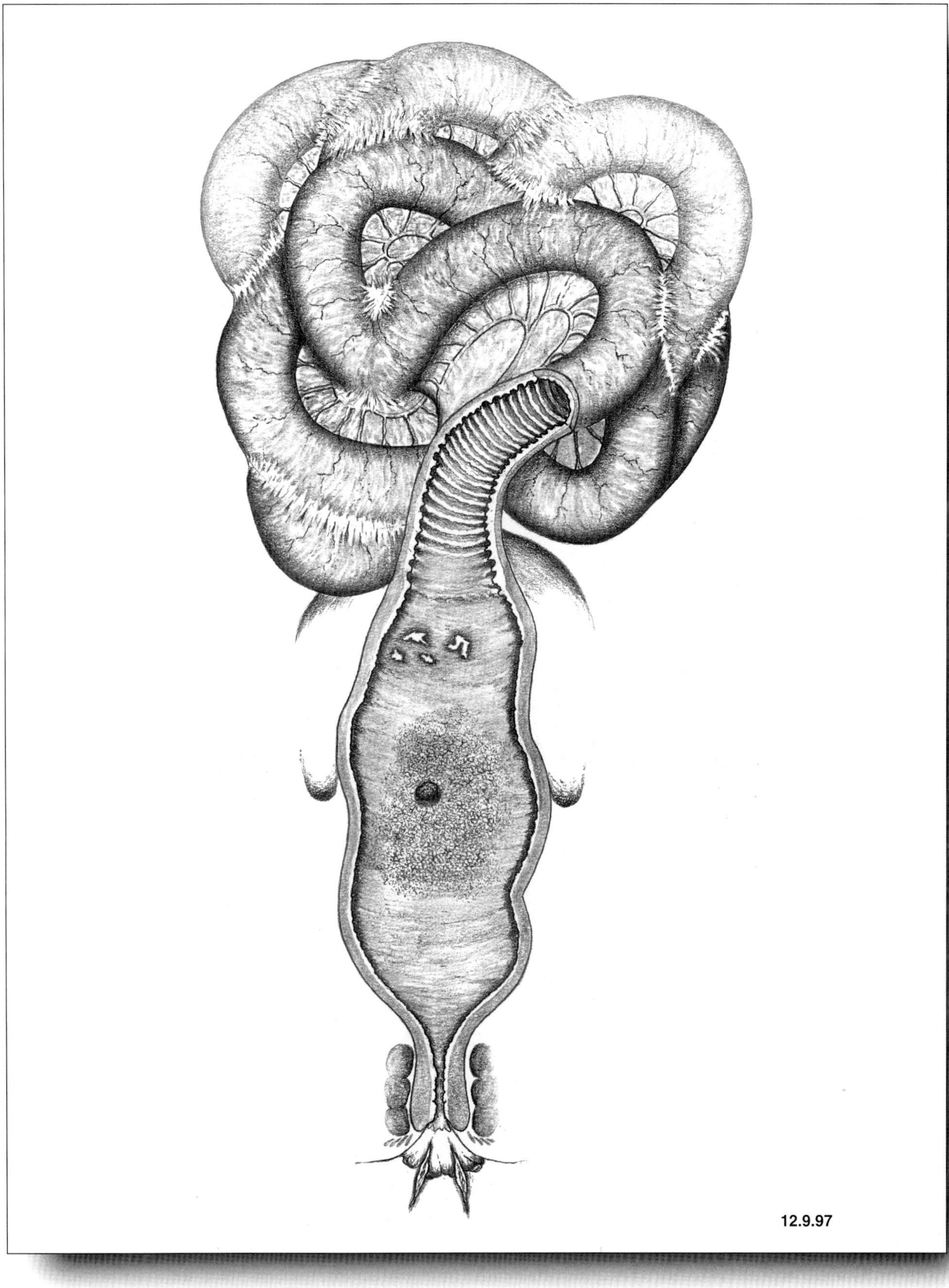

Case 61 (pp. 132–133)

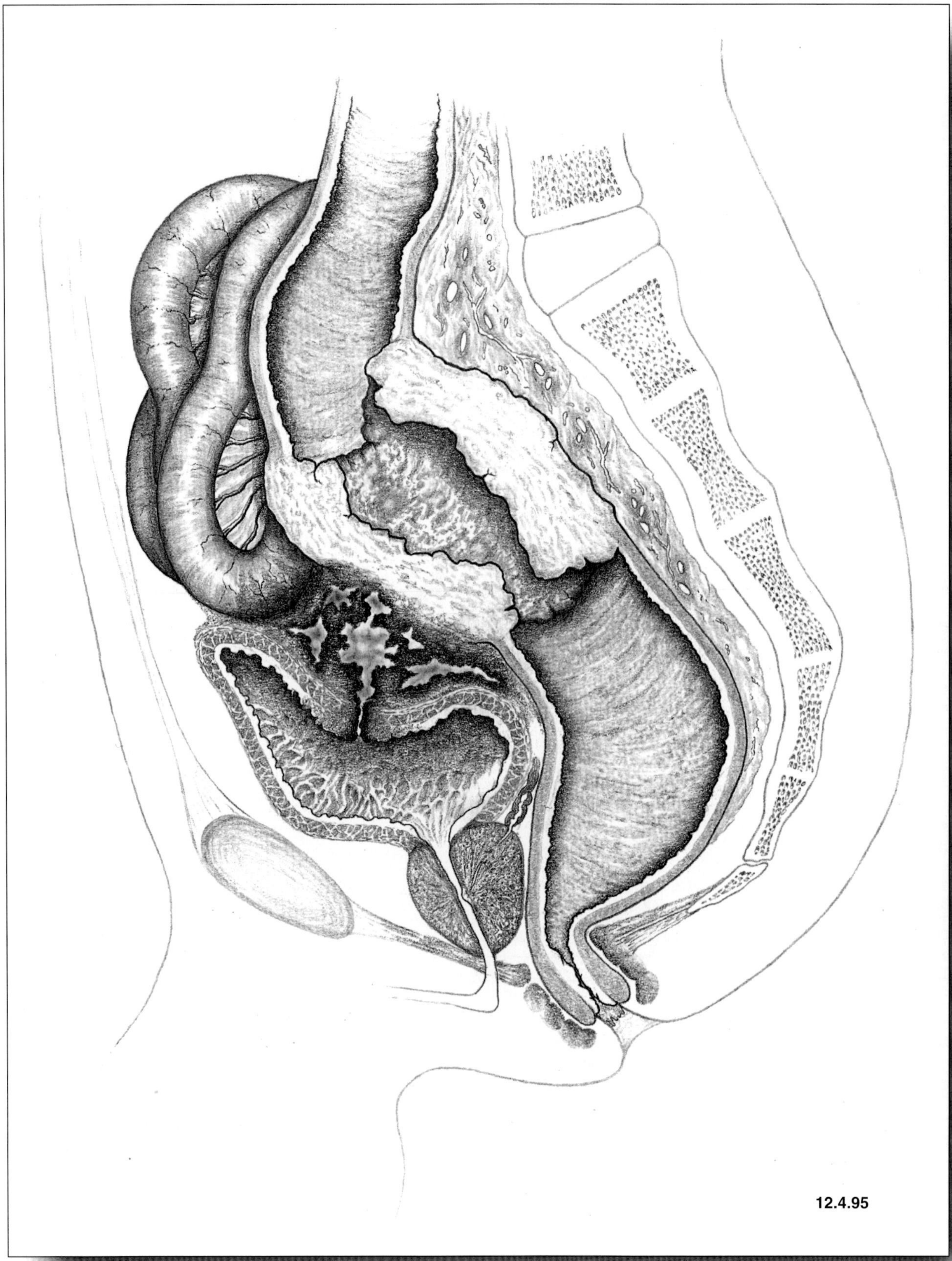

Case 62 (pp. 134–135)

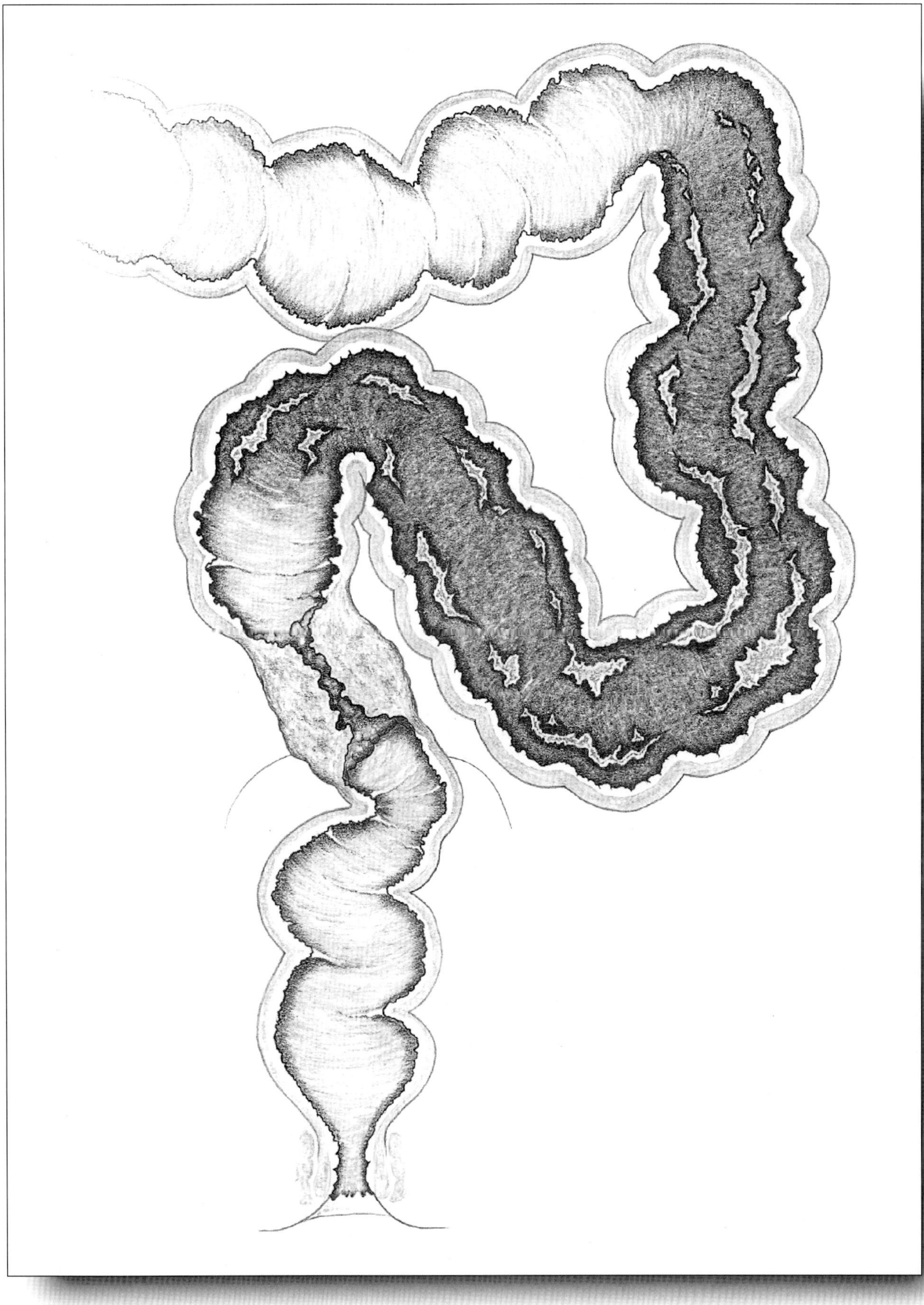

Case 63 (pp. 136–137)

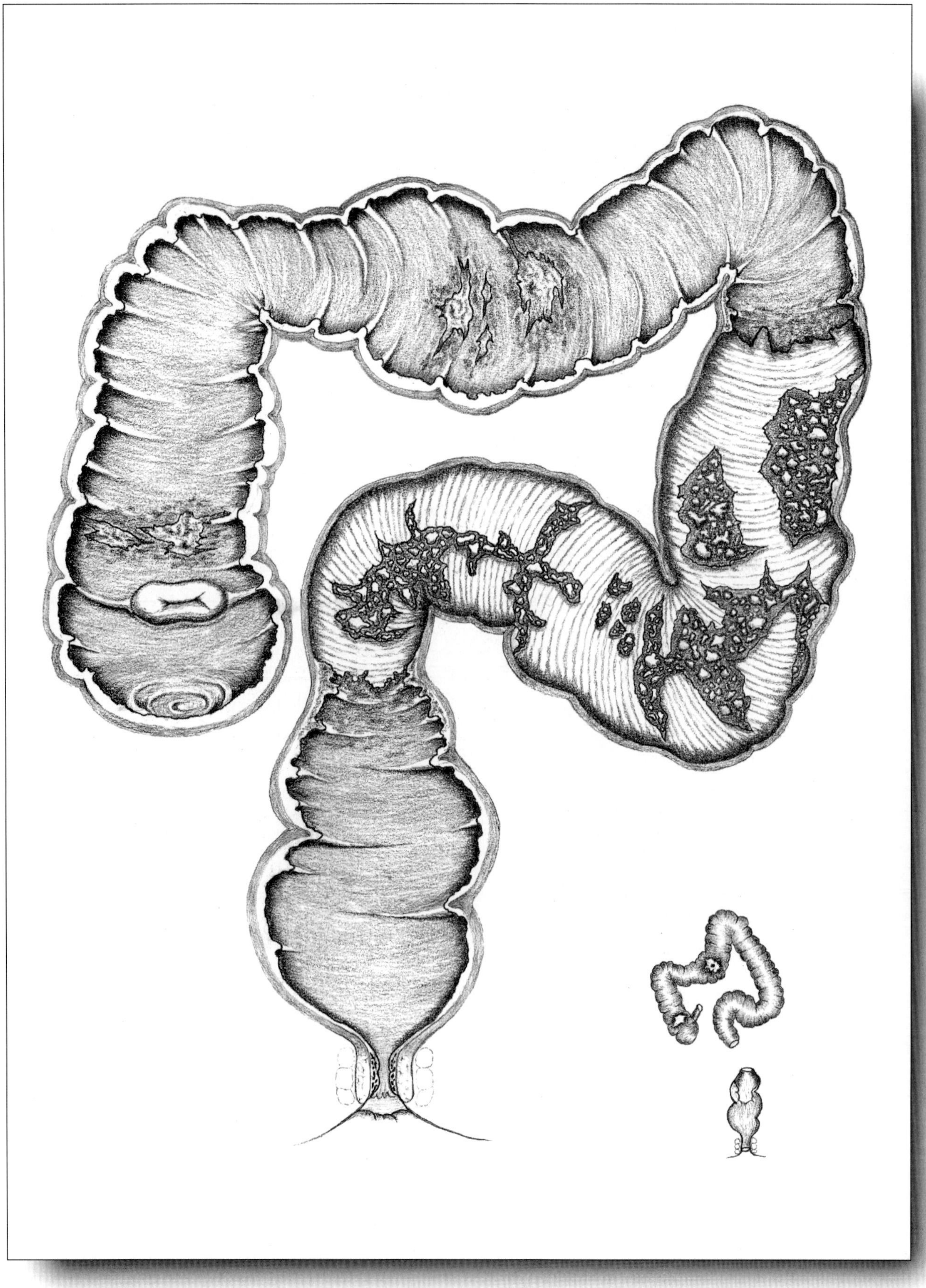

Case 64 (pp. 138–139)

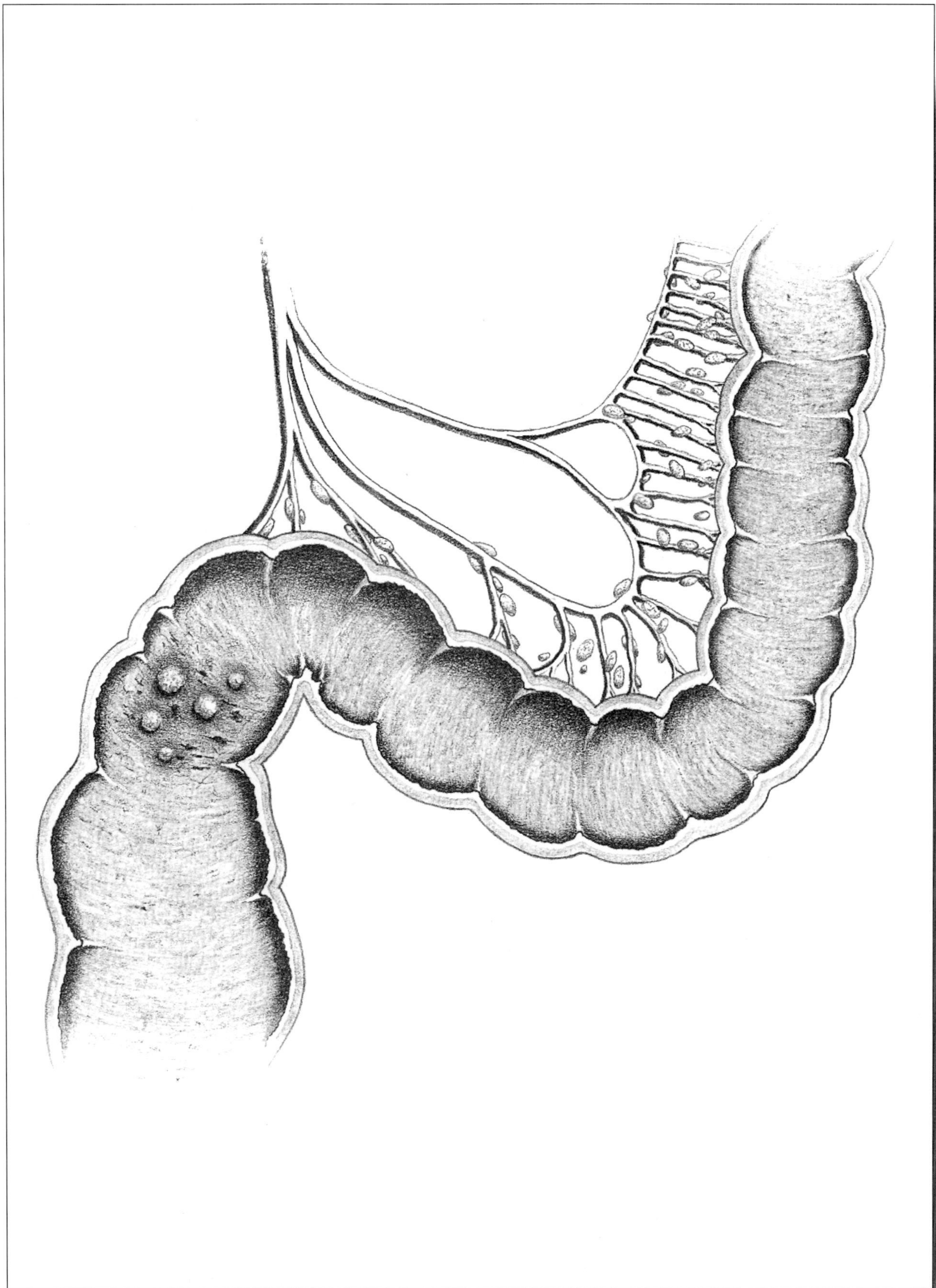

Case 68 (pp. 148–149)

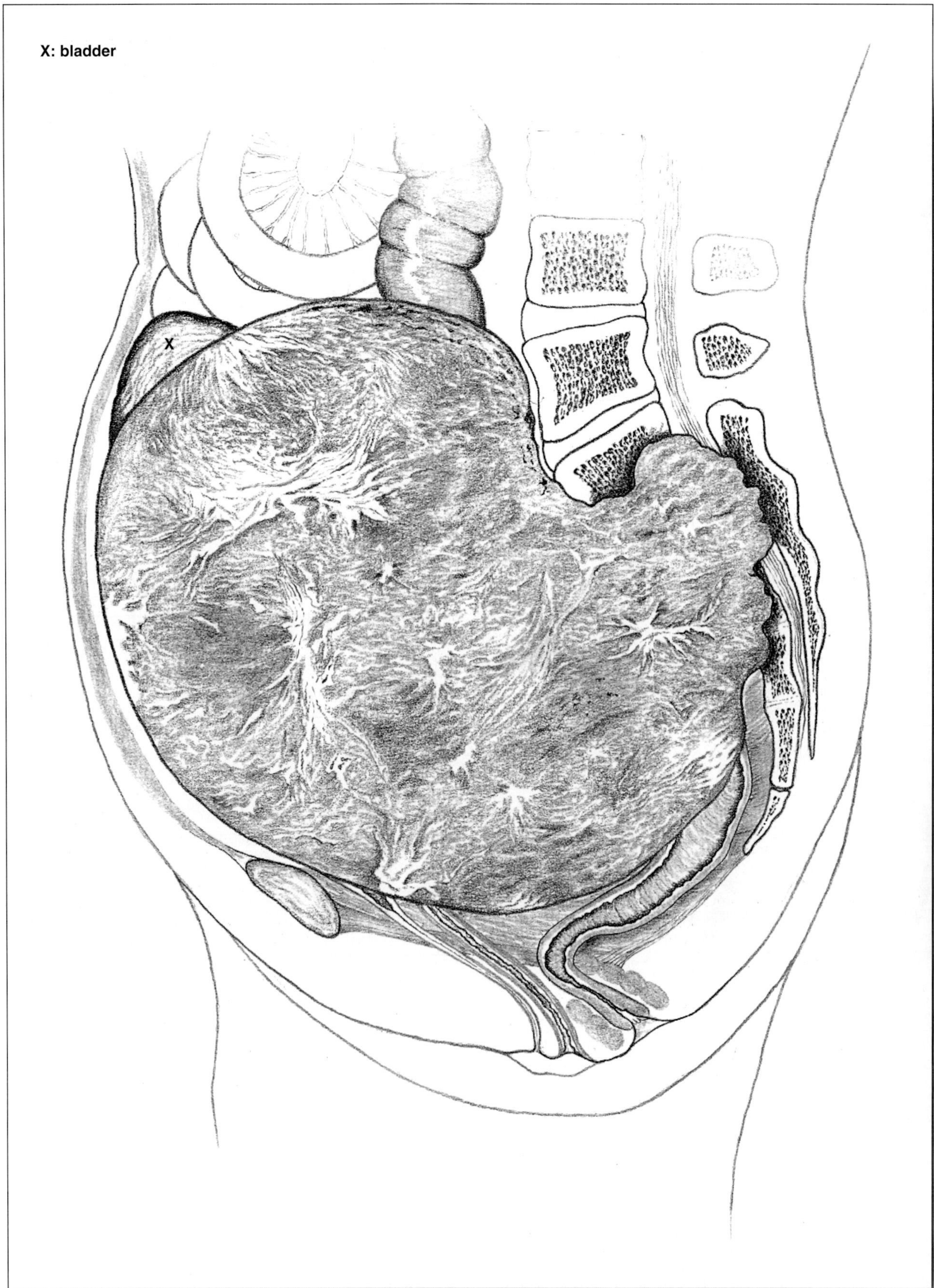

Case 78 (pp. 172–173)

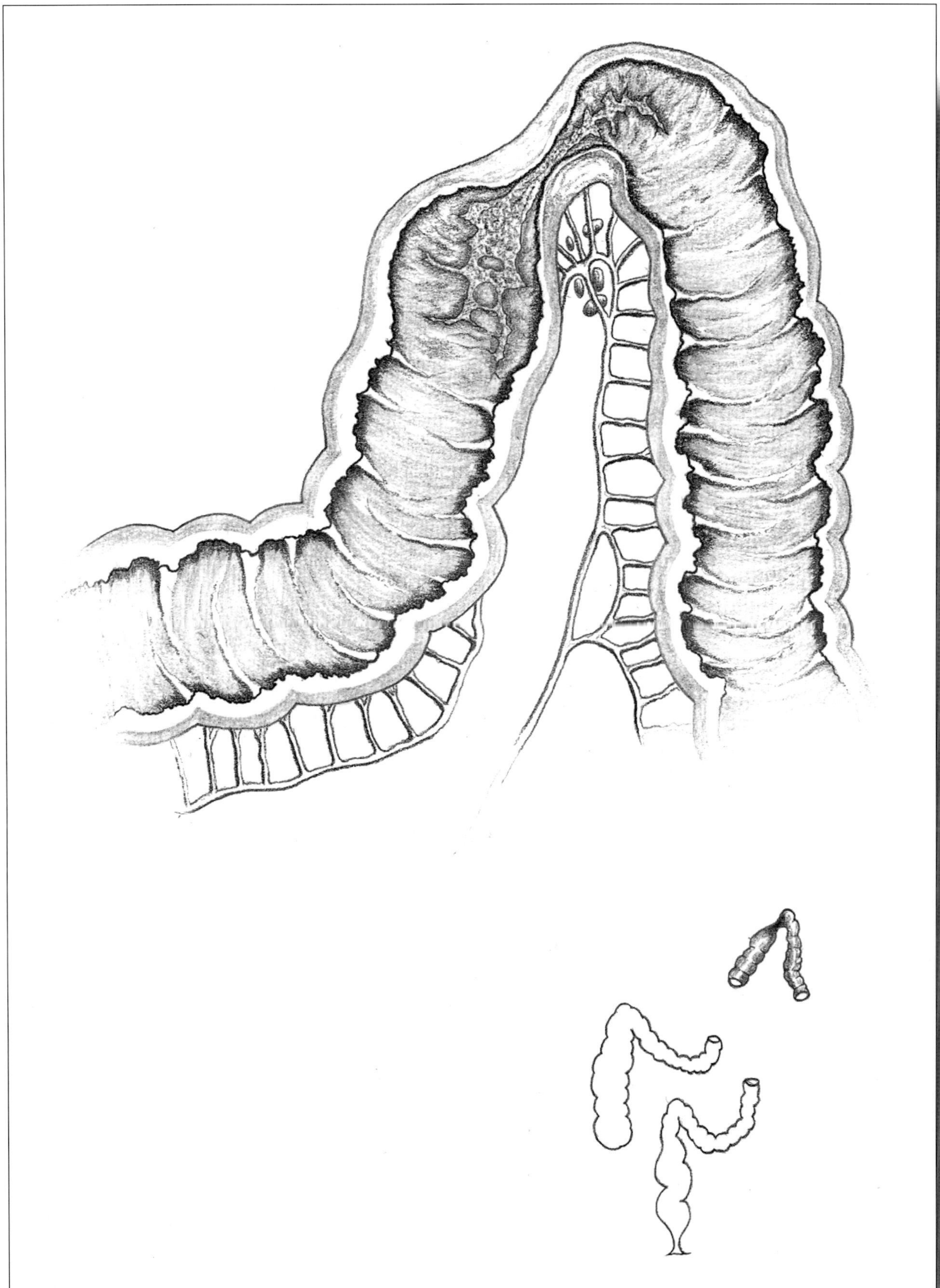

Case 81 (pp. 178–179)

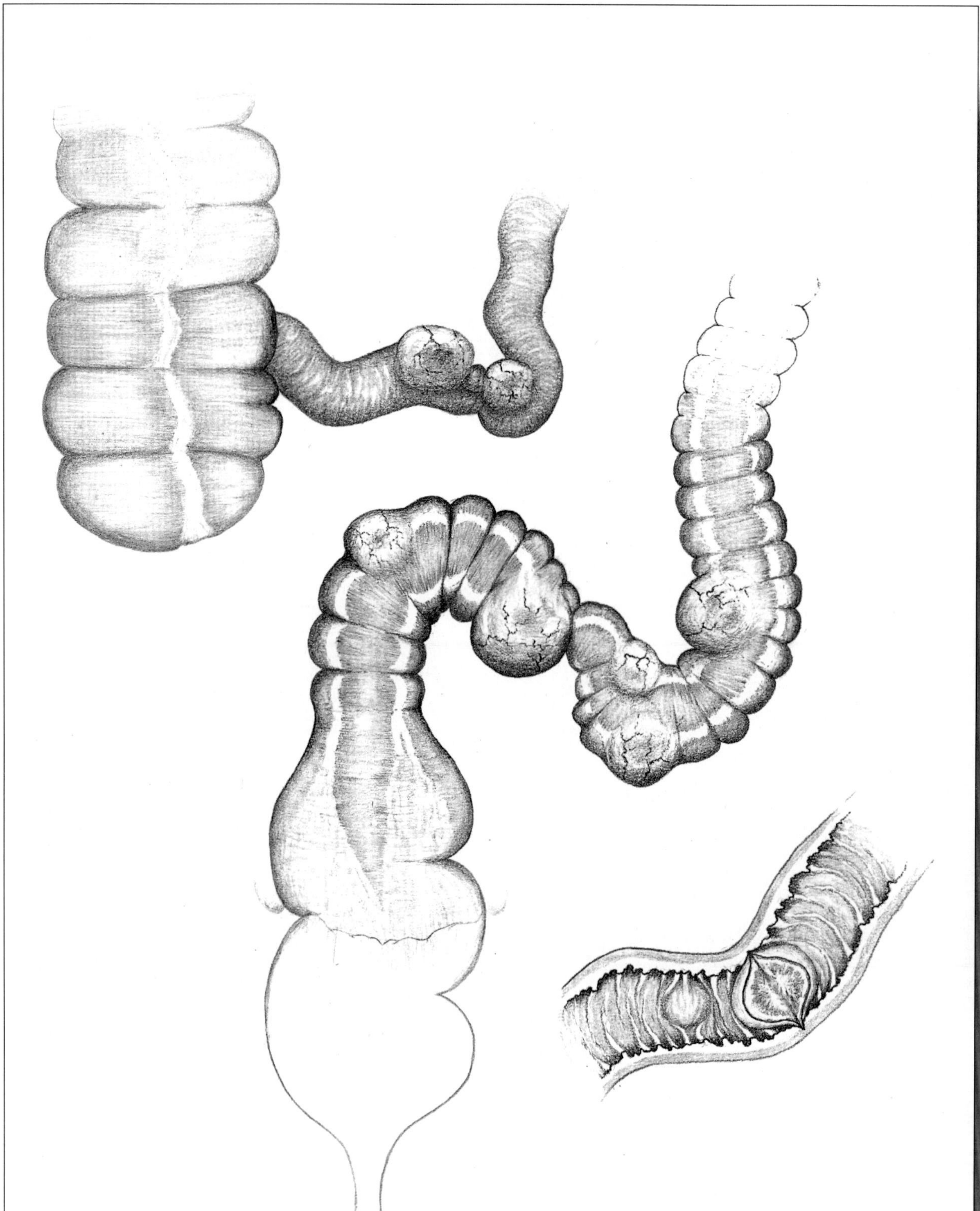

Case 85 (pp. 186–187)

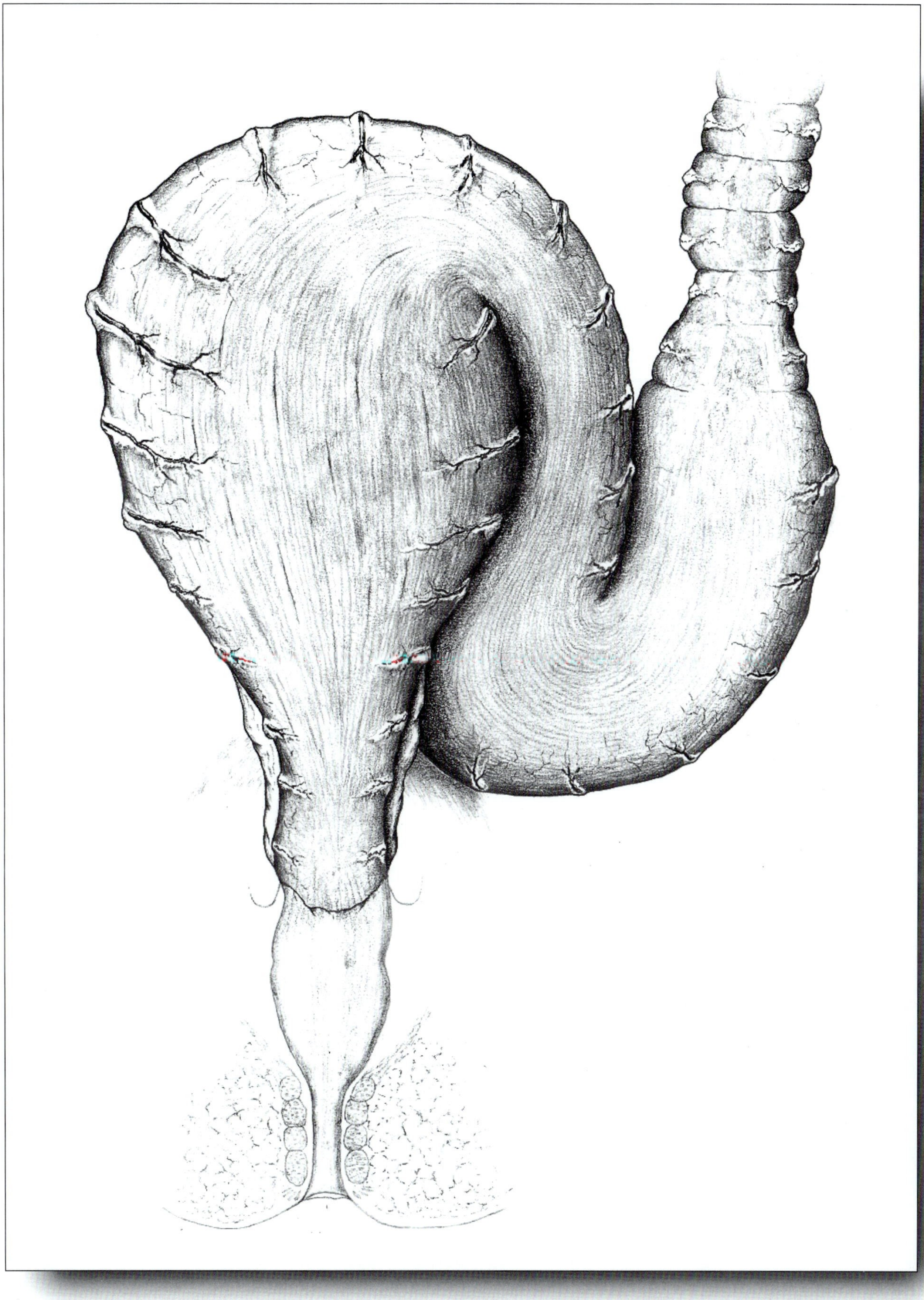

Case 86 (pp. 188–189)

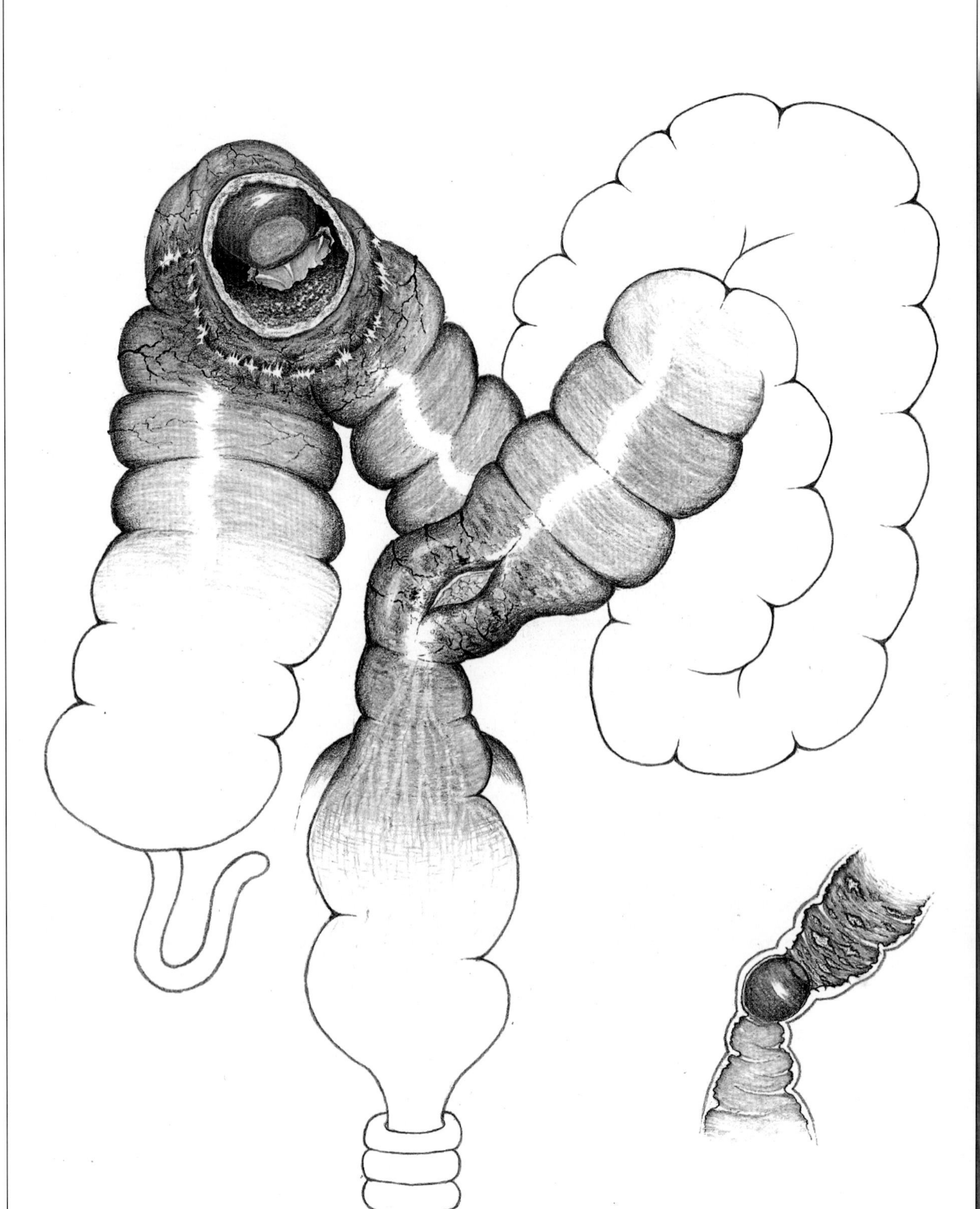

Case 87 (pp. 190–191)

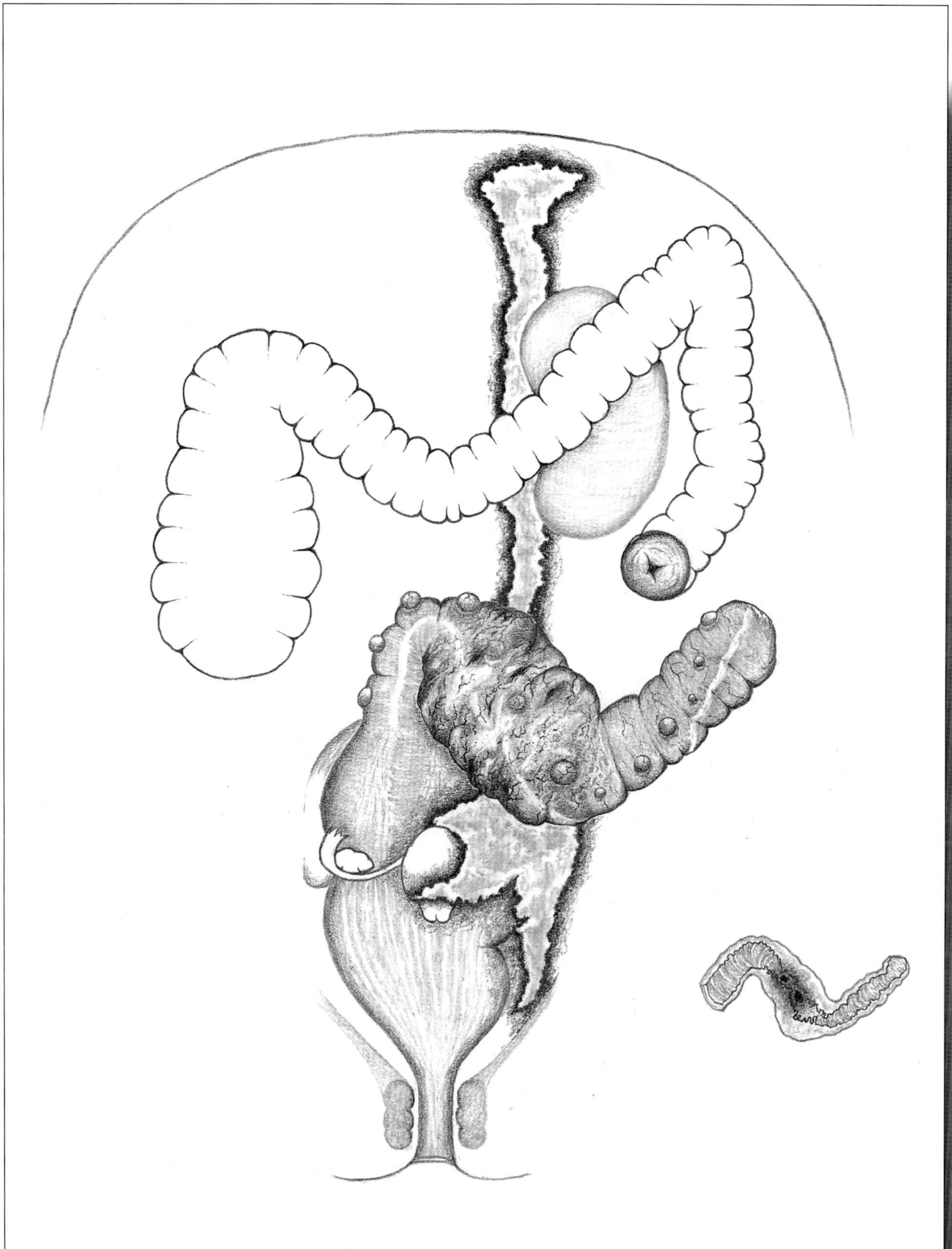

Case 94 (pp. 206–207)

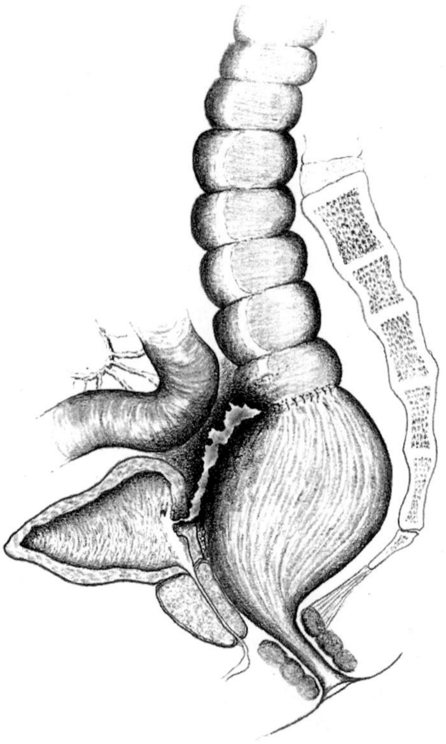

Figure 95.2: Shows the anastomotico-vesical/fistula.

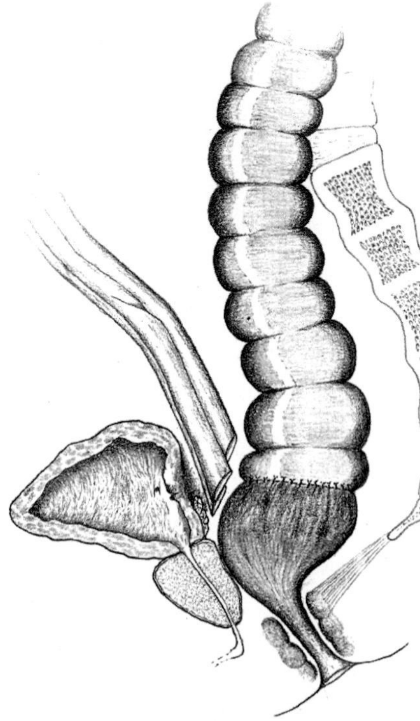

Figure 95.3: The extended low anterior resection (11.1.73).

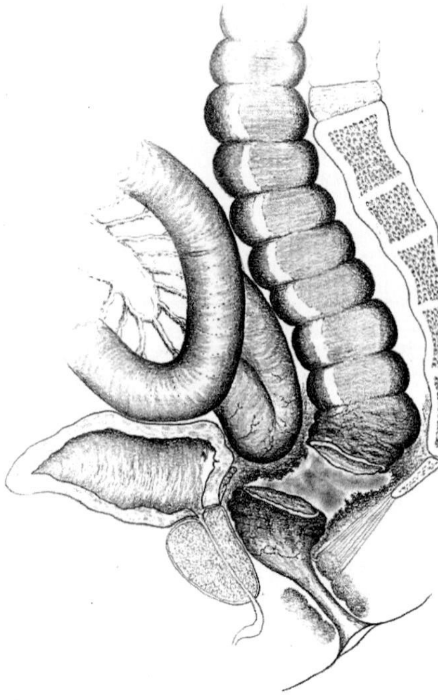

Figure 95.4: Anastomotic dehiscence.

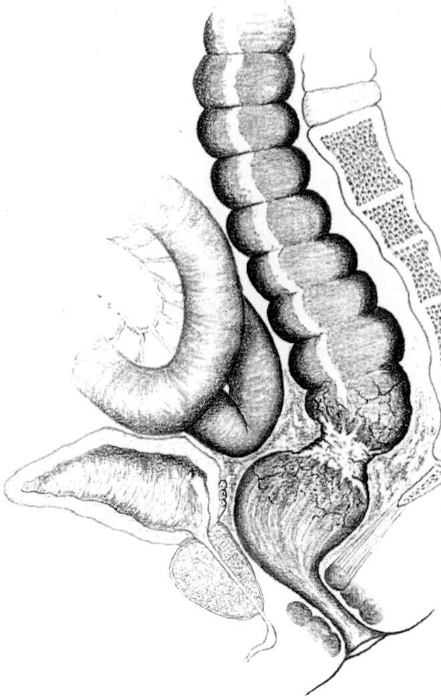

Figure 95.5: Spontaneous auto-anastomosis with stricture.

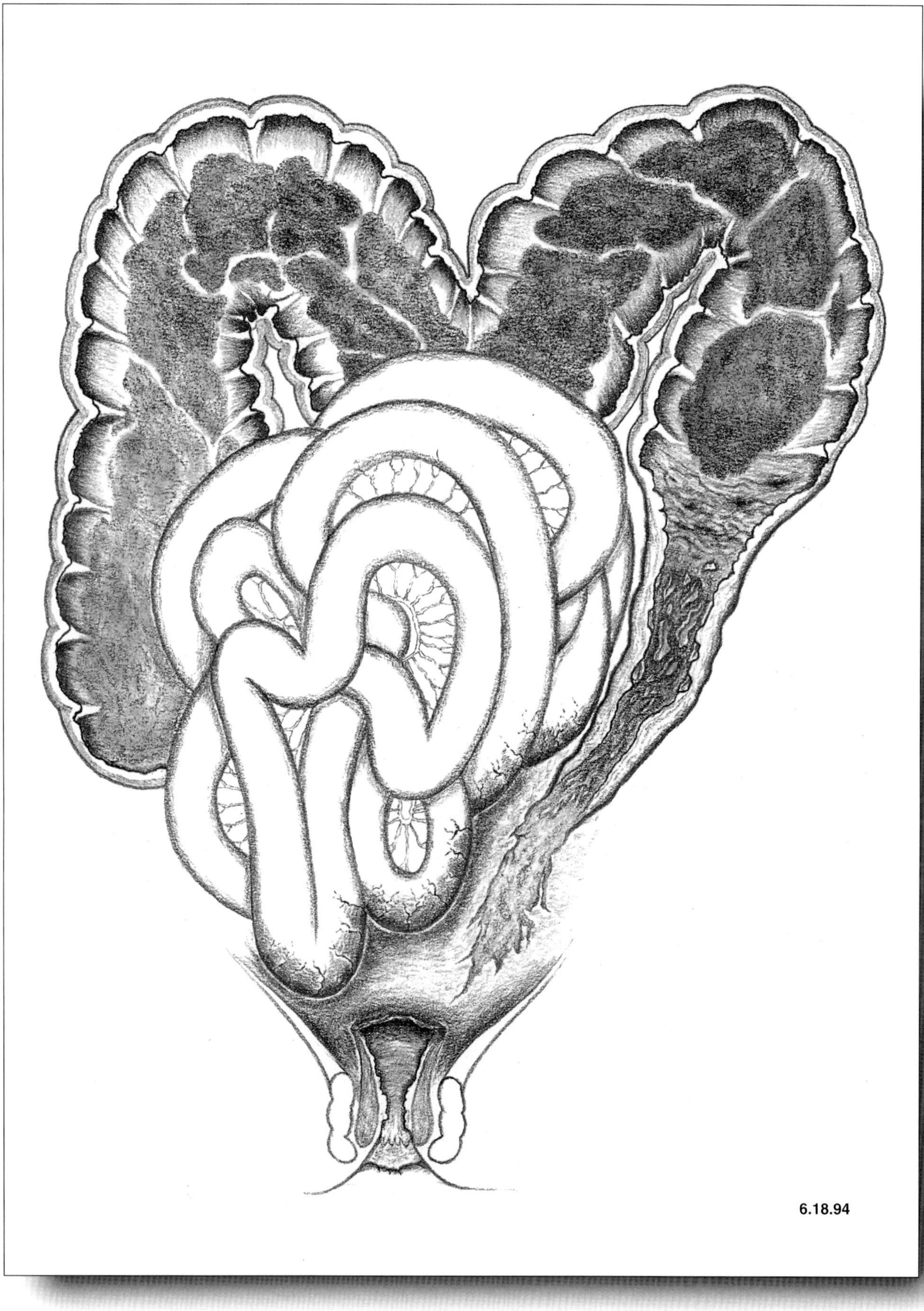

Case 97 (pp. 212–213)

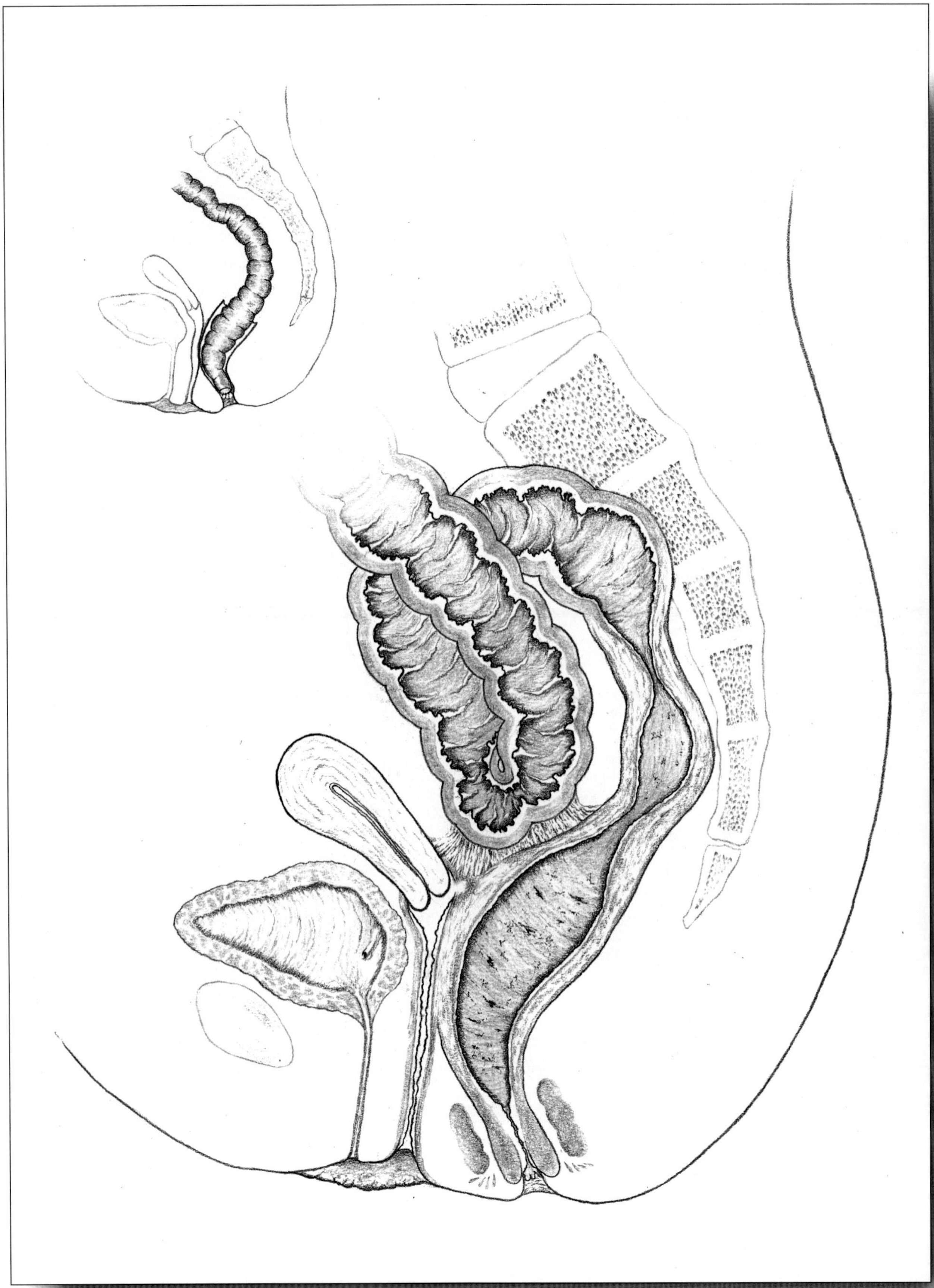

Case 100 (pp. 218–219)

Index